RECONSTRUCTING OBESITY

Food, Nutrition, and Culture

Series Editors: Rachel Black, Connecticut College
Leslie Carlin, University of Toronto

Published by Berghahn Books in Association with the Society for the Anthropology of Food and Nutrition (SAFN).

While eating is a biological necessity, the production, distribution, preparation, and consumption of food are all deeply culturally inscribed activities. Taking an anthropological perspective, this book series provides a forum for thought-provoking work on the bio-cultural, cultural, and social aspects of human nutrition and food habits. The books in this series present timely food-related scholarship intended for researchers, academics, students, and those involved in food policy.

Reconstructing Obesity

The Meaning of Measures and the Measure of Meanings

✛ ✛ ✛

Edited by
Megan B. McCullough and Jessica A. Hardin

berghahn
NEW YORK · OXFORD
www.berghahnbooks.com

Published in 2013 by

Berghahn Books

www.berghahnbooks.com

Library of Congress Cataloging-in-Publication Data

Reconstructing obesity : the meaning of measures and the measure of meanings /
edited by Megan B. McCullough and Jessica A. Hardin. — First edition.
  pages cm.
Includes bibliographical references and index.
ISBN 978-1-78238-141-9 (hardback : alk. paper) — ISBN 978-1-78533-
028-5 (paperback : alk. paper) — ISBN 978-1-78238-142-6 (ebook)
  1. Obesity—Cross-cultural studies. 2. Food habits—Cross-cultural studies.
3. Food preferences—Cross-cultural studies. 4. Body image—Cross-cultural
studies. I. McCullough, Megan B.
  RA645.O23R43 2013
  362.1963'980072—dc23

                                                          2013014897

British Library Cataloguing in Publication Data

A catalogue record for this book is available from the British Library.

ISBN 978-1-78238-141-9 hardback
ISBN 978-1-78533-028-5 paperback
ISBN 978-1-78238-142-6 ebook

For Melvin A. Hardin

Contents

✛ ✛ ✛

Illustrations

✛ ✛ ✛

Figures

Tables

Acknowledgments

✛ ✛ ✛

Volumes begin in conversation with colleagues; this volume is no exception. We would like to thank our colleagues and contributors for coming on this journey with us. Tina Moffat gave us valuable feedback on our introduction. We would also like to thank Leslie Carlin and Rachel Black, co-editors of this series on food and nutrition at Berghahn Books, for their encouragement. We particularly wish to thank Leslie Carlin for inviting us to submit a book proposal and for her feedback and support. Ann Przyzycki DeVita, editor at Berghahn Books, has been supportive of this project, and we thank her for the opportunity to share our work on obesity with a wider audience. Lastly we thank our three anonymous peer reviewers for their comments. Furthermore we owe a great debt to Richard and Ann Lozeau for their hard work. We also extend our appreciation for our friends and families for their support and care. As we have had deeply challenging conversations about anthropology, health, obesity, and the meanings of bodies and personhood, we hope this volume will change other's conversations on the meanings and values attached to culture, health, fatness, and bodies.

Introduction

Reconstructing Obesity

The Meaning of Measures and the Measure of Meanings

Megan B. McCullough and Jessica A. Hardin

✛ ✛ ✛

"That is child abuse!" one my Anthropology of the Body students declared, ruffled and affronted, after learning about gavage, the forced feeding and fattening of young Muslim girls in certain West African subcultures (Popenoe 2005). When thinking about fat, college students articulate very clear ideas about what constitutes a "healthy" body, and their responses to fatness and obesity, words often used interchangeably, range from baffled, outraged, curious, to liberated as they are asked to unpack their ideas about fat, value, and health. When my classes have analytically examined fat and obesity, individually and collectively, students learned to identify tendrils of culturally located morality discourses woven into concepts and beliefs about fatness, including the belief in the United States that all fat equaled ill health. Students struggled to identify and grasp the way fat is culturally gendered and that fat, such as that discussed above regarding gavage, is hard to imagine as something of beauty or value. Similarly in teaching "The Sweetness of Fat" by Sobo (1994), Jessica found that students could only explain Jamaican concepts of health, nurturance, and moral worth embodied in fatness when it was a creation of a precarious economic and agricultural environment. For Jessica's undergraduate students, fatness could only be valued and thinness avoided in an environment of scarcity, thus they constructed a linear and evolutionary perspective in which fatness decreases in value as development and knowledge increases, thereby placing Euro-American cultural understandings of fatness at the top of their progression.

The Centers for Disease Control states that more than one-third of U.S. adults (35.7 percent) are obese and that no state meets the nation's Healthy People 2010 goal to lower obesity prevalence to 15 percent (CDC 2012). Furthermore, the CDC's website states that what they term "obesity-related conditions," including heart disease, stroke, type 2 diabetes, and certain types of cancer, are some of the leading causes of death in the United States. The World Health Organization's overweight and obesity fact sheet notes that worldwide rates of obesity have doubled since 1980 and 65 percent of the world's population live in countries where being overweight and obese kills more people than being underweight (WHO 2012).[1] Research data indicates that obesity rates also run along gendered lines. On its fact sheet, the World Health Organization cites that, "in 2008, more than 1.4 billion adults, 20 and older, were overweight and of these over 200 million men and nearly 300 million women were obese" (WHO 2013). Obesity statistics alone are almost mind numbing in their quantity and scope, not to mention the implications of such statistics on human health.

The medicalization of obesity, combined with ideas about the questionable moral status of fat and fatness, saturates social life in the United States. Images of fat people in public health studies and news reports permeate global and national mediascapes where science and health research is popularized and sensationalized (Campos, Saguy, Ernsberger and Gaesser 2006). These sensationalized narratives run from ranking the world's fattest nations (Streib 2007) to novel obesity-related rankings, such as the recently released study ranking countries that are exercising the least.[2]

There are also a plethora of televised weight loss boot camps and "reality" shows about obesity, along with media reports on health studies or new food or drink legislation that often feature objectified fat bodies; the most disturbing of these are often images of headless, heavy torsos walking down the street or of a large person's midsection sitting in front of huge trays of food in shopping mall food courts, all of which reinforce negative ideas about fat and fat people as abnormal, repulsive, and out-of-control (Brownell et al. 2005; Farrell 2011). Fat women and men are both targeted as out-of-control and unattractive in ways that are similar and in ways that differ according to culturally gendered configurations (Aphramor and Gingras 2009; McCullough, this volume; Royce 2009; Rubin and Josephs, this volume). There is also the bizarre news story that can, for example, argue in a facile manner that fat people are more responsible for global warming than thin ones (Landau 2009).[3]

Such vignettes reflect and reinforce the idea that fat is an acceptable stigma to target, as well portray fat and fat people as blameworthy and unhealthy (Jutel 2006; Saguy and Almeling 2008; Saguy and Riley 2005). Meanwhile news reports of studies that discuss how very difficult and multifaceted sustainable weight loss is and the intricate mechanisms through which the body holds on to fat often do not make it into the popular domain, and if they do, their staying power is limited and critical discussion about the knotty issue of weight loss and the role of biological and genetic processes in sustainability does not ensue (see Becker, this volume).[4]

There is also very little discussion in local, national, and global public spheres on what the social, political, emotional, and health costs are for obese and fat people trying anything and everything they can to be thin, disciplined citizen-subjects (Greenhalgh 2012; Becker, Trainer, McCullough, and Rubin and Joseph, this volume). We do not deny the real social and biological consequences of obesity on individuals, communities, and nations, but we still want more from our students and from ourselves as scholars. Regardless of the fact that research on obesity is often oversimplified in media representations, science, public health, and other health research are also cultural artifacts that are both a scientific product, as well as a social product with unconscious moral and evaluative underpinnings.[5]

Some branches of health research are very interested in context and use it to target research to modify the lives of the subjects. However, health research is often unreflexive in understanding how health research's own models are embedded and imbued with unconscious cultural beliefs in research design and in data analysis. Furthermore, health research is also shaped by the sociocultural environment of its own workplace, work practices, and funding demands.

Our students come to ideas about the questionable moral status of fat and the conflation of obesity with sickness and disease honestly (Bacon 2008; Boero 2007, 2012; Guthman 2011; Koppleman 2009). Obesity interventions and the obesity/weight loss industry are frequently very fear-based and predict social and physical death if weight is not modified and the fat subject disciplined into normalcy. Weight bias is also one of the few areas of health research in which discriminatory aspects embedded in research design and health interventions have not been fully explored or acknowledged (Rothblum and Solovay 2009; Puhl and Brownell 2001). What we feel is missing in this crowded and busy area of study is a lack of attention to the lived experiences of people, how and why they eat what they do, and how people in cross-cultural settings understand risk, health, and bodies. The cultural context in which fat individuals and communities live is not given its due, nor is the production of research on obesity itself seen as a cultural act. By examining select health research, health interventions, and global and local debates about obesity, as well as the lived, embodied experiences of fatness, this volume argues for a more complex vision of what obesity and fatness are and how they are studied.

As anthropologists, we find that the frequent correlation of the words *fat* and *obese* makes their meanings less clear. We find the conflation of fat or obesity with ill health, disease, and sickness worthy of attention. Such repetitive equations indicate to us that there is something deeply unresolved about fatness and obesity in the arena of social life and scientific research in the United States, in global public health, as well as in many cultures around the world. The significance of stigma, inequality, and asymmetrical power relations in obesity research cannot be overlooked because stigmatization is a social experience that threatens positive health outcomes (Yang et al. 2007). Fat and obese as materialized in insults, academic study, medical research, and popular media debates are cultural products, and as such, they prompt in us a series of questions: What is obesity? What is fatness? What is the relationship between health and fat? Is the fat body universally discernible and therefore readable? Are all bodies, cultures, and locations so comparable? And beyond how one measures fat and applies that information, the question remains, how meaningful are such measurements really? Based on what our students have said in class and what we see in popular globalized media, we also have to ask, is all fat bad? What does "fat as bad" mean in different contexts? And if fat does indicate both a moral state and a state of health, how and why is this so? Does such a linkage impede or assist health interventions and does it impede or assist in creating health? Why are not the psychosocial, health, political, and economic costs to fat individuals and obese populations who are fighting to be thin or thinner studied or acknowledged? What is titillating or horrifying about fatness that we wish to measure it, rank it, and talk about it?

A central issue about obesity and fat as an area of research is that the topic itself seems stuck between research practices and paradigms. On the one hand, there are researchers that focus on obesity as a health problem to be solved through scientific research, evidence-based practices, risk assessments, generalizability and well-designed health interventions, and on the other hand, there are paradigms that are deeply critical of how obesity is framed as a social and medical problem. These social science approaches seek to uncover and analyze what they see as the lack of attention to the relationships among fat bodies, inequality, stigma, and morality, or what can also be called the context of everyday life. We invite the reader to join us in rethinking this complex rift and questioning the usefulness of replicating it. This book offers a different vision. Collectively this volume is an experiment at tacking between the various sides to provoke a different set of analytical explorations about obesity research and the health effectiveness of obesity interventions. In aid of this "tacking," each author seriously considers what cultural difference, embodiment, and local knowledge, in all their complexity and untidiness, make in understanding obesity and in the construction of health interventions.[6]

Defining Terms

Work on obesity or on fat embodiment is very prickly and loaded. Definitions and meanings of terms and concepts can be quite slippery as well as deeply political. The struggle over what even to call this social and biomedical phenomenon, *obesity* or *fatness* and how it is researched and analyzed highlights the methodological, theoretical, and applied concerns and questions with which our authors rigorously engage. We consider obesity a medical classification. Fatness is understood as a political labeling of the body that has multiple meanings. On one hand, fat denotes not only weight but also an insulting evaluation of the body and person who is fat, and on the other hand, fat activists use fat to reclaim the word by reaffirming and valuing large size and calling attention to this process of reclaiming. We consider fatness and obesity to be culturally located terms (as are biomedicine and public health) that have complex, multifaceted ontological systems behind their use, engaging with gender, religion, history, race, and social class to name a few. We suggest that terms for various kinds of large embodiment might need to be contextualized in academic, activist, and research work to better understand their use, their fluidity, and their meanings.

Tacking Among Obesities: Local Biologies and Global Assemblages

To facilitate tacking between fatness paradigms and obesity researches, *Reconstructing Obesity* authors draw on cultural and medical anthropological, sociological, and psychological work on embodiment, body size, biosocial dynamics, and body image along with concerns about inequality and unidirectional causation models because this combined approach can assist us bridging the differences in obesity research. This latter method of studying the body accounts for culture and so challenges the universality and naturalizing of body meanings, body size, and body shape. Our work explores how everyday lives, "local moral worlds" (Kleinman 1995), social relationships, and the capacity to act fit into the "local biologies" (Lock 2001) of obese bodies. The concept of local biologies "acknowledges the importance of the biological body as an active agent and the dynamic inter-relationship between culture and biology, such that biological difference can influence individual experience as well as cultural interpretations of experience" (Nichter 2008: 165). We find this concept useful in understanding the complexity of meanings and embodiments with which obesity is suffused, touching as it does on the individual, social, and political body (Scheper-Hughes and Lock 1987). Local biologies highlights the ways social cohesion, history, psychobiological pathways, and material factors cannot be viewed in purely biological terms—local biologies expands and complicates any understanding of biology as "pure" or easily bounded (Nguyen and Peschard 2003: 447–448). Additionally, local biologies assists us in charting the shifting permutations of obesity as it moves between the local and the global, the individual and the social, the normal and the abnormal, the cultural and the scientific (Lock 2001).

Obesity is an increasing global, cultural, and biological phenomenon, as is the stigmatization of obesity (Brewis 2010). To attempt to flexibly frame obesity as a complex local and global issue, we are, as other anthropologists have been (Browner and Sargent 2010), drawn to Collier and Ong's productive concept of "global assemblages" (Collier and Ong 2005). Popular terms such as *globesity* have no analytical complexity, and although the word *global* is implied in this term, this implication has no purchase on power structures or biopolitical governance, nor does it capture the multiple domains and movements at play in obesity research or fat embodiment. We deploy global assemblages alongside local biologies to capture how *obesities* (our term to emphasize its multivalent and polysemic character) have become domains in which the forms and values of individual and collective existence are problematized, and where the convergence of scientific practices and "technological forms, material or transport infrastructures, circuits of interaction and situated values" occurs (Collier and Ong 2005: 11). The concept of global assemblages aids us in tracing obesities as local cultural understandings of how bodies morph in a constant tide of exchange with the global flows of public health, scientific practices, technologies, values, and information. The idea of global assemblages fosters productive exchange about obesity among social science, bicultural research, and health science research. Such divisions between fields hinder both theoretical development and prevention and treatment efforts of what we have come to call obesities. Culture is often little accounted for or is used reductively or instrumentally (or both) in science-oriented obesity studies. Health exists outside of health practitioner-patient interactions, and much of the work in this volume illustrates this point, as well as demonstrates how significant the context of culture is in understanding the global assemblages of obesities.

Bridging Paradigms: Two Reconsiderations and Two Innovations

Drawing on local biologies and global assemblages, we seek to navigate this tacking between obesity research paradigms and fat studies paradigms through the use of two reconsiderations and two innovative theoretical and research-oriented movements that can productively increase dialogue among approaches to studying obesity and fatness and in constructing effective health interventions. We see the two reconsiderations we discuss as recurring in that other scholars and researchers have noted, as does this volume, that obesity does not equal sickness and that there is a moral undercurrent to discussions of and about obesity. Although these reconsiderations continue to be recurring and reiterative, the insights and complexities that these two reconsiderations yield seems never truly to take hold and be incorporated in certain kinds of health research and in public sphere discussions about obesity. The idea that obesity equals sickness is an oversimplified equation, and that moral constructs impact the way obesity research is designed, conducted, and interpreted seems worthy of continual use as an analytical tool because of the ability of discourses of disease and morality to morph into and reappear in many forms in obesity research. Although these thematic ideas have been identified by scholars, their very proliferation and their cultural staying power indicate that that they remain significant in obesity research.

Two Reconsiderations

For the first reconsideration, we note, as many researchers have before us, the notion that obesity equals sickness needs to be unpacked and contextualized. The underlying message from popular media and health studies argues that there are direct, easily identifiable links between obesity and disease or ill health. How can this implied relationship be rendered more complexly in medical studies and in media representations? Can such studies reflect more awareness of how social metaphors shape scientific work? Work on Pacific island populations has provided science and social science, historically and currently, an excellent means of studying the impact of a nutrition transition and its concomitant and developing sociopolitical changes. To acknowledge the importance of this geographical area in obesity research and health science, we include a number of works that address this area as a means of acknowledging the importance of the Western Pacific to obesity research as well as a way in which this volume critically discusses the idea of obesity equals illness. Becker, Hardin, and Rosen touch on or discuss at length the complicated correlations among obesity, illness, and culture. Additionally the issue of individual and collective agency is explored by Becker (this volume) for how it haunts the equation between obesity and sickness in ways that demand further exploration in both the United States and the Pacific.

Second, as Fat Studies and excellent work in psychology, feminist studies, sociology, and anthropology argue, public health messaging, unintentionally, often capitalizes on or perpetuates fat stigma as well as facilitating the internalization of such stigma and the suffering and pain such internalization produces (Brewis 2010; Brewis et al. 2011; Bordo 1993; Boero 2007, 2012; Greenhalgh 2012; LeBesco 2004, 2010; Lewis et al. 2011; Rothblum and Solovay 2009; Saguy and Ameling 2008; Saguy and Riley 2005).[7]

We argue here that when obesity is studied as an obvious, readable category, such medical and public health studies inadvertently universalize and naturalize fat as a global category of the body and a category of the body that universally means the body is troubled. What if we instead tried to imagine a new relationship between the particular and the general by thinking of *obesities* rather than obesity? We want to offer a hybrid model that shifts between scientific and cultural understandings of the body to better grasp the wide range of types, proxies, experiences, and meanings of obesity (Yates-Doerr, McNaughton, Rubin and Joseph, McCullough, this volume). It is our hope that by making such a move the embeddedness of stigma becomes more visible, and in understanding the multiple meanings of obesities, there will be more awareness of culture and stigma in research design and data analysis. Our chapters ground the ways stigma is a moral experience in which stigmatized conditions (obesity, poverty, gender, race, class, etc.) highlight what really matters and what is threatened ("destroying the lived value") for individuals and communities, thereby underlining the experience of stigma in people's daily lives and in their medical care (Yang et al. 2007: 1524).

Two Innovations

Measurements as a way of quantifying obesity need to be problematized in local and global health. How measurements are made and collected need cultural contextualization so that reification is minimized. We understand that public health and health intervention research is oriented toward evidence-based practices, validity, comparability, applicability, and replicability. Most authors in this volume do not take the fat body, or any body, as a given, nor do we see the fat body as universal in meaning or measure, but we understand that this approach may fit quite poorly with health promotion and implementation work. Nonetheless, we ask that health research perhaps consider the multiple meanings of the body and the significance of a communities' or organizations' local moral world (Kleinman 1995). It is not essential that public health, behavioral health, and implementation science engage in interpretive, ontological, or phenomenological explorations of bodies and embodiment as many anthropologists, psychologists, feminist scholars, and sociologists do. However, intervention and health promotion work could benefit from not assuming that an "individual" is universal, rights-bearing, and agentive, but rather see the individual as a culturally located concept best understood in context (Lock and Farquhar 2007). Furthermore theoretical frameworks and/or methodologies that problematize individualism, assumed universalism, and unidirectional causation in understanding disease and ill health are better able to chart structural inequalities as well as the ways subjects are blamed for their own poor health to construct more effective health interventions that account for stigma and social hierarchies (Nguyen and Peschard 2003). When a health promotion or implementation project processes data on context (often understood as the environment in which the research is conducted), we hope that complexity of context (including the anomalies) could be more thoroughly incorporated in analysis through an anthropological emphasis on understanding what constitutes an individual, local cultural knowledge, social relevance, and cultural variation. We hope such considerations will be of service in designing and enriching health implementations, interventions, and promotions that attempt to account for the complexity of obesity (such as the systems model) and therefore improve health care effectiveness (Browson, Colditz, and Proctor 2012: 181–182).

Moffat and Galloway's study of a school's health food initiative (this volume) demonstrates not only how qualitative and quantitative research work together (which is common in public health and hybrid implementation work) but also how exceptions in the qualitative data were not quickly categorized as a barrier or an outlier but rather richly worked through. We invite the reader to join us in pondering what kind of impact measurement and evidence-based assessment has, and we wish to explore how and why large embodiment has come to be conceived of almost solely in terms of disease in public health and intervention work and we further invite readers to examine how this happens. We also ask that readers keep in mind that while there may be scientific evidence about health and how that is interpreted, applied, and processed varies greatly across and within cultures. All ten chapters in this volume explain what might be missed in this process of universalizing measurements and minimizing local context as way to understand health.

While many approaches to the study of obesity, including biocultural models, public health interventions, biomedical studies, and constructionist/fat studies analyses, posit fatness as a recognizable and discernible state, as well as a distinguishable category, we seek to ascertain the category of fatness, large body size, disordered eating, and obesity *in situ*.[8] Our second innovation seeks to account for the context of bodies, food histories, and epidemiological change to show how large bodies are differently conceived of as normal, or sick, or something more ambiguous.

We find the use of culture in much obesity research too instrumental, or rather "thin," and often Eurocentric. Culture as a concept in many biocultural, public health, and intervention work perspectives is limited to *lifestyle* choices. This term has become a culturally neutral representative of environmental features like patterns of behaviors, beliefs, material culture of diet and food production, and body ideals. Rock (2003) argues that lifestyle should not be conflated with culture and defines lifestyle as "an assemblage of bodily practices that are amenable to quantification. As such, lifestyles can be shown to co-occur with other things, such as certain diseases, in patterned ways across space and over time" (Rock 2003: 56). When lifestyle is conflated with culture, then culture is operationalized as limited to adaptive or maladaptive features and assumes an instrumental quality where the only determinant of health and health choices is related to outcomes; however, we know from other ethnographic studies that health choices are made for myriad reasons—not only based on epidemiological outcomes (Klaits 2010; Galloway and Moffat, Rosen, Trainer, Garth, Hardin, McNaughton, this volume). People's choices are deeply felt, held, and practiced so viewing them as maladaptive is missing their significance in the construction of personhood and their longevity in social life.

We are also uneasy with the way the fat body is universalized (often for activist purposes) and not as culturally located as is necessary to understand the multiple meanings of fat locally and globally within constructionist work on fatness. We consider gender crucial in these formulations of the body and explicitly note here that we see gender constructs as an inherent and integral part of culture and meaning-making. Meleo-Erwin (2012) makes the argument that some fat studies scholars and some fat activists are normalizing fatness in troubling ways that may limit understandings of fat as a kind of normativity rather than approach fatness as a critical politics of embodiment wherein normal is questioned and there is a more complicated understanding of how fatness is experienced in the world (2012: 388). We appreciate this point but wish to modify it here also to include not only an understanding of body normativity as unstable but to note that cultural specificity also renders the fat body a problematic mode of subject-making.

The notion of the individual itself needs to be better understood in health interventions, as this construction limits health practitioners from understanding bodies as social. Social bodies are linked in meaning and experience to others, and we find it troubling that research ranging from biomedical to fat studies places an emphasis on the individual body as well as normalizing the fat body as an obvious body category. Here, Becker, Hardin, and Rosen's work (this volume) reminds us that many cultural groups understand personhood as the relation of the self to the social self and to the social body. Garth's chapter (this volume) reminds us that bodies are historically produced and linked through stories and experiences to other bodies and modes of being in the present. Rubin and Joseph's work (this volume) demonstrates how particular subcultures, such as African-American women, understand their own individualness and body size differently from mainstream American understandings, and therefore obesity research frequently "traps" them between concerns over obesity as a risk factor on the one hand and praise for a positive body image on the other.

Health and Obesity: A Critical Approach

Weight does have a multifaceted and complex impact on health outcomes.[9] There are now and will be in the future, complex, painful, and expensive implications for people's health status globally related to obesity. To deny that members of cultures and subcultures are at risk for certain diseases, and that structural violence and inequalities as well as individual agency (no matter how limited) may produce obesity among other health issues, is to negate the validity of people's everyday realities. To nullify the structures that unite health and power is to reinforce further the status quo that blames people for their poor health rather than accounting for the social embeddedness of health (Williams 2002). However, it is also important to recognize how obesity is constructed as a health problem through rigorous work on the moral assumptions and stigmatizing characterizations implied or buried in research and intervention practices. All research is, after all, also a cultural product in addition to being health research or that of psychology or anthropology. Furthermore, ignoring, minimizing, or being unable to come to terms with how emic cultural knowledge about food, bodies, health, beliefs, social practices, and moral values impacts health-seeking behaviors and health care delivery makes for less effective interventions.

In bringing together our model of tacking between and among obesity research and fatness study paradigms, along with our two reconsiderations and two innovations for obesity research, we advance the argument that bringing biocultural, health science, and constructionist approaches toward a more integrated discussion of obesity encourages work on obesity to move in comparative and culturally grounded directions. By seriously accounting for culture and engaging in a comparative framework, this interdisciplinary approach to obesities challenges an individually oriented unit of analysis and, in turn, offers ethnographically grounded theoretical and applied frameworks for examining obesities.

Part I: Global Health, Naturalizing Measures, and Universalizing Effects

Becker, Yates-Doerr, and McNaughton engage with illness as an obesity outcome and with the role of obesity measures in different ways, each challenging a reductive or universal relationship among body size quantification, interior states of the body, and health.

The Comaroffs (2006) suggest that in the modern nation-state, statistics and figures are often reified in complex ways (see also Hacking 1991). They argue that "quantifacts" and "mythostats" function as "assertions of the real" (Comaroff and Comaroff 2006: 209). The Comaroffs warn us that such formulations of statistics:

> …render large abstractions concretely meaningful to personal experience, speaking with authority about the connection of human beings to otherwise incomprehensible phenomena.… Viewed thus, the statistic is a medium of communication and a species of commodified knowledge, one whose value and veracity accumulates as it circulates. Part fetish, it has also become a term in the ordinary language of being (Comarofff and Comaroff 2006: 209–210).

Drawing attention to the ways that statistics about obesity reify the universality of fat is not to contend with their "truth value," but to draw attention to the fact that obesity statistics offer a rather limited way to conceive of and to understand the meanings and significance of obesity and fatness. We argue that mythostats and quantifacts, if not contextualized, can obscure the everyday experiences and local biologies (Lock 1993; 2005) of actual bodies and peoples that these numbers are supposedly representing. Numbers often do not solely measure actual health nor do they measure the way cultural groups themselves understand and define health (Bacon 2008). Becker, Yates-Doerr, and McNaughton examine the constructions and uses of measurements in the diagnosing of obesity and in the gauging of success in public health interventions so that the use of statistical data becomes a less fetishized and therefore a more accurate part of the obesity puzzle. We suggest that the processes of quantifiable knowledge gathering and analysis need to be culturally unpacked and the meanings these statistics generate need their circulations traced and analyzed (Asad 1994).

Becker's groundbreaking chapter subjects the easy popular discourse of obesity equals sickness to scientific rigor. Although she understands obesity and disordered eating as linked to poor health outcomes, she nevertheless shares a discomfort with the reification of quatifacts and mythostats. For example, Becker turns her critical eye on some benchmark health studies and points out where there is not a full accounting of issues such as race, gender, and economic status. Therefore she queries the validity of applying study results universally. Becker elucidates how the naturalization of body weight, the lack of accounting for cultural variation/local context, and the commercialization of weight management combined with moral orientations work together to perpetuate a charged discourse that limits the feasibility and effectiveness of reducing the health issues related to obesity.

The work of Yates-Doerr and McNaughton scrutinizes how measures do their work in social life, and their chapters put quantifiable data into discussion with qualitative data to posit applied recommendations. Both authors particularly, although not exclusively, focus on the notion that obesity equals sickness must be subject to rigorous examination, and that measurements need to be problematized in local and global health and not be made into a mythostat and a quatifact. These three authors directly link our first reconsideration and our first innovation—the idea that obesity is equivalent to ill health and the validity of measurements needs study—to the field of obesity research to chart the fraught territory between the measures of meanings and the meanings of measures.

Part II: Large Embodiment and Histories of Fat

Hardin's and Garth's work builds on the rich tradition of cross-cultural studies of the meanings of body size by drawing attention to the polysemic meaning of body size and sociocultural history in contexts where mythostats and quatifacts heighten attention to the relationship between body size, health, and disease. We see the ethnographic studies conducted by Anderson-Fye (2003, 2004), Becker (1995), Bordo (1993), Kulick and Meneley (2005), Nichter (2000), Popenoe (2003), and Sobo (1994) as exemplifying rich social, cultural, symbolic, and discursive analyses. These scholars reveal how body size is a semiotic category and a signifying practice. The works listed above are often used as evidence for the values of large body size in "fat-tolerant" or "fat-positive" societies, thus marking these societies as "other." We seek to build on exploration of body size preferences and the meanings of body size to further explore bodies and size in context with attention to historical depth, race, gender, embodied experience as well as the individual and social dilemmas surrounding the negotiation of the meaning of body size, health, and food.

Hardin and Garth explore how the meanings of fatness and obesity are informed by public conflict over the biomedical and semiotic control of the diseased obese body among Evangelical Samoans and in the social memory of past food scarcity among Cubans in their current health-seeking behavior. The Samoan and Cuban case studies illustrate how health and health-seeking behaviors exist outside of patient-client/provider interactions. Hardin's and Garth's work shows us how local biologies help us account for the significance of health-seeking behaviors and cultural body beliefs. Given the increasing global concern over obesity, global assemblages helps us understand how obesity interventions travel and in this traveling miss the deep significance of human action in the Samoan and Cuban cases where health-seeking behaviors do not map well or are invisible to health promotion models.

Furthermore, Garth and Hardin richly document the multiple meanings of food itself and the economic landscape of food production and distribution. Such understandings of the biopolitics of food needs both more study in the field of obesity research and then more integration into health intervention work (Benson 2012). Bodies are not universal in meaning and neither is food. Both authors specifically take on the second innovation, the relevance of cultural context to understanding fatness and obesity, by arguing that it is essential to understand that large bodies are differently conceived of as normal, sick, or a range of more complicated and historically centered meanings.

Part III: Cultures of Practice and Conflicting Interventions

Constructionist accounts tend to downplay, as Moffat points out in her review (2010: 12), that weight can actually be associated with health problems (see Boero 2007; de Vries 2007; Rothblum and Solovay 2009). While there are health problems that are associated with obesity or health issues that correlate with populations that may also have high rates of obesity, obesity does not correlate linearly to disease. In this section Rosen, Trainer, and Moffat and Galloway demonstrate the complex ways obesity may and may not necessarily correlate directly with disease. Furthermore, their research highlights the importance of the relationship between locating the cultural context not only for the research subject but also for the culture of the interventions themselves. There is a very strong emphasis in public health, health promotion, behavioral medicine, and implementation science on the effectiveness of an intervention and in locating what parts of the intervention are translational and appropriate for wider application. Rosen, Moffat, and Galloway and Trainer explore how and why certain translational approaches do not work, as well as making some clear suggestions on what could be improved in these models.

Building on a biocultural approach to the study of obesities, these chapters integrate ethnographic and qualitative methods with those of epidemiology, behavioral science, and biocultural anthropology to take the call of translational research (McGarvey 2009) seriously by looking to incorporate local biologies, models of selfhood, and social change into rigorously culturally informed interventions. In health interventions the issue of categories and vocabularies are often unexamined and unquestioned. As Rosen (this volume) notes, anthropologists abjure the application of global terms like *collectivistic, individualistic,* or *community* because they are not culturally located or contextualized. In behavioral medicine such terms as *individual, collectivist,* or *community* are vocabularies so ingrained and accepted as a part of explanatory models that behavioral medicine is almost incapable of working without them. Part of the issue here is that behavioral medicine could benefit from taking into account the ways its approach is culturally located, as Rosen discusses in her work on adapting a diabetes intervention in Samoa.

Harkening back to our concern with the uses of measurements and meanings, Trainer demonstrates how obesity statistics, while revealing the rapid and exponential growth of obesity in the Middle East, do not go far enough in reflecting the economic, social, and cultural diversity of the region. Furthermore, Trainer's work highlights the cost to health and well-being for Emirati girls who may be "thin" according to BMI but are not "healthy." Trainer demonstrates the unintended health consequences for Emirati girls engendered by the combined messages of judgmental and scientific discourses about being overweight or obese (see also Greenhalgh 2012).

Bicultural and behavioral analyses that deeply incorporate culture, as Galloway and Moffat, Rosen, and Trainer do, not only demonstrate the ways that fat etiologies influence food ideologies but that public health initiatives, while intending to target obesity from a multilevel and multisector approach, often miss the point, and the target, when culture is eliminated. Work in the United Arab Emirates, Samoa, and Canada draw on our two innovations (disease as equivalent to obesity, the problematic of measurements and the importance of cultural context) we proposed for obesity research and study how these innovations might be applied in a health intervention or health assessment work.

Part IV: Fat Etiologies, Stigma, and Gaps of Care in Biomedical Models of Obesity

Rigorously exploring the connections between obesity and health problems can be done, as Rubin and Joseph and McCullough demonstrate, in sensitive and sophisticated ways that do not reinforce stigma and prejudice (for example, Bacon 2008; Ernsberger and Koletsky 1999). Part IV examines the relationships between obesity interventions and "the barrage of fat etiologies" (McCullough, this volume) present in everyday American life. Closely examining public health interventions reveals that there is no neat division between where obesity research ends and where popular representations of obesity begin. By exploring intervention approaches, health messaging, and medical care, these chapters reveal that measurement-based understandings of obesity and fatness combined with a lack of understanding of the moral, emotional, and gendered dimensions of stigma do not produce meaningful interventions or appropriate medical care.

The Fat Studies Reader (Rothblum and Solovay 2009) argues that "social problems," such as the "obesity epidemic," are socially constructed and validated through media portrayals of biomedical and public health studies and statistics that circulate as "truth claims" (Bacon 2008; Boero 2007, 2012; Braziel and LeBesco 2001; LeBesco 2010; Moffat 2010; Murray 2008; Nichter 2000; Saguy and Riley 2005; Spector and Kitsuse 2010). Building on work in feminism and fat studies concerned with how scientific truth claims operate to medicalize and stigmatize specific body types and marginalize categories of people for not disciplining themselves to meet societal norms, McCullough and Rubin and Joseph draw on very different methods and approaches to capture the range of stigmatizing experiences and the very real health, social and emotional impact that stigmatizing social practices and stigma laden messaging on obesity engender. We also mean *engender* in the sense that studies about fat and body image are deeply tied to gender and race. Rubin and Joseph's work is an analysis of the lack of discussion between the literature on eating disorders and body image research. They are especially concerned with the position the lack of discussion between eating disorders and body image studies produces for African-American women. McCullough produces a moving reflexive account of an obese pregnancy. Drawing on embodied social experience, McCullough challenges the reader to question the ethics of pregnancy care in which body size and the imagined measures of obesity render the obese maternal body subject to uneven medical surveillance and poor treatment in clinical settings. In doing so, McCullough brings to the fore how and why stigma not only might prevent obese people from seeking help but also the ways in which everyday mistreatment (intentional and unintentional) impacts health outcomes. Demonstrating our theoretically driven second reconsideration and second innovation (the significance of stigma and its reproduction in medical practice and the importance of cultural context), these chapters power-fully articulate how certain forms of fat embodiment elucidate medical imperial-ism and further complicate obesity research and effective health interventions by calling attention to the prevalence of fat stigma at the both the meta and macro levels of social life and medical practice.

Concluding Remarks

Taken together, these chapters productively work to foster interdisciplinary re-search and discussion to successfully de-naturalize and de-universalize obesity in the hopes of loosening the taken-for-granted ground in which stigmatizing assumptions about fatness and obesity are embedded, thereby re-conceiving the singular meaning of obesity and fatness.

As a possible direction for future research, we suggest that the culture of obe-sity research itself is in need of study. Health science and health services research is both situated in culture and produces culture in its work practices and its workplace. Sobo et al. (2008) have pointed out the significance of organizational culture in health service research, such as grant-related timelines, funding appli-cations, administrative burdens, staff turnover, political maneuverings, high work-loads and the pressure to publish, that impact the kind of studies done (not only the kind of work that is funded but the time of the study itself—the emphasis be-ing on short studies with investigators constantly applying for more grant money), and the implementation of research finding. Although the volume's authors do not explore the issue of health science's organizational cultures directly, we note that the issue of culture in obesity research is multifaceted and multidirectional and could benefit from not only more studies that document how cultural ideas about large embodiment seep into research design and interventions but that the way health service and health research is funded and conducted is also pertinent (see Sobo et al. 2008 for a case study). More research of this sort might better help us understand why health promotions, interventions, and implementations fail or are incomplete rather than the tendency to blame sustainability on the individual obese subject or subjects.

Following Asad (1994), we are not concerned with the merits of biocultural versus social anthropology, constructionist work versus health research, and quan-titative versus qualitative (or ethnographic) representations of the social world, but with the effects that such representations have on how obesity is constructed and understood as an epidemic and social problem. The impact of obesity will very likely add to the health burdens of those populations who can ill afford the economic and social costs of poor health. Health interventions and health implementations that merely see culture as adaptive or maladaptive assume an instrumental quality where the only determinants of health and health choices is related to outcomes; we know from ethnographic studies that health choices are made for a myriad of complex cultural, economic, and political reasons that may not correlate with an outcomes based approach. As Becker notes in her chapter, "[T]he interrogation of the tensions between the social and clinical realities of weight disorders is not intended to dismiss their health salience, but rather to expose misguided assumptions that potentially undermine the effectiveness and feasibility of interventions aimed at reducing the health, economic, and social burdens they impose."

Not all approaches to the study of obesity will find relevant or convincing the importance of not universalizing the human body or seeing health as not solely tied to measurement. Measurements and indicators are all too often naturalized (Merry 2011). We understand that measurement is a powerful tool in health science work and that the multiple meanings and effects of measurement are often not acknowledged as having significance other than that necessary to validity and reliability. Implied in the approach to implementing evidence-based practices is an idea of the individual as a rational actor. The suggestion is, if the *facts* about obesity are known then certain behaviors should logically follow. This implied notion of the individual and the concept of rational actors needs the kind of serious examination this volume provides. We recognize that our understanding of fat as multivalent and polysemic will be difficult to operationalize quickly within accepted science and implementation models. We know that our unpacking and revealing fat stigma in popular and scientific discourse may not find purchase with other approaches to obesity research. However, the work in this volume is not only theoretical but also pragmatic.

Approaches to obesity should expand the scope of health intervention, promotion, and implementation beyond the individual to engage deeply with culture to account for gendered dynamics, models of embodiment, histories, globalization, and a host of other factors. Our work explores how everyday lives, local moral worlds, and the capacity to act fit into and forges the local biologies (Lock 2001) of emerging biological assemblages of governance, biomedical research, and the complex structural contributors to health problems (Bharadwai 2010). The cases studies presented here argue that understanding the local biologies of obese subjects and obese populations would actually make a difference in the construction of health intervention and promotion models as well as in augmenting epidemiological work. Our collective work also demonstrates concretely why certain aspects of interventions are not transferable and replicable, and our work reveals the stories beneath and between the interventions and health research discourses. This combination is an invaluable and frequently missing perspective in health promotion, health intervention, and health implementation research.

Notes

1. The Downey Obesity Report from the Robert Wood Johnson Foundation is also a good source of well-reported obesity statistics (Morgan Downey 2011).
2. The following are a small sample of rankings of global obesity rates: http://www.forbes.com/2007/02/07/worlds-fattest-countries-forbeslife-cx_ls_0208 worldfat_2.html; http://www.globalpost.com/dispatch/commerce/091125/obesity-epide mic-fattest-countries?page=0,1; http://www.globalpost.com/dispatch/health/101119/fat-top-10-obese; http://www.infoplease.com/world/statistics/obesity.html; http://www.huff ingtonpost.com/2012/02/22/obesity-rates-rising-developed-fattest-world_n_1294212 .html.
   News story on countries that need to exercise August 2012
   http://www.huffingtonpost.com/2012/07/19/exercise-countries_n_1683435.html.
3. This article claims that fat people use up more of the world's resources and therefore have a larger carbon footprint, but issues of wealth and consumption (wealthy thin people with multiple houses might have a bigger carbon footprint, for example) are underdeveloped, among other issues with this article.
4. The *New York Times*'s Tara Parker-Pope (2011, 2012) wrote an article about the complexity of losing weight and keeping it off, but such research does not often make it into the news nor into popular debates. See also http://www.downeyobesityreport.com/tag/robert-wood-johnson-foundation/ and http://www.nytimes.com/2012/05/15/science/a-mathe matical-challenge-to-obesity.html.
5. Health science and health service research encompass many fields and subfields. We use these two terms to talk about clinical research on obesity as well as quantitative and qualitative research work that include fields such as public health, global public health, behavioral health, health services research, quality improvement research, and implementation science. Health science research is the application of science to health. Health service research is primarily focused on improving health care quality, efficiency, and effectiveness. There is some slippage in terms and meanings. We try to be specific where we can, and although we acknowledge the complexity and variety of these fields, we try to identify and discuss general trends or approaches in understanding obesity that we think bear examination. See also http://www.downeyobesityreport.com/tag/robert-wood-johnson-foundation/ and http://www.nytimes.com/2012/05/15/science/a-mathematical-challenge-to-obesity.html.
6. Clifford Geertz talked about "tacking" in his 1974 essay entitled "'From the Native's Point of View': On the Nature of Anthropological Understanding." Geertz discusses what he calls "dialectical tacking" between local detail and global structure to cover both simultaneously in an attempt to understand the "native's point of view." We are not using the term as Geertz does, but we did derive inspiration from the metaphor of "tacking" in trying to understand the local details and the wider structures of debates in obesity research.
7. Brewis's biocultural anthropological work on the relationships among stigma, measurement, obesity, and culture is a stand out in the field of anthropology (Brewis et al. 2011; Brewis 2010).
8. We understand the "constructionist" position in the study of obesity as research generated out of the social sciences, cultural studies, queer studies, literary studies, and size activists that study fat, not obesity, in part as a rejection of the medicalization of health and the pathologizing of body weight that obesity implies and legitimizes. The work of construc-

tionists is mostly based in the United States, Australia, New Zealand, and Western Europe, specifically Great Britain, as evidenced by the edited volumes *The Fat Studies Reader* (Solovay and Rothblum 2009) and *Fat Studies in the UK* (Tomrley and Naylor 2009) (see also Bordo 1993; LeBesco 2004; Saguy and Ameling 2008; Saguy and Riley 2005). We acknowledge that the term *constructionist* is a rather facile label and that academic work on obesity, which can fall in this very broad category, is extremely varied and wide-ranging. *The Fat Studies Reader* (Rothblum and Solovay 2009) is a defining text for the area of fat studies. For a good anthropological review of this literature see Moffat (2010).

9. Biocultural anthropologists, biologists, and biomedical researchers have demonstrated that there are links among obesity, genetics, and the environment (Brown and Sweeney 2009; McGarvey 1991, 1993, 2009; Popkin 1994; Ulijaszek 2006; Ulijaszek and Lofink 2006). Bringing genetics into the equation does not immediately lead to a new eugenics, as LeBesco has suggested (2009:65–75). Biomedicine and scientific research is carried out by individuals and structures that are products of culture and embedded in larger "cultures of technoscience" (Franklin 2005:73). Therefore, we acknowledge that stigmatizing assumptions may leak into genetic research and that genetic studies are often interpreted and circulated in the media in a limited fashion. We maintain studying the links among obesity, genetics, environment, and socioeconomic status is important and can be used to complicate understandings of obesity and disease rather than be used to further abuse fat bodies or particular cultures or subcultures (Brewis 2010, 2011; McGarvey 1991; Ulijaszek and Lofink 2006).

References

Aphramor, L., and J. Gingras. 2009. "That Remains to be Said: Disappeared Feminist Discourses on Fat in Dietetic Theory and Practice." In *The Fat Studies Reader*, ed. E. Rothblum and S. Solovay. New York: New York University Press, 97–105.

Anderson-Fye, E. P. 2003. "Never Leave Yourself: Ethnopsychology as Mediator of Psychological Globalization among Belizean Schoolgirls." *Ethos* 31, no. 1: 59–94.

———. 2004. "A 'Coca-Cola' Shape: Cultural Change, Body Image, and Eating Disorders in San Andres, Belize." *Culture, Medicine, and Psychiatry* 28, no. 4: 561–595.

Asad, T. 1994. "Ethnographic Representation, Statistics, and Modern Power." *Social Research* 61, no. 1: 55–88.

Bacon, L. 2008. *Health at Every Size: The Surprising Truth About Your Weight.* Dallas: BenBella Books.

Becker, A. E. 1995. *Body, Self and Society: The View from Fiji.* Philadelphia: University of Pennsylvania Press.

Benson, P. 2012. "Political Injustice and Contemporary Capitalism." *American Ethnologist* 39, no. 3: 488–490.

Bharadwaj, A. 2010. "Reproductive Viability and the State: Stem Cell Research in India." In *Reproduction, Globalization, and the State: New Theoretical and Ethnographic Perspectives*, ed. C. Browner and C. F. Sargent. Durham: Duke University Press, 113–125.

Boero, N. 2007. "All the News That's Fat to Print: The American 'Obesity Epidemic' and the Media." *Qualitative Sociology* 30, no. 1: 41–61.

———. 2012. *Killer Fat: Media, Medicine and Moral in the American "Obesity" Epidemic.* New Jersey: Rutgers University Press.

Bordo, S. 1993. *Unbearable Weight: Feminism, Western Culture, and the Body.* Berkeley, Los Angeles, and London: University of California.

Braziel, J. E., and K. LeBesco, eds. 2001. *Bodies out of Bounds: Fatness and Transgression.* Berkeley: University of California Press.

Brewis, A. A. 2010. *Obesity: Cultural and Biocultural Perspectives.* New Brunswick: Rutgers University Press.

Brewis, A. A., D. J. Hruschka, and A. Wutich. 2011. "Vulnerablity to Fat-Stigma in Women's Everyday Relationships." *Social Science and Medicine* 73: 491–497.

Brown, P., and J. Sweeney. 2009. "The Anthropology of Overweight, Obesity, and the Body." *AnthroNotes* 30, no. 1: 6–12.

Brownell, K. D., R. M. Puhl, M. B. Schwartz, and L. Rudd. 2005. *Weight Bias: Nature, Consequences and Remedies.* New York: Guilford Press.

Browner, C., and C. F. Sargent. 2010. "Toward Global Anthropological Studies of Reproduction: Concepts, Methods, Theoretical Approaches." In *Reproduction, Globalization, and the State,* ed. C. Browner and C. F. Sargent. Durham: Duke University Press, 1–18.

Browson, R. C., G. A. Colditz, and E. K. Proctor. 2012. *Dissemination and Implementation Research in Health: Translating Science to Practice.* Oxford and New York: Oxford University Press.

Campos, P., A. C. Saguy, E. O. Ernsberger, and G. Gaesser. 2006. "The Epidemiology of Overweight and Obesity: Public Health Crisis or Moral Panic?" *International Journal of Epidemiology* 35, no. 1: 55–60.

CDC (Centers for Disease Control and Prevention). 2012. "Adult Obesity Facts. Division of Nutrition, Physical Activity, and Obesity, National Center for Chronic Disease Prevention and Health Promotion." Available at http://www.cdc.gov/obesity/data/adult.html, accessed August 15, 2012.

Collier, S. J., and A. Ong. 2005. "Global Assemblages, Anthropological Problems." In *Global Assemblages: Technology, Politics, and Ethics as Anthropological Problems,* ed. S. J. Collier and A. Ong. Malden: Blackwell Publishing, 3–21.

Comaroff, J., and J. Comaroff. 2006. "Figuring Crime: Quantifacts and the Production of the Un/real." *Public Culture* 18, no. 1: 209–246.

Downey, M. 2011. "Conflicts of Interest on Obesity Panel." *The Downey Obesity Report* November 3, 2011. Available at http://www.downeyobesityreport.com/2011/11/conflicts-of-interest-on-obesity-panel/, accessed August 15, 2012

Driefus, C. 2012. "A Mathematical Challenge to Obesity." *New York Times,* May 14. Available at http://www.nytimes.com/2012/05/15/science/a-mathematical-challenge-to-obesity.html Accessed August 15, 2012.

de Vries, C. 2007. "Sleeping Giant: Fact or Fairytale? Examining the Impact of European Integration on National Elections." *European Union Politics* 8, no. 3: 363–385.

Ernsberger, P., and R. J. Koletsky. 1999. "Biomedical Rationale for a Wellness Approach to Obesity: An Alternative to a Focus on Weight Loss." *Journal of Social Issues* 55, no. 2: 221–259.

Farrell, A. E. 2011. *Fat Shame: Stigma and the Fat Body in American Culture.* New York: New York University Press.

Franklin, S. 2005. "Stem Cells R Us: Emergent Forms and the Global Biological." In *Global Assemblages: Technology, Politics, and Ethics as Anthropological Problems,* ed. S. J. Collier and A. Ong. Malden: Blackwell Publishing, 59–78.

Geertz, C. 1974. "'From the Native's Point of View': On the Nature of Anthropological Understanding." *Bulletin of the American Academy of Arts and Sciences* 28, no. 1: 26–45.

Greehalgh, S. 2012. "Weighty Subjects: The Biopolitics of the U.S. War on Fat." *American Ethnologist* 39, no. 3: 471–487.

Guthman, J. 2011. *Weighing In: Obesity, Food Justice and the Limits of Capitalism.* Berkley: University of California Press.

Hacking, I. 1991. "How Should We Do the History of Statistics?" In *The Foucault Effect: Studies in Governmentality,* ed. G. Burchell, C. Gordon, and P. Miller. Chicago: University of Chicago Press, 181–196.

Jutel, A. 2006. "The Emergence of Overweight as a Disease Entity: Measuring Up Normality." *Social Science and Medicine* 63, no. 9: 2268–2276.

Klaits, F. 2010. *Death in a Church of Life: Moral Passion During Botswana's Time of Aids.* Berkeley, Los Angeles, and London: University of California Press.

Kleinman, A. 1995. *Writing at the Margin: Discourse between Anthropology and Medicine.* Berkeley, Los Angeles, and London: University of California Press.

Koppelman, S. 2009. "Fat Stories in the Classroom: What and How Are They Teaching About Us?" In *The Fat Studies Reader,* ed. E. Rothblum and S. Solovay. New York: New York University Press, 213–222.

Kulick, D., and A. Meneley, eds. 2005. *Fat: The Anthropology of an Obsession.* New York: Jeremy P. Tarcher/Penguin.

Landau, E. 2009. "Thinner is Better to Curb Global Warming, Study Says." CNN Health, April 20, available at http://articles.cnn.com/2009-04-20/health/thin.global.warming_1 _obese-people-global-warming-greenhouse-gas-emissions. Accessed July 30, 2011.

LeBesco, K. 2004. *Revolting Bodies? The Struggle to Redefine Fat Identity.* Amherst: University of Massachusetts Press.

———. 2009. "Quest for a Cause: The Fat Gene, the Gay Gene, and the New Eugenics." In *The Fat Studies Reader,* ed. E. Rothblum and S. Solovay. New York: New York University Press, 65–74.

———. 2010. "Fat Panic and the New Morality." In *Against Health: How Health Became the New Morality,* ed. J. M. Metzl and A. Kirkland. New York: New York University Press, 72–82.

Lewis, S., S. L. Thomas, R. W. Blood, D. J. Castle, J. Hyde, and P. A. Komesaroff. 2011. "How Do Obese Individuals Perceive and Respond to the Different Types of Obesity Stigma That They Encounter in Their Daily Lives? A Qualitative Study." *Social Science and Medicine* 73: 1349–1356.

Lock, M. 1993. *Encounters with Aging: Mythologies of Menopause in Japan and North America.* Berkeley: University of California Press.

———. 2001. "The Tempering of Medical Anthropology: Troubling Natural Categories." *Medical Anthropology Quarterly* 15, no. 4: 478–492.

———. 2005. "Medical Anthropology: Intimations for the Future." In *Medical Anthropology: Regional Perspectives and Shared Concerns,* ed. F. Salliant and S. Genest. Malden: Blackwell, 266–288.

Lock, M and J. Farquhar, eds. 2007. *Beyond the Body Proper: Reading the Anthropology of Material Life.* Durham, NC: Duke University Press.

McGarvey, S. 1991. "Obesity in Samoans and a Perspective on its Etiology in Polynesians." *American Journal of Clinical Nutrition* 53, no. 1: 1586–1594.

————. 1993. "Population Change in Adult Obesity and Blood Lipids in American Samoa from 1976–1978 to 1990." *American Journal of Human Biology* 5, no. 1: 17–30.

————. 2009. "Interdisciplinary Translational Research in Anthropology, Nutrition, and Public Health." *Annual Review of Anthropology* 38: 233–249.

Meleo-Erwin, Z. 2012. "Disrupting Normal: Toward the 'Ordinary and Familiar' in Fat Politics." *Feminism and Psychology* 22, no. 3: 388–402.

Merry, S. E. 2011. "Measuring the World: Indicators, Human Rights, and Global Governance." *Current Anthropology* 52, Supplement 3: 583–595.

Moffat, T. 2010. "The 'Childhood Obesity Epidemic': Health Crisis or Social Construction." *Medical Anthropology Quarterly* 24, no. 1: 1–21.

Murray, S. 2008 *The "Fat" Female Body.* New York: Palgrave Macmillan.

Nichter, M. 2000. *Fat Talk: What Girls and Their Parents Say About Dieting.* Cambridge and London: Harvard University Press.

————. 2008. "Coming to Our Senses: Appreciating the Sensorial in Medical Anthropology." *Transcultural Psychiatry* 45, no. 2: 163–197.

Nguyen, V.-K., and K. Peschard. 2003. "Anthropology, Inequality and Disease: A Review." *Annual Review of Anthropology* 32: 447–474.

Parker-Pope, T. 2011. "The Fat Trap." *The New York Times,* December 28, available at http://www.nytimes.com/2012/01/01/magazine/tara-parker-pope-fat-trap.html, accessed August 5, 2012.

————. 2012. "A Mathematical Challenge to Obesity." *The New York Times,* May 14, available at http://www.nytimes.com/2012/05/15/science/a-mathematical-challenge-to-obesity.html, accessed August 5, 2012.

Popenoe, R. 2003. *Feeding Desire: Fatness, Beauty and Sexuality among a Saharan People.* New York: Routledge.

————. 2005. "Ideal." In *Fat,* ed. D. Kulick and A. Meneley. New York: Tarcher/Penguin Books, 9–28.

Popkin, B. M. 1994. "The Nutrition Transition in Low-Income Countries: An Emerging Crisis." *Nutritional Reviews* 52, no. 9: 285–298.

Puhl, R. M., and K. Brownell. 2001. "Bias, Discrimination, and Obesity." *Obesity* 14: 1802–1815.

Rock, M. 2003. "Sweet Blood and Social Suffering: Rethinking Cause-Effect Relationships in Diabetes, Distress, and Duress." *Medical Anthropology* 22: 131–174.

Rothblum, E., and S. Solovay, eds. 2009. *The Fat Studies Reader.* New York: New York University Press.

Royce, T. 2009."The Shape of Abuse: Fat Oppression as a Form of Violence Against Women." In *The Fat Studies Reader,* ed. E. Rothblum and S. Solovay. New York: New York University Press, 151–157.

Saguy, A.C., and R. Almeling. 2008. "Fat in the Fire? Science, the News Media, and the 'Obesity Epidemic.'" *Sociological Review* 23, no. 1: 53–83.

Saguy, A. C., and K. W. Riley. 2005. "Weighing Both Sides: Morality, Mortality, and Framing Contests over Obesity." *Journal of Health Politics* 30, no. 5: 869–921.

Scheper-Hughes, N., and M. M. Lock. 1987. "The Mindful Body: A Prolegomenon to Future Work in Medical Anthropology." *Medical Anthropology Quarterly* 1, no. 1: 6–41.

Sobo, E. J. 1994. "The Sweetness of Fat: Health, Procreation, and Sociability in Rural Jamaica." In *Many Mirrors: Body Image and Social Relations,* ed. N. Sault. New Brunswick: Rutgers University Press, 133–153.

Sobo, E. J., C. Bowman, and A. Gifford. 2008. "Behind the Scenes in Health Care Improvement: The Complex Structures and Emergent Strategies of Implementation Science." *Social Science and Medicine* 67: 1530–1540.

Spector, M., and J. Kitsuse. 2010 [2000]. *Constructing Social Problems.* New Brunswick: Transaction Publishers.

Streib, L. 2007. "World's Fattest Countries." Available at http://www.forbes.com/2007/02/07/worlds-fattest-countries-forbeslife-cx_ls_0208worldfat.html, accessed August 12, 2012.

Tomrley, C., and A. K. Naylor, eds. 2009. *Fat Studies in the UK.* York: Raw Nerve Books.

Ulijaszek, S. J. 2006. "Obesity: A Disorder of Convenience." *Obesity Reviews* 8, Suppl. 1: 183–187.

Ulijaszek, S. J., and H. Lofink. 2006. "Obesity in Bicultural Perspective." *Annual Review of Anthropology* 35: 337–360.

WHO (World Health Organization). 2012. "Obesity and Overweight. Fact Sheet No. 311." Available at http://www.who.int/mediacentre/factsheets/fs311/en/index.html, accessed August 15, 2012.

———. 2013. "Obesity and Overweight. Fact Sheet No. 311" Available at http://www.who.int/mediacentre/factsheets/fs311/en/, accessed May 9, 2013.

Williams, D. R. 2002. "Racial/Ethnic Variations in Women's Health: The Social Imbeddedness of Health." *American Journal of Public Health* 92, no. 4: 588–597.

Yang, L. H., A. Kleinman, B. G. Link, J. C. Phelan, S. Lee, and B. Good. 2007. "Culture and Stigma: Adding Moral Experience to Stigma Theory." *Social Science and Medicine* 64: 1524–1535.

Global Health, Naturalizing Measures, and Universalizing Effects

CHAPTER 1

Resocializing Body Weight, Obesity, and Health Agency

Anne E. Becker

✦ ✦ ✦

In an era of spectacular scientific precision, the operationalization of body weight—as a collection of clinical facts that predict or portend health outcomes—has offered stubborn resistance. Capturing the parameters for obesity, in turn, in nosologic terms for clinical guidance has been both contested and contentious. Surprisingly, or perhaps not, a good deal of ink has been spilled and affect evoked in public and scientific discourse about obesity in the United States. Even outside its increasingly broad sphere of medicalization and medical intervention, weight management has become firmly entrenched as commercial enterprise, moral orientation, social identity, and personal avocation. The stark limitations of its technologies notwithstanding, the market for weight management products is perpetually bullish. On the one hand, consumer enthusiasm to disregard overwhelmingly long odds against sustainable meaningful weight reduction may appear perplexing. On the other, the construct of overweight is a deep reservoir of social metaphors that underwrite its enduring and seductive traction in both lay and scientific discourse. Its complex—but still imperfectly understood—grounding in both biological and social realities, moreover, perpetuates tensions that sustain the plasticity of the construct and its affective charge in this discourse.

Abetted by biomedical technologies that can measure physical proxies of excessive—or inadequate—fatness, corpulence has migrated from a visual and embodied fact toward a signifier of health risk as a "condition" or "phenotype." As a result, obesity has emerged as a construct that quantifies and naturalizes fatness as a condition of medical relevance. This medical relevance—not wholly uncontested in some spheres—has also invigorated its social relevance in ways that could surely be tapped to promote a public health agenda, but unfortunately remain frequently obscure or neglected in prescriptions for prevention or action. Thus, alongside the intellectual exercise of deconstructing and resocializing weight and its management is an urgent pragmatic purpose. The rapid escalation of obesity worldwide has profound implications for population health, not just in high-income regions, but in low- and middle-income countries as well. Disordered eating also has an ever-widening global reach. Precisely because these health conditions easily trace their kinship from normative behaviors—which exhibit striking cultural variation—preventive health interventions and health care delivery must engage local knowledge and social relevance to optimize their feasibility and effectiveness in reducing their associated health burdens.

The Naturalization of Body Weight and Weight Disorders

The present day clinical formulation of the impact of weight on health emerged with powerful influence and concreticity in a swell of clinical empiricism that was, in part, fueled by large population-based studies. Framingham, circa 1948, may have seemed an unlikely birthplace for epic epidemiologic discovery at the time. In hindsight, however, when a small cohort of its residents landed in the eponymous Framingham Study, its 5,209 initial participants have wielded unimaginable epidemiologic leverage. Since that departure point, approximately twelve hundred scientific papers have been published that, in aggregate, have become bedrock to the medical grasp of risk factors for cardiovascular disease, obesity among them (Framingham Heart Study 2011). That the study cohort was "primarily Caucasian" is shrugged off on the study's website, with an immodest claim that "the importance of the major CVD risk factors identified in this group have been shown in other studies to apply almost universally among racial and ethnic groups, even though the patterns of distribution may vary from group to group" (Framingham Heart Study 2011). Whether a few thousand Framinghamers—those who joined the study cohort either upon its launch or since then in one of three generational cohorts plus an omni cohort—fairly represent even their fellow Americans would sustain an interesting debate.

Conversely, that large population cohorts from other regions have not had adequate opportunities to mine their aggregate data suggests a nontrivial critique of the generalization of the clinical relevance of obesity from this modest cohort. With a population now just shy of sixty-seven thousand (U.S. Census Bureau 2009), Framingham is perched at the perimeter of the metro-Boston beltway, a convenience that surely must have endeared it to the ambitious and competitive academic hospitals crowded nearby. The questionable validity of its representation of the biological, social, and psychological complexities of health risks—not only of the U.S. population of which it is a just a fraction of a percent, but also of the rest of the world's nearly 7 billion (The World Bank 2010)—seems to have been brushed off. And yet, available data suggest that the prevalence of obesity varies not just across ethnic groups, but also with socioeconomic factors. These socioeconomic variables, in turn, relate to obesity risk factors in various ways, such as in the nutritional quality of the diet and the accessibility of fresh fruits and vegetables or safe areas for recreational physical activity (Judge et al. 2006). Nonetheless, the Framingham Study cohort has achieved singular prominence for mapping the territory of risk and cardiovascular disease.

Discernment of the epidemiologic significance of fatness to health requires the operationalization and measurement of fatness. Weight is easily measured in most settings[1] but is only meaningful when contextualized against developmental stage, gender, and height. By extension, body mass index (BMI) is a convenient proxy for excessive adiposity in globally wide routine use. BMI is not uncontested as the gold standard proxy for obesity in adults, however (see Yates-Doerr, this volume). For example, whole populations, such as elite athletes (Nevill et al. 2010) and Pacific Islanders (Rush et al. 2009), may be systematically misclassified as obese, notwithstanding normal adiposity. Others have rejected the emphasis on BMI on the grounds that waist to hip ratio is a more salient predictor of health outcomes (Jacobson and Brown 1996). And still others have coined the term "normal weight obesity," proposing that normal BMI can be associated with excessive percentage body fat and thus reframing the "real definition of obesity" (Mayo Clinic 2008). Even when BMI is taken as a conventional proxy for the clinical salience of weight, its dimensional quality (i.e., as a measure generating numeric values along a *continuum*) is problematic for lay interpretation and public health messaging that has routinely relied on *categorical* descriptors to delimit healthful—and unhealthful—body weights.

On September 14, 1995, The *New England Journal of Medicine* published a landmark study titled "Body Weight and Mortality among Women" (Manson et al. 1995). The Nurses' Health Study, from which the study data were produced, yielded findings based on an epidemiologically enviable cohort of just more than 115,000 women followed prospectively over sixteen years, a much larger sample than within all cohorts combined from the Framingham Heart Study. Because these data were collected from a cohort of registered nurses, of which 98 percent were white, a more informative and appropriately conservative title for the study would have announced findings relating BMI to mortality among well-educated and economically well-off white women. In a deft stroke of pen, however, the authors dismissed this major limitation while asserting its virtue by enhancing the "internal validity" (Manson et al. 1995) of the study by removing educational and socioeconomic factors as potential confounding variables. The authors invoked an ideal of value-free science in expounding the importance of understanding the "*true association* [emphasis added] between weight and mortality," curiously juxtaposed with two statements in the article describing U.S. weight standards as "increasingly permissive." (Manson et al. 1995) Whether or not the authors intended to be contemptuous, it might be rather difficult for some not to read values into these statements.

In their rebuttal of a letter to the editor in response to their paper that raised concern about the piece's unwarranted "social prescriptions" and potential associated unintended consequences of reinforcing unhealthful body shape concerns that could exacerbate an eating disorder (Hamburg 1996), the authors responded that "the hyperbole and sensationalism of the media should be dissociated from the science presented by the researchers" (Manson et al. 1995). In an ironic twist, they chased this comment with a shot of their own hyperbole, erroneously asserting that "the leading eating disorder in the United States is obesity, not anorexia nervosa or bulimia" (Manson et al. 1996). Obesity may be prevalent, but it is not an eating disorder, nor is it, indeed, any kind of mental disorder (Marcus and Wildes 2009). This misattribution, however, is a telling illustration of the stunningly polymorphous quality of the obesity construct.

Fat and Fatness as a Polymorphous Social Construct

Amidst a global epidemic of obesity, nowhere is the prevalence higher than in the Western Pacific (Coyne 2000; Hodge et al. 1994). Although the WHO guidelines for a BMI cut-point for obesity (30 kg/m^2) have been critiqued as inappropriate for Polynesians (Rush et al. 2009), there is widespread public health concern about the impact of increasing prevalence and intransigence of obesity on noncommunicable diseases in Pacific populations (National Food and Nutrition Centre 2007; Dalton and Crowley 2000), ushering in an era of the so-called "double-burden" of diseases (Marshall 2004) characterizing both poor populations (including malnutrition relating to diarrheal disease and food insecurity) and affluent populations (including obesity-related chronic medical conditions such as diabetes mellitus, hypertension, coronary artery disease, and some cancers.) Fatness has, therefore, been present in the Pacific island public health discourse alongside health educational campaigns to promote dietary patterns associated with child health. The rapid escalation of obesity in Pacific populations has accompanied an influx of processed foodstuffs, motorized transport, and urban migration: all factors that can plausibly be connected causally to energy imbalance and weight gain. The Obesity Prevention in Communities (OPIC) project has undertaken to identify behavioral risk factors for obesity with the explicit motive to develop effective preventive programs to mitigate risk in the several participating Pacific sites (Swinburn et al. 2007).

Long before fatness was perceived as a proxy for physical health in Fiji, it was a proxy for social health (Mavoa and McCabe 2008; Becker 1995). Traditional aesthetic female body size ideals in Polynesia are famously discrepant from the prevailing late-twentieth-century slender body ideals for most populations of Anglo-European descent. In contrast, body ideals in the Pacific Islands range from robust and muscular to a frankly obese body size (Mackenzie 1985). In Fiji, for example, body weight and weight loss index social connection and neglect, re-spectively (Becker 1995). Relatedly, local explanatory models for the indigenous illness construct, *macake,* which is characterized by poor appetite, locate respon-sibility for a child's weight loss with his or her caregivers (Becker 1995). The diag-nostic label initiates a social commentary that calls out deficits in caregiving and issues a moral prescriptive to redress them. Consumption and sharing of food, moreover, is construed primarily as a social transaction that anchors it in a public domain. Likewise, social commentary—and critique—regarding body weight, size, and even fatness is routine and quite public.

Commentary on body size in adults references not just the density and ca-pacity of an individual's social network to access and deliver adequate food, but also cultural standards for capacity to contribute labor to one's household and community. The locally intensive interest in body size as a social marker sheds light, in part, on the rapid migration of body ideals revealed among ethnic Fijian adolescent girls following the introduction of television to rural Fiji (Becker et al. 2002; Becker 2004). Initially, these young women responded to images and nar-ratives presented in the mostly imported television programming by perceiving themselves as "fat" and, in a remarkable shift, construing "fat" as socially unde-sirable. Conversely, thinness catapulted from a reviled to an admired attribute. The fluidity of body weight ideals is neither unique to Fiji nor historically ex-traordinary, however. Similar shifts are well-documented in American society, for example, during the twentieth century (Brumberg 1989; Bordo 1993) when an increasingly thin and then tubular body shape gained social currency for women (Garner et al. 1980; Wiseman et al. 1992; Silverstein, Peterson, and Perdue 1986; Silverstein et al. 1986). In Fiji, however, the emerging social prestige associated with thinness (relative to conventional standards) was juxtaposed with the per-sistent value of capacity for physical labor—often inferred from body weight. Insofar as thinness appeared to be a sort of gateway to upward social mobility through enhanced access to coveted jobs in the tourism and travel industries, entry into these roles was also read as a threatened departure from kin- and com-munity-based social obligations, sometimes locally equated with selfishness. Put in somewhat of a double-bind, young women also decried being "too fat," given its association there with laziness, and expressed a preference instead for their weight to be "just enough" (see Becker and Thomas, in press).

Therewith, body shape ideals for young ethnic Fijian women have toggled within the timeframe of a few decades from robust (*jubu vina*) to small (*hewa-hewa*) and then back to big enough (*varausia*). In parallel with the collective distaste for embodying either selfishness or laziness—and the attendant uncer-tainties about how embodied experience maps on to unstable social norms for weight—behaviors aimed at weight management have surged among teenage schoolgirls in Fiji. For example, young women reported inducing vomiting and exercising as a means of weight control in unprecedented numbers and actions in a recent study of youth risk behaviors in school-going Fijian adolescents (Thomas et al. 2011). Although not locally recognized as an eating disorder (or as any other kind of disorder), the behaviors bear certain striking similarities to bulimia nervosa as described in the DSM-IV. Of the two symptomatic profiles discerned, one was distinguished by the use of traditional purgatives. In some cases, the purgatives were either administered or encouraged by a mother or other adult relative as a tool for weight management. This profile associated with traditional purgative use, even with its greater continuity with local traditions constituting normative behavior, was in fact associated with greater distress (Thomas et al. 2011). It is noteworthy that prevalent purgative use in this study population was juxtaposed with continued prevalent use of prophylactic traditional remedies for *macake*—aimed at preventing appetite loss. The rapid fluctuation of body ideals paralleled the new moral valence that being "large" had accrued and corresponded to striking uncertainty about ideal body size. Likewise, emergent and novel-for-Fiji weight management behaviors were rationalized by both their relation to health and to social benefits.

The Naturalization of Eating Disorders

I feel FAT!?

I'm 5'3" and 105 lbs. My friends always tell me im not fat, and i know im not fat but i feel fat…like all the time. I feel like i weigh a ton and it makes me extremely depressed. My weight fluctuates alot, so like one day my jeans will fit right and others they'll be more tight. when they're tight im depressed. My friends get mad when i say im fat becasue thy think they're bigger than me so it makes them feel huge. But idk…i cant help it! what do i do?? do u think im fat? [grammatical and spelling errors as well as abbreviations preserved verbatim from the original]

–Anonymous post on Yahoo! Answers (Anonymous a).

The invalidation of embodied experience against fluctuating social norms for ideal body size, so new to Fiji, is an old story elsewhere. In the anonymous posting above, (presumably) a young woman seeks judgment about her fatness from passersby in cyberspace. The inherent fragility of this fatness construct is evoked in one of the posts in response, "Hello body double: I am your exact height and weight…I fluctuate all the time with my jeans too. I just don't obsess over it. We are small though:-)You're not fat! Because then you're calling me fat and I know I'm not" (Anonymous b).

Perhaps the most illustrative examples of the social construction of weight as a proxy for disorder emerge, paradoxically, from the eating disorders literature. Indeed, among the mental disorders, eating disorders allow extraordinary transparency of the cultural processes and social environment that both shape them phenomenologically and moderate risk. Why should this be? In part, this is because eating disorders comprise signs and symptoms that are mostly dimensional in that they lie along a continuum. Inasmuch as these dimensions transect—or at least pass nearby—social norms, which themselves are in perpetual flux, the points of crossover into a pathological domain lack consistency and clarity. For example, the lower boundary of the BMI range deemed "normal weight" for adults at 18.5 kg/m² is quite close to the BMI (17.5 kg/m²) given as an example of low weight consistent with anorexia nervosa (APA 2000). This leaves only a narrow sliver of BMI territory that is neither normal nor in anorexic range. The assignment of particular BMI ranges to categorical designations of underweight, normal weight, overweight, and obesity, moreover, reifies a classificatory scheme that has historically fluctuated (see Yates-Doerr and Rubin and Joseph, this volume). Even more conceptually slippery is how the "intense fear of fatness," requisite to a diagnosis of anorexia nervosa, should be operationalized. How, after all, is fatness construed? Can this construct be meaningfully universalized? Probably not easily because both the intensity of fear and the apperception of fatness—what its salient dimensions are—are on the one hand deeply subjective while also being culturally, or even clinically, co-constructed against the context of local social norms (see also Yates-Doerr, this volume). For instance, some concern with weight gain is arguably socially normative in some contexts and even verges upon sensible given the widespread public health messaging about health risks associated with overweight. Even patients and clinicians with a shared social milieu might view concerns about weight gain quite differently; moreover, a clinician might infer a fear of fatness at the same time as a patient vigorously disavows it (Becker et al. 2009a).

Similarly, the clinical definition of binge eating makes its contextual nature explicit (APA 2000). Binge episodes are classified as "subjective" and "objective," unified by their common sense of lack of control but distinguished by a clinician's subjective determination of how much food constitutes an "unusually large amount given the circumstances" (APA 2000), and yet there is markedly inconsistent operationalization of the number of calories in a binge in the scientific literature (Wolfe et al. 2009). Other diagnostic features that set binge eating apart from normative food consumption would be expected to vary along with cultural mores for meals and diet. For instance, a diagnosis of binge eating disorder requires distress associated with the binge eating behavior. Such emotional distress, in turn, must surely be inextricably tied to the social relevance of overeating, personal agency, and discomfort with breaching social norms governing meal patterns, among other things. In short, a binge episode is not just deeply subjective, but also culturally relative.

Likewise, behaviors consistent with eating pathology in some contexts might be regarded as appropriate weight management strategies in other contexts. Americans are exhorted to increase their level of physical activity, for example, in the context of considerable ambiguity as to what duration, what frequency, and what intensity of physical activity are optimal to achieve or maintain good health (Haskell et al. 2007). As a result, clinicians attempting to ascertain whether physical activity is excessive enough to meet the bar for nonpurging type bulimia nervosa may find it challenging to distinguish health-promoting behavior from eating pathology. This is especially the case when the behavior is ego-syntonic—as it often is among individuals with an eating disorder—and not regarded as excessive at all. If the guidance is confusing for clinicians to apply, it is potentially bewildering to patients and also presents an opportunity for them to rationalize and defend behavior as promoting health when it actually may threaten it (see Rubin and Joseph, this volume, for further discussion of the impact of conflicting health messaging).

Much has been written about historical changes in prevalence of anorexia nervosa in the twentieth century that illuminates the increasing social premium on thinness (Bemporad 1996). The core psychopathology of anorexia nervosa is an intense fear of fatness and body image disturbance. What fatness is feared, however, is curiously unspecified. Standardized assessments have sought to measure this construct in "drive for thinness" (Garner et al. 1983) and "importance of body weight" (Fairburn et al. 2008), but the operationalization of the essence of this drive has nevertheless proven elusive. In fact, a score reflecting the absence of any body weight or shape concerns on the gold standard self-report assessment for eating disorders (the EDE-Q) appears to be rare even among healthy young women (Mond et al. 2006). Moreover, the relative absence of weight concerns has been reported among individuals presenting with symptoms otherwise resembling anorexia nervosa (Dalle Grave et al. 2008), raising doubt about its centrality to anorexia nervosa (Palmer 1993). That the prevalence of anorexia nervosa is closely tied to specific historical and cultural contexts suggests that fatness—however it may be locally defined—and fear of it must be constructed relative to contemporaneous local social norms. For example, the intense fear of fatness requisite to a diagnosis of anorexia nervosa was found to be absent in a substantial percentage of Hong Kong Chinese patients presenting with an eating disorder otherwise entirely consistent with anorexia nervosa (Lee et al. 1993). Sing Lee, who coined the term "non-fat phobic anorexia nervosa," has pointed out that the local salience of a rationale for entrenched food refusal may explain this cross-cultural phenomenologic difference (Lee 1995; 1991). Tellingly, the percentage of Hong Kong Chinese presenting with "fat phobia" has increased over the last decade (Lee et al. 2010). But what dimension of "fat" is invoked within this criterion? Fat attaches to astonishingly different definitions (Lee et al. 2001), and these are not necessarily fixed even within the same individual (Becker et al. 2009b). Even if fat phobia were equated with fear of weight gain, which it is often understood to be, present diagnostic criteria and clinical guidance do not make explicit how much weight gain (or how much fear) would constitute enough to judge this criterion as present or how this hypothetical amount could be adjusted for local social norms.

The American Psychiatric Association's (APA) editions of Diagnostic and Statistical Manuals of Mental Disorders (DSM) reflect a series of high watermarks for expert consensus about nosology and diagnostic criteria for mental illness over a period of decades. Although highly sought after, the materialization of biomarkers for mental illness has been maddeningly slow, leaving diagnostic assessment to behavioral, affective, and cognitive signs and symptoms that can be observed, reported, or elicited. When the APA's DSM-5 goes to press in 2013, the best available evidence to inform clinicians on how to recognize an eating disorder will still not be drawn from a representative sample of the globe's population. A well-documented publishing bias favors epidemiologic studies and clinical trials conducted in North American and Western European populations. By contrast, more than 90 percent of the world's population is represented in fewer than 6 percent of publications in leading psychiatric journals (Patel and Sumathipala 2001). Thus, the reification of presentations of illness most common to North American and European populations is almost inevitable. Superimposed upon this study population selection bias is a strong incentive to tweak eligibility criteria in clinical trial design so as to optimize detection of a signal of effect against background noise inhering in phenomenologically diverse study participants. In other words, outlier clinical presentations are preferentially excluded from eligibility for study participation, rendering clinical trial data representative of—and most relevant to—the common presentations. As a result, cultural diversity in clinical presentation is minimally visible in the scientific literature on eating disorders, their etiology, and their treatment. The ensuing artificial homogeneity is ultimately naturalized in prevailing clinical wisdom.

A second dimension of weight relevant to anorexia nervosa also illustrates its clinical construction. The formal diagnostic criterion for underweight in anorexia nervosa does not specify a fixed particular percentage of expected body weight, body mass index (BMI), or BMI centile required to establish the diagnosis, but rather provides an example to guide clinicians in evaluating the relevance of weight to the full clinical and social context for any particular patient. Embedded in the DSM-IV's criterion A for anorexia nervosa is the parenthetical guidance: "(e.g., less than 85 percent expected)" (APA 2000). Despite the intention that the *salience* of weight in assessing anorexia nervosa be evaluated within the invariably rich clinical context that renders it meaningful to health, this criterion has instead routinely been interpreted as a specific cut-point or threshold weight for anorexia nervosa. There are various unintended consequences that follow from this misinterpretation because body weight typically fluctuates even for normal weight individuals. With rigid application of this criterion for anorexia nervosa, an individual could be seen to meet diagnostic criteria for anorexia nervosa in the morning and yet miss meeting these criteria in the afternoon (Thomas et al.

2010). Further, even if 85 percent were the best cut-point available, the norms against which it should be measured are uncertain (Thomas et al. 2008).

Clinical Construction of Personal Agency Over Weight Control

> Most obese persons will not stay in treatment. Of those who stay in treatment, most will not lose weight, and of those who do lose weight, most will regain it.
> —Albert Stunkard (Stunkard 1958).

If the clinical construction of obesity reached its heyday as epidemiologic data sets identifying prospective risk factors for cardiac disease, the public imagination was also enlivened by the parallel scientific and lay discourse positing dietary modulation of health risk. Notwithstanding that the diet heart hypothesis fell rather flat in randomized controlled trials (De Lorgeril et al. 1997), the quest for a healthful diet gained traction with the American lay public and clinicians alike. The scientific prominence of this hypothesis and all the implications for behavioral control of health risk surely must have fortified the valuation of a healthful body and diet among the lay public. Widespread interest in achieving health through cultivation of good habits and sterling deployment of judicious dietary restraint also coincided with aesthetic preferences for more slender bodies in the United States (Becker 1995).

The titanic commercial success of the weight management industries rely on the seemingly inexhaustible consumer optimism in personal agency vis a vis weight control. Even as the pharmaceutical industry has energetically pursued development and brought to market a number of agents with either disappointing or only modest effectiveness for weight reduction, sales of diet and weight control products in the lay domain, including, diet books, diet foods, dietary supplements, and fitness equipment, remain brisk. For example, Americans expended a nearly unimaginable estimated $1.6 billion on weight loss supplements in 2005 (Pillitteri et al. 2008). But this figure pales in comparison to the estimated more than $60 billion spent on the full gamut of weight loss products and services last year (Marketdata Enterprises, Inc. 2011). Also a well of deep confidence in personal agency is the allure of narratives of self-transformation that inhere in weight control marketing and in reality television shows. As one vivid illustration, during the week of July 11, 2011, approximately 2.5 million viewers tuned in to ABC to view *Extreme Makeover, Weight Loss Edition,* recording it as the tenth most highly rated show among eighteen- to forty-nine-year-old viewers during that week (USA Today 2011). Notwithstanding an abundance of rhetoric pitching the theoretical benefits of one dieting approach over the other, there is a stunning lack of differentiation among the Ornish, Zone, Weight Watchers, and Atkins diet approaches when evaluated head to head in a study featuring a randomized controlled trial design (Dansinger et al. 2005). By contrast, the high attrition and low adherence were profound. Forty-two percent of study participants did not complete the full twelve months of the study, and 21 percent did not stay in the trial for even two months. No serious adverse effects were reported to explain this, and the most common reason for dropout that respondents gave was that the diet was "too hard to follow." The most clinically useful finding was arguably that there was a strong association between adherence and success (Dansinger et al. 2005). Interestingly, the adherence itself—often colloquially attributed to willpower—may actually be strongly influenced by physiologic factors, such as a diet's impact on hunger and metabolism rather than just a behavioral commitment (Ludwig and Ebbeling 2010).

Although widespread buy-in to the payoffs of weight management could theoretically be harnessed to great benefit in designing interventions that rely on active patient participation for their impact, sustained weight loss has proven dismally elusive to the vast majority of those attempting it. In the pre–bariatric surgery era, recidivism rates following obesity treatment ranged up to 97 percent (Ayyad and Anderson 2000; Kramer et al. 1989), and even more recent data are equally underwhelming about the sustainability of weight loss (Kraschnewski et al. 2010). In fact, Dr. Albert Stunkard's pessimistic summary of the outlook for weight maintenance, quoted above, appears to stand a half century later.

Attached to the assumption that weight control is within personal agency is the attribution of individual responsibility for becoming obese. Even if "at odds with compelling scientific evidence" of genetic vulnerability to obesity, the narrative conceptualizing weight management as a matter of personal will and cultivation of good habits surely fuels the unapologetic stigma affixed to obesity in the United States (see Friedman 2004). Socioeconomic status is inversely associated with waist to hip ratio (Brunner et al. 1997), and prospective data demonstrate that overweight in adolescence is associated with lower education and lower chance for women to marry in young adulthood (Gortmaker et al. 1993). Even being in the presence of an obese individual has been shown to be potentially stigmatizing (Hebl and Mannix 2003). Negative attitudes reflecting a weight bias have been documented among health care personnel (Puhl and Heuer 2009), and the judgmental language emanating from the clinical and scientific communities is unmistakable as well.

The creep of contempt for perceived personal failure to keep weight gain in check is also evident in statements peppering the public health discourse. British Member of Parliament, Mrs. Milton, recommended that NHS clinicians use the term "fat" in lieu of "obese" to achieve greater emotional impact on patients and promote their taking "personal responsibility" for their lifestyles (Martin 2010). The *New York Times* reported on a study linking specific food consumption habits to long-term weight outcomes. Their interview with lead study author Dr. Dariush Mozaffarian yielded two statements, "'The notion that it's O.K. to eat everything in moderation is just an excuse to eat whatever you want'" and "'Physical activity in the United States is poor, but diet is even worse'" (Brody 2011), that reflect his dim view of American predilections.

Another high-impact medical journal, *JAMA*, published a commentary in mid-July 2011 that issued an almost unfathomable proposal for addressing severe childhood obesity, that "as an alternative therapeutic approach, placement of the severely obese child under protective custody warrants discussion" (Murtagh and Ludwig 2011). The authors lay out an argument rationalizing this recommendation as a means of minimizing health risk, but curiously fail to review the data either for the efficacy or adverse psychological impact of this Draconian approach. The authors equated "having excessive junk food in the home or failing to model a physically active lifestyle" to parenting deficiencies that contribute to child obesity (Murtagh and Ludwig 2011). This recommendation reveals potentially unwarranted assumptions about parental agency as well as a flimsy construction of poor parenting. What might be read as a vituperative edge in this article supports that, even stipulating to and setting aside the concrete health and social benefits of maintaining a healthful body weight, the dogma relating to weight control verges on morally prescriptive.

A Counterdiscourse to the Health Benefits of Weight Management

What is now known should be sufficient to end the opprobrium of the obese. To end the stigma of obesity, the scientific community must communicate more effectively a growing body of compelling evidence indicating that morbid obesity is the result of differences in biology and not a personal choice.
— Jeffrey M. Friedman (Friedman 2004).

The rich counterdiscourse to obesity-related stigma invokes social justice as well as empirical support for potentially insurmountable biologic and social obstacles to weight control. Included among these is a powerful critique likening the social prejudices and penalties associated with obesity to other forms of discrimination, sometimes dubbed "weightism" (e.g., Steiner-Adair 1978; Puhl et al., 2008). Compelling evidence also supports biologic inertia to weight reduction efforts (Friedman 2004) and the impact of a "toxic food environment" on obesity risk (Brownell and Horgen 2004). In addition, a key advocacy strategy has impugned the relevance of obesity to health (see also Rubin and Joseph, McCullough, this volume). A vehement counterdiscourse to the conflation of weight with health conveys its key message that the relation between weight and health is misunderstood (Bacon 2011a). For instance, the organization, Health at Every Size (HAES), contests the ascribed benefits of weight loss to health and draws attention to the emotional and psychological perils encountered by individuals pursuing a self-defeating course of weight control and inevitable regain. The attendant risks are also considerable: body disparagement and development of unhealthful dietary patterns that undermine weight loss and even potentially result in net weight gain. The movement's homepage presents ideology based on a realistic and contextualized appraisal of the impact of the diet industry on Americans as well as a critique of narrowly defined health outcomes emphasized in the public health discourse. They describe the "collateral damage" in promotion of dieting and conclude that "Fighting fat hasn't made the fat go away. And being thinner, even if we knew how to successfully accomplish it, will not necessarily make us healthier or happier. The war on obesity has taken its toll." (Bacon 2011b). Perhaps telling of the David and Goliath dynamic in play, their website has logged only just more than twenty-five hundred signatures to date (Bacon 2011b), and the corresponding book is ranked beyond eleven thousandth in sales at Amazon.com in contrast to four diet or weight loss books ranked in the top thirty (Amazon. com 2011). Likewise, if book sales are a good metric for public hunger for dieting tips, a search of Amazon's books using the keyword "diet" returns a staggering fifty-six thousand entries (Amazon.com 2011).

Misattribution of Health Agency and its Implications for Public Health Messaging about Obesity and for Resocializing Weight Disorders

> Most of the preventable diseases that are cutting healthful years off lives could be eliminated if people had access to better health information.
> —Former United States Surgeon General, Vice Admiral Richard H. Carmona, MD, MPH, FACS (Carmona 2005).

Whereas broad access to health information and health literacy have indisputable social benefits in mitigating obesity risk (Kennen et al. 2005; Sharif and Blank 2010), a strategy premised on better distribution of better science is inadequate to contend with the complex and myriad biosocial factors that can and do derail intention. Although behavioral theories of change acknowledge that the proximity of benefits can override motivation and that executive function moderates the relation between intention and outcome (Huizinga et al. 2008; Hall et al. 2008), these approaches tilt toward vesting individual actors with responsibility—and autonomy and agency—to manage behaviors which are, in part a social fiction. This model that posits health as the outcome of a rational self-steward fails to consider adequately how health behaviors are governed by social contexts as well as by independent decision or action (Christakis and Fowler 2007; Brownell and Horgen 2004; Burke et al. 2009). Overcoming behavioral inertia, moreover, is also influenced by experience in and valuation of decision making (Linbladh and

Lyttkens 2002), which is itself highly social context dependent. Thus, the prevailing clinical ethos that conflates health literacy with health agency fails to discern fully the complexity of motivation, evanescent social norms, and the tremendous power of social environment, including social structural impediments to practicing healthful behaviors.

As the high rate of weight loss recidivism suggests, even a strong motivation to control weight is apparently no match for the multiple factors that consistently override intentions to adhere to a regimen of diet and physical activity that would presumably support a hypothetically optimal body weight. Whether dietary mishaps are attributed to physiologic drive or social structural factors that limit access to affordable and healthful foods, therapeutic strategies for managing overweight that assume personal health agency set up expectations for unrealistic outcomes. Even obesity interventions that are not primarily centered on behavioral weight loss strategies, such as pharmacologic and bariatric surgical treatment, require adherence to dietary restraint for their success.

To benefit meaningfully from health literacy approaches to obesity, health consumers need to be well-equipped to access and interpret health data, as well as to formulate and pursue a personal health agenda. But realistically, numerous social barriers will continue to preempt and constrain personal health agency among many health consumers, even within high-income countries. However sophisticated and critical they are as consumers, there is no reason to think that Americans will not continue to spend billions of their dollars on diet products that are destined to fail them, but considering the long odds against achieving sustained weight loss with diet and exercise, this optimistic appraisal of self-agency appears sadly miscalculated. In other regions of the world, there may be additional major cultural barriers to health interventions that rely on self-agency for positive outcomes. As Rochelle Rosen writes in this volume, a diabetes self-management model adapted and implemented in American Samoa as "Diabetes Care in American Samoa" may have been poorly conceived in its premise that individuals would choose self-promotion of their health at the expense of dissonance with local cultural norms. She also writes that insofar as social well-being is intrinsic to health, diet, and physical activity, changes that compromise such social integration may be unsuccessful. Similarly, to the extent that sickness can be understood to index or embody poor social health among ethnic Fijians (Becker 1995), self-promotion of health has varying cultural legitimacy. Thus implementation of health promotion strategies—including those aimed at obesity prevention—that may have reasonable consonance with local expectations and possibilities for health autonomy and agency in high-income regions may still have considerable difficulty gaining the traction requisite to adherence and good outcomes in low-resource settings.

And finally, health agency is continually challenged by social environmental factors that may conflict with a public health agenda. For example, corporate actions aimed at increasing sales profits from processed food exports to regions of the Western Pacific set the stage for degradation of the food environment (Hughes and Lawrence 2005) that, in turn, favors obesigenic diets and for exporting media products that contribute to disordered eating behaviors (Becker et al. 2011). The obesity and nutritional interventions focused on health literacy may have insubstantial impact when both competing cultural priorities and corporate interests override their influence on individual behavior. Thus, a health promotion strategy built on a platform of self-agency fails to recognize the torrent of social factors that obstruct not just efficacy of interventions, but that also impede health agency.

As this volume goes to press, it is informative to consider another high-profile proposed obesity intervention that has met with both approbation and criticism, thereby illuminating radically divergent perspectives on personal agency vis-à-vis health. In May 2012, New York City Mayor Bloomberg proposed a ban on large-sized sugary sodas sold in restaurants, movie theaters, and by street vendors (Grynbaum 2012). Preeminent Harvard nutritional epidemiologist Walter Willet hastily declared support of this ban as "a valuable and creative step in the right direction that deserves the support of everyone who cares about the well-being of our children and all Americans" (Willet 2012). Whereas others joined in praising a policy that would restructure a food environment that presently encourages and enables overconsumption (Bittman 2012; Lieberman 2012), others opposed it. The Center for Consumer Freedom, for example, ridiculed the mayor's proposed policy intervention in an ad depicting him as a nanny (Dicker 2012). The *New York Times* ran an editorial titled "A Ban too Far," countering that "The administration should be focusing its energies on programs that educate and encourage people to make sound choices" and concluding that "Promoting healthy lifestyles is important. In the case of sugary drinks, a regular reminder that a 64-ounce cola has 780 calories should help. But too much nannying with a ban might well cause people to tune out." (*New York Times* 2012). In a letter to the editor, one writer responded that "the continued focus on simply informing and educating consumers is doomed to failure and diminishes this important policy and the influence it could have on obesity" (Elbel 2012). The churn inspired by Mayor Bloomberg's proposed ban on sales of large servings of soda in New York City illustrates the polarization of views about whether individuals can adequately manage their own consumption to safeguard their health.

Conclusions

In aggregate, the chapters in this volume offer a thoughtful and highly useful critique of the understanding and dimensions of obesity that are socially constructed. And yet, even if there are discernibly socially constructed understandings of obesity and of disordered eating, the potential biological impact of weight disorders—at either end of the spectrum—is undeniable. Their associated health burdens, in turn, have the potential to impose substantial economic and social burdens on individuals, caregivers, and health care systems—some of which are among the most vulnerable. Thus, the interrogation of tensions between the social and clinical realities of weight disorders is not intended to dismiss their health salience, but rather to expose misguided assumptions that potentially undermine the effectiveness and feasibility of interventions aimed at reducing the health, economic, and social burdens they impose (see also Rubin and Joseph, this volume). Socioculturally informed implementation research is essential, therefore, to ensure that health interventions are maximally beneficial as they are deployed for these biosocially complex conditions. Such research should especially evaluate aspects of interventions that may not be transferrable or effective without keen understanding of and adaptation to local contexts. For example, in the face of social structural barriers to health, assumptions about personal health agency may be naïve and thus may misguide strategies for health promotion. And finally, obesity discourse and interventions need to be monitored and evaluated to prevent unintended adverse consequences—such as the stigmatization of overweight, shaming and demoralization, or disordered eating—that may emerge despite noble social and clinical goals to promote health and well-being.

Notes

1. See Yates-Doerr's critique of the routine assumption that weighing is straightforward, chapter 2, this volume.

References

Amazon.com, Inc. 2011. Search Results: Diet Books. Available at http://www.amazon.com/s/ref=nb_sb_ss_i_3_1 0?url=search-alias percent3Dstripbooksandfield-keywords=diet+books andsprefix=diet+books, accessed July 28, 2011.

American Psychiatric Association. 2000. *Diagnostic and Statistical Manual of Mental Disorders, 4th ed., Text Revision.* Arlington, VA: American Psychiatric Association.

Anonymous a. "I Feel FAT!?" *Yahoo answers,* available at http://answers.yahoo.com/question/index?qid=20080324152923AARvihZ, accessed August 3, 2011.

Anonymous b. "Hello Body Double." *Yahoo answers,* available at http://answers.yahoo.com/question/index?qid=20080324152923AARvihZ, accessed August 3, 2011.

Ayyad, C., and T. Andersen. 2000. "Long-Term Efficacy of Dietary Treatment of Obesity: A Systematic Review of Studies Published between 1931 and 1999." *Obesity Reviews: An Official Journal of the International Association for the Study of Obesity* 1, no. 2: 113–119.

Bacon, L. 2011a. *Health at Every Size: The Surprising Truth about your Weight.* Available at http://www.lindabacon.org/HAESbook, accessed July 28, 2011.

———. 2011b. *Health at Every Size.* Available at http://www.haescommunity.org, accessed July 28, 2011.

Becker, A. E. 1995. *Body, Self, and Society: The View from Fiji.* Philadelphia: University of Pennsylvania Press.

———. 2004 "Television, Disordered Eating, and Young Women in Fiji: Negotiating Body Image and Identity during Rapid Social Change." *Culture Medicine and Psychiatry* 28, no. 4: 533–559.

Becker, A. E., R. A. Burwell, S. E. Gilman, D. B. Herzog, and P. Hamburg. 2002. "Eating behaviours and attitudes following prolonged television exposure among ethnic Fijian adolescent girls." *The British Journal of Psychiatry* 180: 509–14.

Becker, A. E., A. Perloe, and K. Eddy. 2009a. "Clarifying Criteria for Cognitive Signs and Symptoms for Eating Disorders in DSM-V." *International Journal of Eating Disorders* 42, no. 7 (November): 611–608.

Becker, A. E., J. J. Thomas, and K. M. Pike. 2009b. "Should Non-fat-phobic Anorexia Nervosa be Included in DSM-V?" *International Journal of Eating Disorders* 42, no. 7: 620–635.

Becker, A. E., and J. J. Thomas. In press. "Eating Pathology in Fiji: Phenomenologic Diversity, Low Visibility, and High Vulnerability." In *Revisioning Psychiatry: Cultural Phenomenology, Critical Neuroscience, and Global Mental Health,* L. Kirmayer, R. Lemelson, C. Cummings, eds. Cambridge: Cambridge University Press.

Becker, A. E., K. Fay, J. Agnew-Blais, N. A. Khan, R. H. Striegel-Moore, and S. E. Gilman. 2011. "Social Network Media Exposure and Adolescent Eating Pathology in Fiji." *British Journal of Psychiatry* 198, no. 1: 43–50.

Bemporad, J.R. 1996. "Self-Starvation through the Ages: Reflections on the Pre-history of Anorexia Nervosa." *International Journal of Eating Disorders* 19, no. 3: 217–237.

Bittman, M. 2012. "What is Food? The Opinionator." *The New York Times,* June 5, available at http://opinionator.blogs.nytimes.com/2012/06/05/what-is-food/?hp, accessed June 6, 2012.

Bordo, S. 1993. *Unbearable Weight: Feminism, Western Culture, and the Body.* Berkeley, Los Angeles, and London: University of California.

Brody, J. E. 2011. "Still Counting Calories? Your Weight-Loss Plan May Be Outdated." *The New York Times,* July 18, available at http://www.nytimes.com/2011/07/19/health/19brody.html.

Brownell, K., and K. B. Horgen. 2004. *Food Fight: The Inside Story of the Food Industry, America's Obesity Crisis, and What We Can Do About It.* Chicago: Contemporary Books.

Brumberg, J. J. 1989. *Fasting Girls: The History of Anorexia Nervosa.* New York: Plume.

Brunner, E. J., M. G. Marmot, K. Nanchahal, M. J. Shipley, S. A. Stansfeld, M. Juneja, and K. G. Alberti. 1997. "Social Inequality in Coronary Risk: Central Obesity and the Metabolic Syndrome, Evidence from the Whitehall II Study." *Diabetologia* 40, no. 11: 1341–1349.

Burke, N. J., G. Joseph, R. J. Pasick, and J. C. Barker. 2009. "Theorizing Social Context: Rethinking Behavioral Theory." *Health Education and Behavior* 36, no. 5 (Suppl.): 55S–70S.

Carmona, R. H. 2005. "Improving Americans' Health Literacy." *Journal of the American Dietetic Association* 105, no. 9: 1345.

Christakis, N. A., and J. H. Fowler. 2007. "The Spread of Obesity in a Large Social Network Over 32 Years." *New England Journal of Medicine* 357, no. 4: 370–379.

Coyne, T. 2000. *Lifestyle Diseases in Pacific Communities.* Noumea: Secretariat of the Pacific Community.

Dalle Grave, R., S. Calugi, and G. Marchesini. 2008. "Underweight Eating Disorder without Over-evaluation of Shape and Weight: Atypical Anorexia Nervosa?" *International Journal of Eating Disorders* 41, no. 8: 705–712.

Dalton, A., and S. Crowley. 2000. "Economic Impact of NCD in the Pacific Islands (With Special Reference to Obesity)." Proceedings of the Workshop on Obesity Prevention and Control Strategies in the Pacific, September 26–29, Apia, Western Samoa.

Dansinger, M. L., J. A. Gleason, J. L. Griffith, H. P. Selker, and E. J. Schaefer. 2005. "Comparison of the Atkins, Ornish, Weight Watchers, and Zone Diets for Weight Loss and Heart Disease Risk Reduction: A Randomized Trial." *Journal of the American Medical Association* 293, no. 1: 43–53.

De Lorgeril, M., P. Salen, I. Monjaud, and J. Delaye. 1997. "The 'Diet Heart' Hypothesis in Secondary Prevention of Coronary Heart Disease." *European Heart Journal* 18, no. 1: 13–18.

Dicker, R. 2012. "'Nanny Bloomberg' Ad in *New York Times* Targets N.Y. Mayor's Anti-soda Crusade." *The Huffington Post,* posted June 4, available at http://www.huffingtonpost.com/2012/06/04/nanny-bloomberg-ad-in-new_n_1568037.html, accessed June 6, 2012.

Elbel, B. 2012. "Bloomberg's Supersize Soda Ban, Letters to the Editor." *The New York Times,* June 1, available at http://www.nytimes.com/2012/06/02/opinion/bloombergs-supersize-soda-ban.html, accessed June 10, 2012.

Fairburn, C. G., Z. Cooper, and M. E. O'Connor. 2008. "Eating Disorder Examination (Edition 16.0D)." In *Cognitive Behavior Therapy and Eating Disorders,* ed. C.. G. Fairburn. New York: Guilford, 265–308.

Framingham Heart Study. 2011. ed. Esta Shindler, available at http://www.framinghamheart study.org, Accessed July 14, 2011.

Friedman, J. M. 2004. "Modern Science Versus the Stigma of Obesity." *Nature Medicine* 10, no. 6: 563–569.

Garner, D. M., P. E. Garfinkel, D. Schwartz, and M. Thompson. 1980. "Cultural Expectations of Thinness in Women." *Psychological Reports* 47, no. 2: 483–491.

Garner, D. M., M. P. Olmstead, and J. Polivy. 1983. "Development and Validation of a Multidimensional Eating Disorder Inventory for Anorexia Nervosa and Bulimia." *International Journal of Eating Disorders* 2, no. 2: 15–34.

Gortmaker, S. L., A. Must, J. M. Perrin, A. M. Sobol, and W. H. Dietz. 1993. "Social and Economic Consequences of Qverweight in Adolescence and Young Adulthood." *New England Journal of Medicine* 329, no. 14: 1008–1012.

Grynbaum, M. M. 2012. "New York Plans to Ban Sale of Big Sizes of Sugary Drinks." *The New York Times,* May 5, available at http://www.nytimes.com/2012/05/31/nyregion/bloomberg-plans-a-ban-on-large-sugared-drinks.html, accessed June 10, 2012.

Hall, P.A., G. T. Fong, L. J. Epp, L. J. and Elias. 2008. "Executive Function Moderates the Intention-Behavior Link for Physical Activity and Dietary Behavior." *Psychology and Health* 23, no. 3: 309–326.

Hamburg, P. 1996. "Body Weight and Mortality among Women: Correspondence." *New England Journal of Medicine* 334, no. 11: 732.

Haskell, W. L., I. M. Lee, R. R. Pate, K. E. Powell, S. N. Blair, B. A. Franklin, C. A. Macera, G. W. Heath, P. D. Thompson, and A. Bauman. 2007. "Physical Activity and Public Health: Updated Recommendation for Adults from the American College of Sports Medicine and the American Heart Association." *Medicine and Science in Sports and Exercise* 39, no. 8: 1423–1434.

Hebl, M. R., and L. M. Mannix. 2003. "The Weight of Obesity in Evaluating Others: A Mere Proximity Effect." *Personality and Social Psychology Bulletin* 29, no. 1: 28–38.

Hodge, A. M., G. K. Dowse, P. Toelupe, V. R. Collins, T. Imo, and P. Z. Zimmet. 1994. "Dramatic Increase in the Prevalence of Obesity in Western Samoa Over the 13 Year Period 1978–1991." *International Journal of Obesity Related Metabolic Disorders* 18, no. 6: 419–428.

Hughes, R. G., and M. A. Lawrence. 2005. "Globalization, Food and Health in Pacific Island Countries." *Asia Pacific Journal of Clinical Nutrition* 14, no. 4: 298–306.

Huizinga, M. M., S. Pont, R. L. Rothman, E. Perrin, L. Sanders, and B. Beech. 2008. "ABC's and 123's: Parental Literacy, Numeracy, and Childhood obesity." *Obesity Management* 4, no. 3: 98–103.

Kennen, E. M., T. C. Davis, J. Huang, H. Yu, D. Carden, R. Bass, and C. Arnold. 2005. "Tipping the Scales: The Effect of Literacy on Obese Patients' Knowledge and Readiness to Lose Weight." *Southern Medical Journal* 98, no. 1: 15–18.

Jacobson, T. A., and S. Brown. 1996. "Body Weight and Mortality among Women: Correspondence." *New England Journal of Medicine* 334, no. 11: 732.

Judge, A. M., J. J. Thomas, and A. E. Becker. 2006. "Ethnic Disparities in Overweight and Obesity in the U.S.: A Review of Socio-cultural Contributions." In *New Developments in Obesity Research*, ed. L. F. Ditmier. New York: Nova Science Publishers, 85–119.

Kramer, F. M., R. W. Jeffery, J. L. Forster, and M. K. Snell. 1989. "Long-term Follow-up of Behavioral Treatment for Obesity: Patterns of Weight Regain among Men and Women." *International Journal of Obesity* 13, no. 2: 123–136.

Kraschnewski, J. L., J. Boan, J. Esposito, N. E. Sherwood, E. B. Lehman, D. K. Kephart, and C. N. Sciamanna. 2010. "Long-term Weight Loss Maintenance in the United States." *International Journal of Obesity* 34, no. 11: 1644–1654.

Lee, S. 1991. "Anorexia Nervosa in Hong Kong: A Chinese Perspective." *Psychological Medicine* 21, no. 3: 703–711.

———. 1995. "Self-starvation in Context: Towards a Culturally Sensitive Understanding of Anorexia Nervosa." *Social Science and Medicine* 41, no. 1: 25–36.

Lee, S., T. P. Ho, and L. K. G. Hsu. 1993. "Fat Phobic and Non-fat Phobic Anorexia Nervosa: A Comparative Study of 70 Chinese Patients in Hong Kong." *Psychological Medicine* 23, no. 4: 999–1017.

Lee, S., A. M. Lee, E. Ngai, D. T. S. Lee, and Y. K. Wing. 2001. "Rationales for Food Refusal in Chinese Patients with Anorexia Nervosa." *International Journal of Eating Disorders* 29, no. 2: 224–229.

Lee, S., K. L. Ng, K. Kwok, and C. Fung. 2010. "The Changing Profile of Eating Disorders at a Tertiary Psychiatric Clinic in Hong Kong (1987–2007)." *International Journal of Eating Disorders* 43, no. 4: 307–314.

Lieberman, D. E. 2012. "Evolution's Sweet Tooth, Op-Ed." *The New York Times,* June 5, available at http://www.nytimes.com/2012/06/06/opinion/evolutions-sweet-tooth.html?hp, accessed June 6, 2012.

Lindbladh, E., and C. H. Lyttkens. 2002. "Habit Versus Choice: The Process of Decision-making in Health-related Behaviour." *Social Science and Medicine* 55, no. 3: 451–465.

Ludwig, D. S., and C. B. Ebbeling. 2010. "Weight-loss Maintenance—Mind over Matter?" *New England Journal of Medicine* 363, no. 22: 2159–2161.

Mackenzie, M. 1985. "The Pursuit of Slenderness and Addiction to Self-control." In *Nutrition Update, vol. 2,* ed. J. Weininger and G. M. Briggs. New York: John Wiley and Sons, 174–194.

Manson, J. E., M. J. Stampfer, G. A. Colditz, D. J. Hunter, S. E. Hankinson, C. H. Hennekens, and F. E. Speizer. 1995. "Body Weight and Mortality among Women." *New England Journal of Medicine* 333, no. 11: 677–685.

Manson, J. E., W. C. Willett, and F. E. Speizer. 1996. "Body Weight and Mortality among Women: The Authors Reply." *New England Journal of Medicine* 334, no. 11: 732–633.

Marcus, M. D., and J. E. Wildes. 2009. "Obesity: Is It a Mental Disorder?" *International Journal of Eating Disorders* 42, no. 8: 739–653.

Marketdata Enterprises, Inc. 2011. "Diet Market Worth $60.9 Billion in U.S. Last Year, But Growth is Flat, Due to the Recession." Press release, May 5, .pdf available at www.market dataenterprises.com/pressreleases/DietMkt2011PressRelease.pdf.

Marshall, S. J. 2004. "Developing Countries Face Double Burden of Disease." *Bulletin of the World Health Organization* 84, no. 7: 556.

Martin, D. 2010. "Obese? Just Call Them Fat: Plain-speaking Doctors Will Jolt People into Losing Weight, Says Minister." *Mail Online,* available at http://www.dailymail.co.uk/news/article-1298394/Call-overweight-people-fat-instead-obese-says-health-minister.html, modified July 29, 2010.

Mavoa, H. M., and M. McCabe. 2008. "Sociocultural Factors Relating to Tongans' and Indigenous Fijians' Patterns of Eating, Physical Activity and Body Size." *Asia Pacific Journal of Clinical Nutrition* 17, no. 3: 375–384.

Mayo Clinic. 2008. "Normal Weight Obesity: An Emerging Risk Factor for Heart and Metabolic Problems." Available at http://www.mayoclinic.org/news2008-rst/4738.html, last modified March 27, 2008.

Mond, J. M., P. J. Hay, B. Rodgers, and C. Owen. 2006. "Eating Disorder Examination Questionnaire (EDE-Q): Norms for Young Adult Women." *Behaviour Research and Therapy* 44: 53–62.

Murtagh, L., and D. S. Ludwig. 2011. "State Intervention in Life-threatening Childhood Obesity." *Journal of the American Medical Association* 306, no. 2: 206–207.

National Food and Nutrition Centre. 2007. *2004 Fiji National Nutrition Survey—Main Report.* Suva, Fiji: National Food and Nutrition Centre.

Nevill, A. M., E. M. Winter, S. Ingham, A.Watts, G. S. Metsios, and A. D. Stewart. 2010. "Adjusting Athletes' Body Mass Index to Better Reflect Adiposity in Epidemiological Research." *Journal of Sports Sciences* 28, no. 9: 1009–1016.

New York Times. 2012. "A Ban Too Far, Editorial." *The New York Times,* May 31, available at http://www.nytimes.com/2012/06/01/opinion/a-soda-ban-too-far.html?_r=1, accessed June 6, 2012.

Palmer, R. L. 1993. "Weight Concern Should Not Be a Necessary Criterion for the Eating Disorders: A Polemic." *International Journal of Eating Disorders* 14, no. 4: 459–465.

Patel, V., and A. Sumathipala. 2001. "International Representation in Psychiatric Literature: Survey of Six Leading Journals." *British Journal of Psychiatry* 178: 406–409.

Pillitteri, J. L., S. Shiffman, J. M. Rohay, A. M. Harkins, S. L. Burton, and T. A. Wadden. 2008. "Use of Dietary Supplements for Weight Loss in the United States: Results of a National Survey." *Obesity* 16, no. 4: 790–796.

Puhl, R. M., T. Andreyeva, and K. D. Brownell. 2008. "Perceptions of Weight Discrimination: Prevalence and Comparison to Race and Gender Discrimination in America." *International Journal of Obesity* 32, no. 6: 992–1000.

Puhl, R. M., and C. A. Heuer. 2009. "The Stigma of Obesity: A Review and Update." *Obesity* 17, no. 5: 941–964.

Rush, E. C., I. Freitas, and L. D. Plank. 2009. "Body Size, Body Composition and Fat Distribution: Comparative Analysis of European, Maori, Pacific Island and Asian Indian adults." *British Journal of Nutrition* 102, no. 4: 632–641.

Silverstein, B., B. Peterson, and L. Perdue. 1986. "Some Correlates of the Thin Standard of Bodily Attractiveness for Women." *International Journal of Eating Disorders* 5, no. 5: 895–905.

Silverstein, B., L. Perdue, B. Peterson, L. Vogel, and D. A. Fantini. 1986. "Possible Causes of the Thin Standard of Bodily Attractiveness for Women." *International Journal of Eating Disorders* 5, no. 5: 907–916.

Sharif, I., and A. E. Blank. 2010. "Relationship Between Child Health Literacy and Body Mass Index in Overweight Children." *Patient Education and Counseling* 79, no. 1: 43–48.

Steiner-Adair, C. 1978. "Weightism: A New Form of Prejudice." *National Anorexic Aid Society Newsletter* 10, no. 4.

Stunkard, A. 1958. "Physical Activity, Emotions, and Human Obesity." *Psychosomatic Medicine* 20, no. 5: 366–372.

Swinburn, B., J. Pryor, M. McCabe, R. Carter, M. de Courten, D. Schaaf, and R. Scragg. 2007. The Pacific OPIC Project (Obesity Prevention in Communities)—objectives and designs. Pac Health Dialog, 14: 139–46.

Thomas, J. J., C. A. Roberto, and K. D. Brownell. 2008. "Eighty-five Percent of What? Discrepancies in the Weight Cut-off for Anorexia Nervosa Substantially Affect the Prevalence of Underweight." *Psychological Medicine* 39, no. 5: 833–843.

Thomas, J. J., S. S. Delinsky, S. A. St. Germain, T. J. Weigel, P. G. Levendusky, and A. E. Becker. 2010. "How Do Eating Disorder Specialist Clinicians Apply DSM-IV Diagnostic Criteria in Routine Clinical Practice? Implications for Enhancing Clinical Utility in DSM-5." *Psychiatry Research* 178, no. 3: 511–517.

Thomas, J. J., R. D. Crosby, S. A. Wonderlich, R. H. Striegel-Moore, and A. E. Becker. 2011. "A Latent Profile Analysis of the Typology of Bulimic Symptoms in an Indigenous Pacific Population: Evidence of Cross-cultural Variation in Phenomenology." *Psychological Medicine* 41, no. 1: 195–206.

USA Today News. 2011. Nielsen ratings for week of July 25. Available at http://www.usatoday.com/life/television/news/nielsens-charts.htm.

U.S. Census Bureau. 2009. "National and State Population Estimates: Annual Population Estimates 2000 to 2009." Available at http://www.census.gov/popest/states/NST-ann-est.html.

Willet, W. 2012. "Bloomberg's Supersize Soda Ban, Letters to the Editor." *The New York Times,* June 1, available at http://www.nytimes.com/2012/06/02/opinion/bloombergs-supersize-soda-ban.html, accessed June 10, 2012.

Wiseman, C. V., J. J. Gray, J. E. Mosimann, and A. H. Ahrens. 1992. "Cultural Expectations of Thinness in Women: An Update." *International Journal of Eating Disorders* 11, no. 1: 85–89.

Wolfe, B. E., C. W. Baker, A. T. Smith, and S. Kelly-Weeder. 2009. "Validity and Utility of the Current Definition of Binge Eating." *International Journal of Eating Disorders* 42, no. 8: 674–686.

World Bank. 2010. "Population, Total." Available at http://data.worldbank.org/indicator/SP.POP.TOTL.

CHAPTER 2

The Mismeasure of Obesity

Emily Yates-Doerr

⁜ ⁜ ⁜

> The spirit of Plato dies hard. We have been unable to escape the philosophical tradition that what we can see and measure in the world is merely the superficial and imperfect representation of an underlying reality. Much of the fascination of statistics lies embedded in our gut feeling... that abstract measures summarizing large tables of data must express something more real and fundamental than the data themselves.
> —Stephen Jay Gould, *The Mismeasure of Man* (1981)

In *The Mismeasure of Man*, now written three decades ago, Stephen Jay Gould illustrated the fallacies of reducing the "wondrously complex and multifaceted set of human capabilities" into a standardized measure of intelligence (1996: 24). In this chapter, I draw from Gould's emphasis on the fallacy of reification, applying his argument to the measurements of obesity rather than intelligence. Whereas Gould critiqued the use of skull size and IQ tests to record intelligence, my concern lies with the presupposition that *health* can be located in the metrics of body size that have come to dominate the dietary ideals promoted by the field of public health. I argue that metrics of weight and size are neither representative nor metonymic of health, and though they may be well-suited to some needs—indeed, they form the basis of much international research on metabolic illness—they occupy too much public attention.

This chapter catalogs three techniques for measuring obesity in clinical practice, comparing the different forms of knowledge about obesity produced by each. It then draws attention to a non-numerical understanding of fatness to ask what kinds of experiences of the body become foreclosed by contemporary concern for obesity metrics. Unlike *The Mismeasure of Man*, which is interested in the "unconscious fraud" found in the science of intelligence measurement, scientific fraud does not play a part in my chapter. Although I am concerned with "liars," I do not set out to unravel scientific accuracy on its own terms. Instead, my argu-

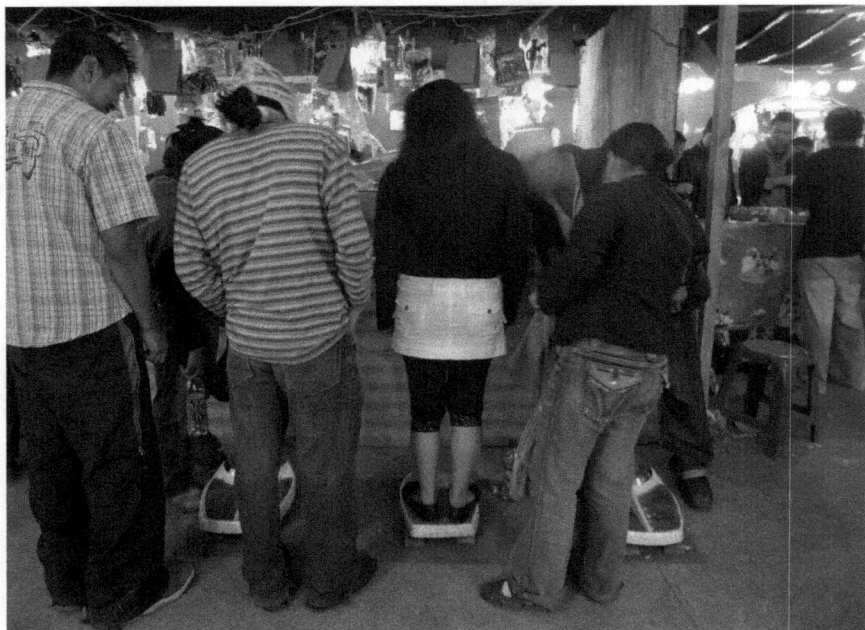

Figure 2.1. Body weight scales have proliferated in the Guatemalan highlands, accompanying nutrition education that links weight to health. Photograph by Emily Yates-Doerr.

ment that measures cannot be trusted runs deeper than fraud—be it intentional or not. In analyzing not just the inaccuracies of measurement, but the impossibilities of measurement, I follow Gould's warning about the powerful temptation of reification: "The idea that we have detected something 'underlying' the externalities of a large set of correlation coefficients, something perhaps more real than the superficial measurements themselves can be intoxicating" (1981: 239).

Through cataloging various numerical methods for assessing obesity—from waist circumference to body mass index to bioimpedance analysis—I suggest that the public health community has become swept up with the idea that measurements can reveal the interior health of the body. In their concern for ever more accurate measures of body size, the representational quality of numbers—and the experiences and people they purport to represent—become easily forgotten.

Body Mass Index

Julia Monterrosa first came to the highland Guatemalan hospital where I was carrying out fieldwork because of her headaches.[1] The attending doctor asked her a few quick questions—there were many people waiting to be treated—and then sent her away with a slip for laboratory blood work and a referral to the hospital's "outpatient obesity/nutrition clinic." She might need to lose some weight, he told her.

A few days later, after waiting several hours in the hospital lobby, the nutritionists of the clinic called her into the consultation room, requesting to see the results of her blood work along with her identity card, where her weight and height were written. They then asked her to take off the jacket and sweater that shielded her from the chill of the Guatemalan highland morning and to step on the scale. Julia placed her hand against the wall for balance and began to lift herself up when the nutritionists stopped her—they had forgotten to calibrate the scale and it might not be accurate (in Spanish, *exacta*).

It took some time to level the scale to zero. The machine was old, having arrived to the hospital years earlier in a crate of used medical equipment donated from Spain. Once the beam had stabilized at the center point, they asked her step onto the scale again. She balanced on the platform, albeit a bit shakily, as they moved the weights right and then left, whispering between themselves as the level balanced and they settled upon a number. The scale was in kilos, so they converted this before announcing the result: 130 pounds.

"No, that can't be," said Julia, easing herself off of the scale. "I just had my weight measured at the pharmacy yesterday and it was 120."

The nutritionists made a few more calculations, before one of them continued, ignoring her protest: "Ma'am, we take your weight and the height from your card and calculate your body mass index. I am sorry to tell you that you have the diagnosis of overweight (*sobrepeso*)." They pointed to a chart displaying information from the World Health Organization (WHO) that indicated that an adult with a BMI between 25 and 29.9 was considered overweight and between 30 or higher was considered obese. "You want to be at a healthy weight," one of the nutritionists explained, signaling the BMI range between 18.5 and 24.9. "Excess weight causes many kinds of illness. In your case it might be causing your headaches."

Julia protested again. "But this can't be. Look at my card. My card also says 120. This scale is a liar."

"Ma'am, scales don't lie," the second nutritionist explained.[2]

Abdominal Circumference

"Scales don't lie" was the exact phrase I had heard the previous weekend at a meeting for scientists who were studying metabolic illness. Yet they also qualified this with an important caveat: "But they can be hard to standardize." Many of the women treated for metabolic illness in Guatemala wore heavy *huipiles* (woven blouses) that would substantially change one's measured weight. The typical adjustment the public health community advised was to subtract between five and eight pounds from the weight reported by the scale—but sometimes public health workers subtracted ten, and sometimes they forgot to do this at all.

One of the topics of the meeting was the shortcomings of the BMI. Though BMI represents the ratio of weight to stature (it is calculated by dividing weight in kilos by height in meters squared), it says nothing about one's distribution of weight. The concern was that while BMI could assess "excess body mass," it left unrecorded a variable the scientists thought more closely correlated to metabolic health: the presence of centralized abdominal fat, which they viewed as more dangerous than fat found elsewhere on the body. The scientists in the room referenced studies, such as one conducted by Moreno et al. (2002), that tested different anthropometric predictors of metabolic illness in children.[3] When correlating metabolic illness with waist circumference, BMI, and triceps/subscapular skinfold ratios, this study found waist circumference to be more tightly correlated with illness than were the other methods:

> A large waist circumference reflects high total body fatness and is also recognized as a good measure of abdominal fat, particularly the most metabolically active intra-abdominal fat, in both adults and children. From our results, simple waist circumference measurements appear to have a similar performance to that of BMI in screening for the metabolic syndrome. Moreover, a single measurement, not a ratio, reduces the chance of error (Moreno et al. 2002: 1311).

To be clear: the scientists I worked among in Guatemala were primarily concerned with cataloging and tracking regional and national trends and did not typically use these numbers to speak of an individual's "health." But elsewhere—in hospitals and public health circles, for example—the reliance on body size measurements to indicate or predict a person's wellbeing was becoming widespread (see figure 2.1). This tendency to transport body size metrics from the field of epidemiology to the realm of personal care was increasingly common outside of clinics and sites of formalized health education. Many women I knew during my fieldwork in Guatemala used the tape measure from their sewing kit to keep track of their weight. While they could not afford the home scales that are typical in the United States, the tape measurer, normally intended for fabric, cost nothing extra. And even women who did not read or write with ease—women for whom a WHO fact sheet about BMI would be meaningless—could follow their doctors' directive to measure the size of their stomachs.

Though the scientists were not themselves presuming to measure health, their reasons for adopting this technique for measurement paralleled the reasons given by doctors and their patients. As they wrote in their study of the efficacy of waist circumference: "The measurement of abdominal circumference is simple and practical" (Alvarado et al. 2010: 19). Whether waist was measured at the narrowest point or at the umbilical level, this method provides "an advantage over techniques for measuring body-fat that require privacy and precision equipment" (Alvarado et al. 2010: 19).

Measuring Health

The two examples presented above illustrate different techniques for measuring obesity. In the first, obesity was determined through what the scientists I worked with called the "Quetelet BMI." In the 1830s Adolphe Quetelet, a Belgian statistician widely regarded as the father of quantitative social sciences, developed a mathematical model for determining the "average man" (*l'homme moyen*), tracing mean values of measured variables along a normal distribution curve (also known as a bell curve). Trained in astronomy, he sought to assess population-wide indicators of weight and height through laws of proportionality. Quetelet himself was not interested in the deviations or risk factors that would come to dominate later interest in obesity (Hacking 2007). Instead, as historian Theodore Porter writes: "He revered statistical laws partly as a source of metaphysical consolation—tokens of stability in a time of revolution—and partly as evidence that this domain could be made properly scientific" (1995: 16). It was only toward the turn of the twentieth century that a so-called scientific association of excess weight with poor health began to emerge, and this association was driven less by concerns of public health than by the concerns of life insurance companies. As Porter explains this, "In estimating risk from height and weight, insurance companies were not drawing on established medical knowledge. Information on build became a reliable basis for projecting differential mortality only as the result of efforts by the companies themselves" (2000: 241).

By the start of the twentieth century many U.S. life insurance companies had defined overweight as "an excess accumulation of body fat," using correlations of weight with height in their determinations of what constituted excessive fat. While these companies generally held that *over*weight was not healthy, the precise cutoffs used to distinguish normal weight, overweight, and obesity remained considerably fluid through the twentieth century. Different industries as well as different governmental organizations employed a variety of methods for measuring a healthy body size—some as simple as a graph of recommended weight for age—as well as different demarcations for determining when, exactly, someone's body size was healthy.

In 1972 an influential paper first-authored by epidemiologist Ancel Keys compared various ways of measuring obesity against one another. This paper ultimately selected the Quetelet index because, of all the different methods tested, it was best at representing different geographical regions in like terms (1972:

330). In other words, the standard it created made population X, population Y, and population Z look, in numerical terms, most like one another so that they could be most easily compared to one another. It is important to note that Keys, as with Quetelet, was not interested in finding a metric that would compare an individual against a normal curve but sought to find a means of calibrating vast amounts of data about body size to make comparisons between populations: business professionals in St. Paul, Minnesota, Bantu working-class South Africans, and Japanese fisherman. Keys renamed the Quetelet Index the body mass index—BMI.

The BMI became a gold standard for assessing relative overweight and obesity following the publication of Keys's paper. Still, it was not until 1998 that the WHO and the National Institutes of Health standardized these terms as underweight: BMI <18.5; overweight: BMI 25 to <30; and obesity: BMI ≥30 (see also Rubin and Joseph, this volume).[4] Even then, scientists could not show that a diagnosis of overweight had a direct impact on death rates—only that it correlated with other risk factors for poor health (Flegal et al. 2005). And some countries, such as Japan and Singapore, have since altered the designations to more closely match their epidemiological risk profiles, shifting the presence of overweight and obesity downward so that the diagnoses fall at lower BMIs.

Whereas Keys primarily saw the BMI as a demographic tool, the implementation of the formula has since shifted. Today the BMI is not limited to population-level comparisons, but is commonly used to make assessments about individual health. Above, Julia's personal BMI was calculated by the nutritionists, who warned her on the basis of the number that her BMI might be causing her headaches. Julia protested, suggesting that her weight had not recently changed and they must have been calculating it incorrectly. But the nutritionists, though they often had to recalibrate and adjust the scale, ignored the possibility of measurement error. After all, a reason that the BMI has spread so widely is due to its "simplicity of calculation" (Keys et al. 1972: 341). This simple calculation then leads to cleanly organized fact sheets, such as those offered by the WHO. "What are the common health consequences of overweight and obesity?" the WHO fact sheet about obesity asks. The answers it provides are directed toward concerns of health:

> Cardiovascular diseases (mainly heart disease and stroke), which were the leading cause of death in 2008; diabetes; musculoskeletal disorders (especially osteoarthritis—a highly disabling degenerative disease of the joints); some cancers (endometrial, breast, and colon). The risk for these noncommunicable diseases increases with the increase in BMI.[5]

Once this seemingly simple measurement is made, who is Julia to argue with the facts?

The second example—waist circumference—presents a different set of concerns. Whereas WHO officials might be content to rely on scales, the scientists I worked with were more dubious about their utility. Though "scales do not lie," human error can bring doubt to their results. Given that Guatemalan scales were typically old or expensive, researchers saw clear advantages in the use of the single measurement of waist circumference that bypassed weight and height. That this single measure also targeted abdominal adiposity, which they held to be a better predictor of morbidity than weight alone, was also beneficial. Accordingly, one Guatemalan public health worker who I spent time with refused to speak of "overweight." In his words, "You can't change your height, so when you rely on the BMI, people tend to focus on weight. But weight itself is not necessarily the problem. We need to be more precise in our language and our measures." Aiming to shift attention away from the "imprecise" measure of weight and toward the presence of fat, he spoke of "over*fat*" instead of "over*weight*." Reasoning that fat was a better indicator of health than was the general measure of weight, he also advocated the use of abdominal circumference instead of the BMI.

Still, measuring waist circumference was not without challenges. There was, for example, the problem of what researchers referred to as the "cultural norms of modesty." When working with Guatemalan children, researchers had to wait to take their measurements until the day of gym class, when children wore uniform T-shirts that were thinner than other clothes. With adults, researchers encountered the bulk of *huipiles* that would throw off measurements—should three centimeters be subtracted to adjust for the fabric? Or five? Or one? There was additionally the concern about where exactly on the body one could find the "natural waist"—the site the researchers wanted to measure. Theoretically, it was measured at the narrowest point along the lower torso, just above the iliac crest, which would be encountered by running a "constant-tension tape" along the lower abdomen, stopping where the tape provided resistance. Point to your belly button, the researcher could ask, looping the tape just above the spot where the person's finger rested. But in practice, breathing might change the number, and with round stomachs the narrowest point was not always at the "natural waist."

While ease of application was a reason that many championed the technique of waist circumference, others were concerned about its potential for inaccuracies. In the Netherlands, where I interviewed several public health nutritionists, I heard numerous complaints about imprecision in the traditional methods of measuring obesity. As one nutrition scientist explained, "We use BMI and abdominal circumferences as proxies for poor health. But these are such crude measures. Really we should be using techniques such as bioimpedance or DEXA scans.[6] These methods will tell us a lot more about what's happening within a person's body. They give us a better sense of *true* obesity."

As I will explore further in the next section, the idea that a person had a true level of obesity that could be revealed by increasingly accurate devices of measurements was prevalent within public health debates about obesity measurements. Rather than view obesity as a sociomaterial construction that could be produced in different ways by varying devices of measurement, it was treated by public health workers that I spoke with in both Guatemala and Europe as an underlying bodily trait that could be objectively reported—if only the right tools could be developed and applied.

Bioelectrical Impedance Analysis (BIA)

After a second doctor I interviewed during postdoctoral research in Europe referred me to the Internet when I asked for clarification about his explanation of bioelectrical impedance analysis, I decided to take the advice seriously.[7] After all, although there are clearly limits to drawing material for ethnographic analysis from online performances, BIA patients (and prospective patients) also told me they commonly used the Internet to find information about devices for weight or fat assessment. Additionally, many of the ideas of accuracy that I came across in online depictions of the BIA echoed ideas present in my conversations with doctors and health workers. The following explanation of BIA from an online video—one of the first results when searching the phrase in Google—provides a nice entry into the social imaginaries surrounding this technology.[8]

"Hello everyone, I am going to take my body fat via bioimpedance." A man— let us call him Juan—is holding his smartphone to a mirror, while projecting the image to an audience through the Internet. "As you can see, I have a set of abs so I'm definitely in single digits," he says, patting the well-defined muscles in his stomach. "Now then, I'm going to use this scale which uses bioimpedance as a conductor which transmits electrical signals, down, and then up and then back down and tells you how much fat, and how much water and how much you weigh and stuff." He then presents his audience with a challenge: "Whoever guesses right online about how much my body fat might be via bioimpedance, right here, will win a free protein container. So let's do it three times and take the average of the three."

Juan sets the camera down to continue the experiment, picking it up only after he has stepped on the scale to show those watching its response. "7.3 percent body fat," he says and then points the camera at the scale, offering visible proof of the number. He repeats the process two more times, and both times the scale repeats the number: 7.3 percent. "This has a 2 percent error rate for bioimpedance, but this method is actually really accurate," he reports. Nonetheless, despite the alleged accuracy when it comes to the meaning of the measurement, confusion remains: everyone who responded to his challenge with a guess of his body fat percentage had underestimated: 3 percent, 4 percent, 4.4 percent, 1 percent,

4.1 percent, 4 percent, 4.3 percent. "It looks like nobody got it right," Juan says before turning off the camera.

Bioelectrical impedance analysis (BIA)—which measures the resistance to conductivity of tissue when an electric current is passed through it—was a body fat assessment strategy that many public health scientists touted for its accuracy. "I like this because it's truly scientific," one woman who went to a weight-loss clinic in Amsterdam that used a bioimpedance monitor in its fitness program explained. When I asked her to tell me more, she said that its results were "trust-worthy" (unlike Julia, above, she did not worry that the scale was a liar). Doctors who promoted BIA would explain to prospective patients that this form of body assessment would fill in missing data, helping them make diagnoses and treatment plans that were more complete than they would be otherwise. As one Italian doctor explained, "It can give us a lot of great information about your body composition. With this information we're better able to make up a treatment plan targeting your needs. You see, it gives us the critical information about your muscle mass, fat mass, and phase angle." A brochure for bioimpedance that I came across at one clinic summarizes the technique:

> Bioimpedance is a means of measuring electrical signals as they pass through the fat, lean mass, and water in the body. Through laboratory research we know the actual impedance or conductivity of various tissues in the body, and we know that by measuring the current between two electrodes, and applying this information to complex proven scientific formulas, accurate body composition can be determined.

Health scores accompanied the numbers produced by BIA machines so as to explain the significance of the results. As we saw in the failure of Juan's audience to approximate his body fat percentage scores adequately—viewing him as fit, they all underestimated his body fat—the numbers themselves must be put into context to be made meaningful, and these scores help provide this context. Although widely agreed upon standards do not exist, the charts that many clinics use cross-reference exam results with gender and age to provide cutoff points for "excellent," "good," "fair," or "poor." One company that markets bioimpedance scales explains this process as follows:

> We continue to refine our body composition technology with modern day algorithms derived from databases encompassing thousands upon thousands of physical measurements. Extrapolated data includes body composition profile, total body fat, total body water, fat free mass, body mass index, basal metabolism or resting energy expenditure. A personal, informative, colorful 5-page professional printout assessment is available that provides accurate individual

Body Composition Analysis but also dietary guidance recommendations related to weight loss control.[9]

In contrast to the measuring tape used by many Guatemalan women, BIA required elaborate technology. Although some bathroom scales claiming to measure fat percentages through bioimpedance advertised their "low error rate," many of the researchers I spoke with dismissed these methods as "unreliable." Even though scales could consistently reproduce the identical results—within 2 percent of one another, as Juan had stated—researchers were doubtful that the resultant number corresponded with a person's "real" body fat percentage and also pointed out that most bathroom bioimpedance scales measure bone density, relying on their own formulas to make body fat percentages meaningful. The instruments commonly advocated by European scientists I spoke with were much more intensive than Juan's bathroom scale. Indeed, the requirements for "reliable" BIA were extensive enough to transform "person" into "patient" because measurements had to be taken by an expert, often in a clinical setting. As one researcher explained, to measure bioimpedance correctly the subject "needs to lie completely still for ten minutes before electrodes are strapped to the wrist, hand, and feet—equidistantly from one another." He clarified that it was not difficult, but it was also not something one could do without guidance.

Many scientists who advocated the use of abdominal circumference and BMI for measuring obesity praised these methods for their simplicity. From an entirely different angle, the BIA was also described as "simple." One doctor explained that the potential for human error seen in other methods—i.e., the concern that scales would not be correctly calibrated to zero or that natural waist would not be correctly located—was mitigated by a reliance on the sophisticated design of the machine: "We just press the button, and it does the measuring. In a few seconds we have the information. We put this into our computer and it will give us everything we need to know to get started with the treatment program."

This purported simplicity of BIA, however, came at a significant economic price. The WHO, in pointing out that there are more accurate techniques for assessing obesity than the BMI, also acknowledges that "the cost of such technologies and the practical difficulties involved in applying them limit their usefulness" (2000: 7). Whereas bathroom scales marketed with bioimpedance capabilities can be found online for as little as $100, not only did scientists discount these as being unreliable, but the public hospitals where I carried out much of my fieldwork in Guatemala had no budget for even the "inexpensive" scales. Meanwhile "professional" BIA machines could cost upward of $5,000, making the technique, despite its theoretical accuracy, ineffective for most health clinics in the world.[10]

In sites where it was used, the high cost of the equipment was justified through numerous promises. For example, one company that sells high-tech bioimpedance scales called "inner scan body composition monitors" reports that the scans will give both doctors and patients greater knowledge of, and greater control over, their bodies. An advertisement pamphlet explains:

> Tanita knows you inside and out, so you can have more information about your body than ever before. Not just body fat and body water, but total body composition: Bone mass, metabolic age, muscle mass, basal metabolic rate indicator, visceral fat and physique rating. … Know all this and you have an amazingly accurate picture of your true fitness level. …

This "amazingly accurate" knowledge was advertised as offering increased personal control over the body. In the words of one health worker, "Bioimpedance can be used to monitor fat and muscle. When people know their body composition, they can more easily maintain healthy cells." In the words of a bioimpedance proponent, "Any diet or fitness program needs this information."

When talking about BMI, doctors and scientists were always quick to mention that it takes the ratio of weight and height as a *proxy* for health, but that there was much that it did not measure. Many referred to the situation of the Olympic wrestler whose relatively high weight is made up not of unhealthy fat, but of "healthier" (and heavier) muscle. "According to the BMI, this athlete could be categorized as obese!" they would say to illustrate the shortcomings of the index. "Not all pounds are equal" was a common critique made of the BMI. Meanwhile, BIA was repeatedly emphasized as being more accurate, more sophisticated, more replicable (and thus more predictable and reliable), and as overall providing a truer assessment of the body than the ostensibly cruder measures of BMI or waist circumference. The ability to assess the specificities of bodily substance (fat, muscle, bone) took away guesswork. As a technique of "surgery without the scalpel,"—as it was advertised—this was an instrument that would reveal interiors, removing mystery about the inner workings of the body. This ability to monitor one's body would, in turn, improve the health of those using it. BIA offered the possibility of going beyond "superficial and imperfect" representations, getting close to the body's "underlying reality" (Gould 1981: 239).

Limitations to Measurement

Above I have described three techniques for the measurement of obesity, detailing the methodological strengths and weaknesses of each. BMI is the mostly widely established strategy for assessing obesity and has the incumbent advantage. Though its emergence as a front-runner following Keys's 1972 article was less than certain, it has since gained momentum. Today it is the method of determining a diagnosis of obesity employed by clinics ranging from city centers in

Europe to rural mountain clinics in Guatemala. Many people know their BMI, and the calculation of weight and height—though certainly not without situational divergences so that someone's weight might be significantly different from one scale to the next—can be done on a pocket calculator.

Abdominal circumference, which requires no scale at all, was also advocated for its simplicity. This technique is not without inconveniences: the person taking the measurement will come in contact with the body of the person being measured, which can challenge norms of modesty in some places; bulky clothing can interfere with the number; and the location of what they called the natural waist may not be obvious. But researchers generally liked that it targeted abdominal adiposity, citing current research that suggests that its single measurement is comparable to—or better than—BMI at indicating or predicting metabolic illness.

In the words of one French researcher I spoke with, the internal scans offered by BIA present "a new frontier" of obesity measurement. It opens up the human body, allowing researchers and patients previously unobtainable insight into cellular composition and, presumably, function. It promises to move beyond the potential superficiality of indirect measurements to yield knowledge about an internal reality that remained, until now, only known in the abstract.

It is notable that whether their chosen method for assessing obesity was BMI, abdominal circumference, or bioimpedance, scientists and health workers defended their choice through the measurement's accuracy. Whether discussing BMI, waist circumference, or BIA, the phrase "This is more accurate" is scattered throughout my field notes. Journal articles defending the use of each particular method invariably cite the method's accuracy. Used in conjunction with exactitude and reliability, these references to accuracy implied an ability to gain correct and precise knowledge about a person's objective level of obesity. Historians of science Lorraine Daston and Peter Galison have drawn attention to the flexibility of the notion of objectivity, which can refer to "everything from empirical reliability to procedural correctness to emotional detachment" (1992: 82). The term *accuracy*, which is used in conjunction with each of these versions of objectivity, is a similarly amalgamated concept.

According to the OED, the word *accuracy* emerged in the second half of the seventeenth century along with experimental science and an emphasis on exactitude in record keeping. The term made headlines in 1850, when James Joule set out to convince the scientific community of his methods for determining heat by using extensive tables of numbers to prove the accuracy of his laboratory measurements. As historian of science Otto Sibum explains, "Absolute standards were imposed in order to make local knowledge work elsewhere. Instruments of precision controlled skill and became representatives of accuracy" (1995: 74). Accuracy in the case of measuring what would become known as caloric heat was achieved by standardizing differences in both climate and research skill so as to make results in one place comparable with those in another. A slightly different version of accuracy is seen in the concerns about whether a warhead can hit its target (Mackenzie 1999). Here, the concern for accuracy imagines that the most accurate measures best indicate an object's distance, size, etc. This is the accuracy professed by skilled mapmakers whose accurate representations are purported to best guide the viewer along an intended route.

But though the different techniques of obesity I have outlined above operate in different ways, enacting different forms of accuracy, when applied to the realm of personal health care, they share an assumption that health can be located in the tissues of the body and that accurate measurements of these tissues can be used for both comparative purposes and to assess an individual against a norm.

In Guatemala I encountered a different way of understanding fatness, in which one person's corporeality was incomparable to another's. I present this account here in an attempt to open up discussions of obesity foreclosed by a focus on accurate metrics. It asks us to rethink our assumptions about the metric-based character of obesity; it also asks us to consider whether there might be forms of accuracy that have nothing to do with replicability or mechanical precision. Although my focus here is on Guatemala because this is where I have done research, I am not interested in emphasizing the distinction between Guatemalan and so-called Western understandings of weight in this account. Following presentations of my research to U.S. and European audiences, audience members often suggest that their own understandings of weight are less precise than it might appear given a public health promotion of metrics. Moreover, in both Guatemalan and the U.S. variegated understandings of and desires for fatness and thinness often coexist. Rather than suggest categorical distinctions between Guatemalan and Western visions of fatness, my research, by pointing to the nuances and complexities surrounding fatness in one region, opens up the possibility that these complex experiences of body size exist elsewhere as well.

Nevertheless, because the idea of fatness that I will draw attention to is substantially different from the indices of obesity I described above, I want to present a brief summary of a longstanding vision of dietary health in the Guatemala region where I conducted fieldwork. Alternatively referred to as humoral or indigenous medicine, it is no longer widely or systematically used today. But given its historic influence, and its resonance with the view of fatness that I outline below, it is helpful to summarize it briefly. In this logic of dietary health, a person's well-being could not be abstracted from a specific meal or from the meal's interactions with the body at the moment of eating. Instead, well-being was conceived through sensory characteristics of foods and their immediate interaction with a body that was, necessarily, situated in a specific environment at a specific time. The classic descriptions of humoral/indigenous practices given by anthropologists Robert Redfield and Alfonso Villas Rojas specify that it would be a mistake to try to overlay categories onto these practices because the "categories are blurred and run into one another" (1971: 160). Guatemala's humoral systems were necessarily expansive, drawing upon an understanding of balance that comprises textures, colors, and tastes. Abstract—that is, distanced or universalized—guidelines are anathema to these practices of dietary health, which depended upon listening to and making decisions around the circumstances surrounding a particular body and its immediate ecological contexts. Anthropologist Susan Weller describes the desire of health care professionals to create rules out of humoral medicine–i.e., orange juice is *cool*, measles are *hot* (1983: 256). Although they sought to establish these rules to simplify and expand the delivery of health care services, this led to widespread misunderstanding about the workings of humoral medicine, which resists classification. From a humoral approach, an individual food would never—could never—be understood as healthy or unhealthy on its own; rather, its health is determined through its relation to the different foods consumed and the state of the individual at the time of consumption.

Similar to this refusal to make situated knowledges about food and health abstract, I saw in my research that fatness was also not something that Guatemalans necessarily associated with measureable size and definitive body weight categorization. Instead fatness related to a specific and mobile state of a person's body. Calling someone fat could be a way of saying he or she was happy and blessed in life. This sense of the term has the connotations of ephemerality also seen in beauty—something that was, indeed, related to fatness. "*Donde no hay gordura, no hay hermosura*" is a local expression that translates loosely to "Where there is no fat, there is no beauty." Likewise, "*Tan bonito el gordito*" (or, "What a beautiful little fattie") was a rhyme I heard several times. The use of these statements illustrates a sense among many of the people I met that fatness was desirable. For many, fatness was also healthy.[11] When traveling to Guatemala's rural communities I often heard some form of the following expression, spoken here by a middle-aged *campesina*: "*Ser gordo es ser sano*" ("In the countryside, to be fat is to be healthy"). From the perspective of the field of public health, it can be easy to dismiss this idea: to hear it and to think it provides evidence of the erroneous—and provincial—thinking of someone who does not understand the consequences of weight gain. But I came to understand that when people were saying "to be fat is to be healthy," their meaning was literal: they were not mistakenly considering obesity to be healthy, but they were understanding health as a quality of the body that could not be directly assessed through body size.

Whereas obesity, as discussed in public health, is typically contingent upon both body size metrics and the occurrence of illness, the understanding of fatness I describe here, while related to food and more loosely related to size, more generally encompassed an experience of abundance. One could be fat in a moment, the way one might feel content— for example, when surrounded by friends and family at a meal where food and conversation were plentiful. To be fat ("*ser gordo*") meant life was going well, and on several occasions I heard someone who did not *look* fat in shape to me (accustomed, as I was, to associating fat with size and measure) claim to be fat. When I heard someone refer to another as fat, I would try to ask for clarification about how they came to this assessment. Although people did not generally understand my question—they did not, after all, treat fatness as a *thing* to be assessed—their responses emphasized relationships, suggesting to me that intimate knowledge of a person would produce this kind of understanding. Unlike weight that can be determined by a stranger, fatness—in the sense in which I am describing it here—must be made through dialogue and interaction and could only be understood through effort, time, contact, and the strength of intimate relations. In contrast to the BMI designation of healthy weight—which is a *standard* in the dual use of the term, i.e., both an "exemplar measure" and a "value which is treated as invariable" (OED)—fatness could not be determined through a scale.[12] Instead, an understanding of fatness and an evaluation of the quality of food that followed required extensive knowledge of a person's life and of the specific contexts in which this food was eaten. Fatness was not a condition, but a fluid experience. It could not be measured.

Conclusion: The Inadequacies of Numerical Accuracy

At the American Anthropological Association meetings in 2010, I presented a summary of my research on fatness in Guatemala on a panel containing several other papers that critiqued public health nutrition's reductive measurement-focused approach to the complex problem of international obesity. Many of the papers were based on fieldwork undertaken in places where people suffered from a range of dietary-related disorders: diabetes, hypertension, metabolic syndrome, etc. On the whole, we were not discounting the suffering experienced by those with these illnesses. We were, rather, interrogating the way that this suffering was often reduced to the problem of weights and measures—and we raised concerns about how this might exacerbate, and not treat the illnesses experienced by those with whom we lived and worked (see especially Hardin and Rubin and Joseph in this volume).

During the discussion held after we had presented our papers it was clear that a vocal contingent of our audience was disinterested in our challenge to the goal of creating single, universal standards for assessing dietary related illness (see also McCullough, this volume, for analysis of these events). Presuming that obesity was a condition that existed independently from the specific measurement practices that brought it into being, their concern lay in finding more accurate obesity standards. One man suggested that we abandon the BMI because abdominal fat was a better index of health (presumably the we he spoke of was the public health community and anthropologists whose primary goal was the collection anthropometrical information). Another person declared that it was premature to see abdominal fat measurements as a panacea and took the position that BMI was too entrenched to be abandoned. The audience discussion shifted focus away from the inadequacies of any measurement system—and from our interest in evoking other ways that people might know and relate with obesity—to the problem of finding the best measurements of obesity. In this shift, the concerns presented by our papers were largely ignored.

In the years I have been studying obesity, I have seen this happen often. In discussions, numbers hold remarkable weight. Many reasons exist for this. When it comes to assessing physical health or measuring weight, waist centimeters, or BIA, reading scores take less time to assess than does the process of becoming familiar with people's lived experiences of eating and movement. To know fatness, as my Guatemalan interlocutors spoke of it, was to have contact, proximity, and a kind of expertise dependent on interpersonal investment. Clearly there are reasons why a country whose overburdened, underfunded health care system would desire fast and inexpensive health care strategies. It takes but a moment to step on a scale or measure one's waist. It takes much longer to develop the kind of intimacy necessary to make a determination of the kind of fatness I described in Guatemala above. Though I would hesitate to convert this intimacy into a price—to make this form of expertise comparable with the cost of a BIA instrument, for example—it certainly requires commitments of time and energy that Guatemala's official public health infrastructure may not be prepared to handle.

The translation of bodily experiences into numbers may also be desirable because of the detachment and the ostensible objectivity or safety offered by metrics. The argument might go: "In making differences comparable, universes are brought together." But the universality achieved by numbers is only possible with a flattening, a silencing of diversity. Donna Haraway explains this well, writing: "Science has been about a search for translation, convertibility, mobility of meanings and universality—which I call reductionism—which one language (guess whose) must be enforced as the standard for all the translations and conversations" (1988: 580). With numbers, other knowledges about bodies become harder to see, and though they certainly do not disappear, they become more difficult for scientists and public health workers to value.

I suggest that numerical connotations of most uses of accuracy further contribute to this devaluation. When accuracy refers to an ability to hit an external target, to precisely follow a formula, or to find replicable results, it makes sense that the methods we follow to achieve accuracy will push us toward a world of measurements and standards. Yet we must also remember that whether the assessment of metabolic health is made through weight, width, or composite indices, all of these numbers remain abstract representations. Quetelet, in his framing of the idea of the average man understood that this measure was an abstraction. Yet he held that "Abstraction was essential to social science. Real individuals were too numerous and diverse for psychological study to contribute much to an understanding of the social condition" (Gigerenzer 1989: 38). Although the method of abstraction might have its place in epidemiology (indeed, the field would not exist without this), this method is less obviously accurate in the realm of dietary health, where accuracy—if we shift the term away from mechanical connotations—might depend upon staying close to people, bodies, and experiences as they are lived. We must remember that the attempt to diagnose and treat Julia's headache through a graph of international standards made very little sense to her. She, like many patients, did not return in my remaining months in the clinic, and I cannot say whether her headache was *caused* by weight or even if the scale used to report her weight was accurate (whether she was *truly* 120 or 130 pounds). But this is not a failure on my part, but rather is a part of the story. Cause and effect, as lived, do not manifest with clear directionality the way numbers and formulas would have us believe. There is no true accuracy existing within measures, and, in this sense, all scales that are used to diagnose problems of health are liars.

The three metric-based methods for assessing obesity I have described above do not have identical effects. They follow different techniques, operate around different distinctions, and produce different versions of obesity.[13] These various measurements and their corresponding classifications of overweight and obesity do not just produce different categories of people (cf. Hacking 1986) but produce different ontologies of the body. When using BMI, because height is fixed, people's attention tends to focus upon their weight. When using abdominal circumference, the focus shifted to concern for stomach fat (hence the attention to over*fat* instead of over*weight*). And with bioimpedance, the object of interest is the previously invisible interior cellular composition of the body.

Yet despite their differences, all of these practices of measuring—in contrast to the notion of fatness I saw in Guatemala—presume that the health of the body can be known by calculating the composition of the body. They reify health, purporting to quantify something that may not, if my Guatemalan interlocutors are to be taken seriously, lay embedded within a substance and that may not be revealed through a metric. They transform people's experience of their bodies into a proxy of weight, centimeters, or fat percentages, and then they replace the experience with the proxy, leaving people to ask "What is my size?" rather than looking toward less fungible qualities of eating. They also encourage the public health community to look for better, more precise, and more accurate measures of health at the cost of ignoring those experiences and practices related to weight, eating, and health that cannot be fixed into metrics.

In his critique of the powerful influence that the normal curve has had on scientific thought, Gould writes:

> The primary desideratum in all experiments is reduction of confusing variables: we bring all the buzzing and blooming confusion of the external world into our laboratories and, holding all else constant in our artificial simplicity, try to vary

just one potential factor at a time. But many subjects defy the use of such an experimental method—particularly most social phenomena—because importation into the laboratory destroys the subject of the investigation (1994: 139).

Many Guatemalans were attuned to this destruction. For them, the act of measuring the human body and relating this measurement to health was incomprehensible. This was something one did with commodities bought and sold—sacks of corn or sugar in the market. But humans? Many people laughed at the request that they wrap a tape measurer around themselves, seeing this as ridiculous because they did not control their size. Some people became angry. This anger is no doubt complex, defying any singular analysis or source. But I think it can be linked, in part, to the way the act of measurement separates the person from the environment—the tape measure literally binding the body into a circumference whole, the scale reporting a specific weight. During the moment of measurement the fluid connections between skin and surroundings become frozen. The waist becomes both literally and figuratively demarcated from the world, bounded by a single measurement that in turn individualizes the body. BMI and BIA scores, when translated into the realm of population health, require "thousands upon thousands of physical measurements" to be made intelligible, but at the end of the measurement an individual body is labeled with a single number or score. In this way, body weight measurement is not only an act of reporting, but an enactment of health that many people in my fieldwork found objectionable.

Science studies scholar Donald Mackenzie has argued that although accuracy is no "mere fiction," it is also always thoroughly political (1999: 356). Sociologist Steven Epstein makes a similar claim in pointing out that Quetelet's *l'homme moyen* (average man) "was 'normal' in the double sense; he was the midpoint of natural variation, but also the way that people were supposed to be" (2009: 38). Epstein suggests that, similarly, standards today are not only invoked to strengthen biological and cultural norms, but to also justify the correction of existing deviations. If we could measure health, then the correction of such "deviation" would be most likely celebrated. But we can never measure health; we measure body size and take this as a substitution for health. Though health can supposedly be seen in the standards and graphs that accompany the instruments for body size measurements, health, like Gould's notion of intelligence, is multifaceted, nebulous, and always in flux.

I conclude by drawing attention to the WHO's own answers to the question: "Why classify overweight and obesity?" In their obesity fact sheet they suggest that classification is valuable because it allows:

- meaningful comparison of weight status within and between populations;
- the identification of individuals and groups at increased risk of morbidity and mortality;

- the identification of priorities for intervention at individual and community levels; and
- a firm basis for evaluating interventions (2000:7).

Certainly this chapter cannot unravel all of these explanations for the utility of obesity classification—the use of measurements is far too ingrained within the field of public health. Instead, I hope to create space for additional questions to be inserted into each of these ostensibly canonical bullet points. Meaningful comparisons for whom, and to what end? How are increased risk of morbidity and mortality determined; what remains unspoken and what concerns are not attended to by using weight as a key determinant of health? How will priorities for intervention be determined on the basis of size? How can calculating weight ever say anything about the evaluation of interventions? How useful are the methods of measuring body size, when transported from the realm of international comparative research projects into the realm of personal and public health? What happens when the statistical projections of body weight indices replace the interpersonal attention that might be provided in situated clinical care?

It is my hope that by asking these questions we might challenge an easy translation between obesity classification for the purposes of epidemiological research and obesity classification for the purposes of an individual's health. In drawing attention to the translation of bodies into numbers, we might also begin to consider other, nonmetric ways of relating to size, weight, and fat. Quetelet's approach to knowledge may have become the basis for worldwide standards of obesity, but there are many other versions of obesity—and health—yet to be explored.

Notes

1. I have been conducting ethnographic fieldwork in Guatemala since 2000, with an intensive period of research between January 2008 and April 2009. Numerous organizations have funded my research, including the Wenner-Gren, Fulbright Hays, the SSRC/Ford Foundation, and the Tinker Foundation. New York University has also provided me with several research and writing grants. Emily Martin, Tom Abercrombie, Rayna Rapp, Sally Merry, and Renato Rosaldo advised my dissertation research, and I am grateful for their endless support. I am currently conducting research in the Netherlands on an ERC funded project supervised by Annemarie Mol. I thank all the members of the Eating Bodies project for their ongoing collaboration.
2. For a more detailed and nuanced view of the work of the nutritionists see Yates-Doerr (2012); for an overview of how many of these technologies of measurement intertwine with concerns of gender and reproduction see Yates-Doerr (2011).
3. In this particular study, the presence of metabolic syndrome was assessed through the presence of four or more risk factors, determined by rates of systolic and diastolic blood pressure, glucose, uric acid, fasting insulin, triglycerides, and HDL-C. However, it should be noted that the metabolic syndrome refers to a cluster of symptoms and is itself a contested diagnostic category (Brietzke 2007; Seidell 2007).

4. As reported in mainstream media outlets around the United States, because the demarcations for overweight and obesity shifted downward, "Millions of Americans became 'fat' overnight—even if they didn't gain a pound." See http://www.cnn.com/HEALTH/9806/17/weight.guidelines/, last accessed April 15, 2011.

5. http://www.who.int/mediacentre/factsheets/fs311/en/index.html, last accessed April 15, 2011.

6. Although I do not have space to explore Dual Energy X-ray Absorptiometry or DEXA scans here, brochures for DEXA scans described them as "very accurate and precise," claiming they were fast becoming the new "gold standard" because they "provided a higher degree of precision in only one measurement" and have the ability to "show exactly where fat is distributed throughout the body."

7. My research on international and public health nutrition in Europe was conducted through a postdoctoral fellowship based in Amsterdam, with research conducted throughout Western Europe. During this fellowship I have followed the development and circulation of ideas about global health nutrition, also interviewing several nutrition scientists—some of whom serve on advisory boards of the World Health Organization and the Food and Agriculture Organization—nutritionists, nutrition students, and doctors.

8. http://www.youtube.com/watch?v=TaxCELxwmas, last accessed April 15, 2011.

9. http://www.bodycompscale.com/, last accessed April 15, 2011.

10. The word *ineffective* might look strange here, given the technique's mechanical achievements. But I mean it quite literally—bioimpedance is *ineffective* in places where it cannot function.

11. Several theories, both economic and evolutionary, have been put forth about why this might be the case, some of which are summarized in Hardin, this volume. I do not have space to explore the validity of these theories, which is largely irrelevant to my interest here—i.e., *that* people in Guatemala saw fatness as healthy, not why this was the case.

12. My Guatemalan informants were unaware of a formalized Health at Any Size movement and had not heard of fat activism, but for an interesting comparison between their practices and these movements in the United States and Europe, see Rubin and Joseph, this volume. For a nice complement to Guatemalan notions of feasting and sociality, compare the examples I have presented with the descriptions of feasting and fasting in Samoa provided by Hardin, this volume.

13. I borrow the idea of versions from Annemarie Mol, who writes that versions, which are simultaneously physical and social "emerge in different circumstances.… Versions of the body are performed, orchestrated enacted. They are done in practices" (Mol 2010).

References

Alvarado, V. J., E. Mayorga, S. Molina, and N. W. Solmons. 2010. "Correspondence of Two Procedures to Measure Abdominal Circumference in a Convenience Sample of Urban, Middle-class Schoolchildren in Guatemala City." *Asia Pacific Journal of Clinical Nutrition* 19, no. 1: 14–21.

Brietzke, S. A. 2007. "Controversy in Diagnosis and Management of the Metabolic Syndrome." *Medical Clinics of North America* 91, no. 6: 1041–1061.

Daston, L., and P. Galison. 1992. "The Image of Objectivity." *Representations* 40: 81–128.

Epstein, S. 2009. "Beyond the Standard Human?" In *Standards and Their Stories: How Quantifying, Classifying, and Formalizing Practices Shape Everyday Life,* ed. M. Lampland and S. L. Star. Ithaca: Cornell University Press, 35–53.

Flegal, K. M., B. I. Graubard, D. F. Williamson, and M. H. Gail. 2005. "Excess Deaths Associated with Underweight, Overweight, and Obesity." *Journal of the American Medical Association* 293, no. 15: 1861–1867.

Gigerenzer, G. 1989. *The Empire of Chance: How Probability Changed Science and Everyday Life.* Cambridge, New York: Cambridge University Press.

Gould, S. J. 1981. *The Mismeasure of Man.* New York: Norton.

———. 1994. "Curveball." *The New Yorker,* November 28, 139–149.

———. 1996. *The Mismeasure of Man.* Revised and expanded edition, New York: Norton.

Hacking, I. 1986. "Making Up People." In *Reconstructing Individualism: Autonomy, Individuality, and the Self in Western Thought,* ed. T. C. Heller, M. Sosna, and D. E. Wellbery. Stanford: Stanford University Press, 226–236.

———. 2007. "Where Did the BMI Come From?" In *Bodies of Evidence: Fat Across Disciplines.* Newnham College, Cambridge University.

Haraway, D. 1988. "Situated Knowledges: The Science Question in Feminism and the Privilege of Partial Perspective." *Feminist Studies* 14, no. 3: 575–599.

Janssen, I., P. T. Katzmarzyk, and R. Ross. 2004. "Waist Circumference and Not Body Mass Index Explains Obesity-related Health Risk." *American Journal of Clinical Nutrition* 79, no. 3: 379–384.

Keys, A., F. Fidanza, M. J. Karvonen, N. Kimura, and H. L. Taylor. 1972. "Indices of Relative Weight and Obesity." *Journal of Chronic Diseases* 25, no. 6–7: 329–343.

Mackenzie, D. 1999. "Nuclear Missile Testing and the Social Construction of Accuracy." In *The Science Studies Reader,* ed. M. Baigioli. New York: Routledge, 342–357.

Mol, A. 2010. "Layers or Versions? Human Bodies and the Love of Bitterness." In *Routledge Handbook of Body Studies,* ed. B. Turner. New York: Routledge, chapter 8.

Moreno, L. A., I. Pineda, G. Rodriguez, J. Fleta, A. Sarria, and M. Bueno. 2002. "Waist Circumference for the Screening of the Metabolic Syndrome in Children." *Acta Pædiatrica* 91, no. 12: 1307–1312.

Porter, T. M. 1995. "Statistical and Social Facts from Quetelet to Durkheim." *Sociological Perspectives* 38, no. 1: 15–26.

———. 2000. "Life Insurance, Medical Testing, and the Management of Mortality." In *Biographies of Scientific Objects,* ed. L. Daston. Chicago: University of Chicago Press, 226–246.

Redfield, R., and A. Villa-Rojas. 1971. *Chan Kom, a Maya Village.* Chicago: University of Chicago Press.

Seidell, J. C. 2007. "The Metabolic Syndrome Does Not Exist [Article in Dutch]." *Ned Tijdschr Geneeskd* 151, no. 14: 812.

Sibum, H. O. 1995. "Reworking the Mechanical Value of Heat: Instruments of Precision and Gestures of Accuracy in Early Victorian England." *Studies in History and Philosophy of Science Part A,* 26, no. 1: 73–106.

Smith, S. C., and D. Haslam. 2007. "Abdominal Obesity, Waist Circumference and Cardiometabolic Risk: Awareness among Primary Care Physicians, the General Population and Patients at Risk in 'the Shape of the Nations Survey.'" *Current Medical Research and Opinion* 23, no. 1: 29–47.

Weller, S. C. 1983. "New Data on Intracultural Variability: The Hot-Cold Concept of Medicine and Illness." *Human Organization* 42, no. 3: 249–257.

WHO (World Health Organization). 2000. *Obesity: Preventing and Managing the Global Epidemic.* Geneva: World Health Organization.

Yates-Doerr, E. 2011. "Bodily Betrayal: Love and Anger in the Time of Epigenetics." In *A Companion to the Anthropology of the Body and Embodiment,* ed. F. E. Mascia-Lees. Malden, MA: Wiley-Blackwell, chapter 16.

———. 2012. "The Weight of the Self: Care and Compassion in Guatemalan Dietary Choices." *Medical Anthropology Quarterly* 25, no. 1: 136–158.

CHAPTER 3

"Diabesity" and the Stigmatizing of Lifestyle in Australia

Darlene McNaughton

✛ ✛ ✛

A forty-year-old friend was in hospital after having her first child. Like most women, she had gained approximately 30 kg during her pregnancy, placing her pre-delivery weight at around 95 k. One of the nurses working on the maternity ward came into the room my friend shared with several other mothers and their newborns. The nurse was looking for a woman who had gestational diabetes. My friend explained that the nurse looked around the room and then came straight over to her bed and asked, "Are you the woman with gestational diabetes?" She wasn't. It was the younger (mid twenties) and physically much smaller woman in the bed across the room.

At a recent lunch time gathering, another friend, also in her forties, revealed that she had been diagnosed with type 2 diabetes mellitus—something she was not expecting and was clearly surprised by. "How can I have diabetes," she said. "I'm not overweight, I've never been overweight. In fact I've always been small, like all my life. I eat well and I exercise, I mean, I drink a bit, sure, hell we all have our vices, but I'm not fat, never have been. So how is it that I have bloody diabetes!"

We find ourselves in a time where governments, health education campaigns, the medical establishment, and the media frequently remind, expect, and even admonish us to be deeply concerned about our health (Lupton 1995; Petersen and Lupton 1997). We are told that new knowledge is revealing a growing array of potential risks to our well-being, the threat of which can only be alleviated or avoided if we are vigilant and take greater personal responsibility for our health (Brandt and Rozin 2007). As Robert Crawford (1994) has shown in his seminal analysis, in recent decades health has been constructed as a precarious thing and the boundaries between it and illness presented as shifting, permeable, and under constant threat by the potential for illness, rather than illness itself.

Crawford (1994) also notes that in this coalescing of illness potential and medicine on the one hand, and personal responsibility and morality on the other, that health has also become a metaphor for self-control, self-denial, and will-power. In this framing, health is a moral discourse, an opportunity to reaffirm the values by which the self is separated from the other (Crawford 1994: 1352). This emphasis on personal responsibility and culpability sees those deemed to be at risk commonly imagined as ignorant, irresponsible citizens, who lack self-control and self-discipline and require intervention (Bell et al.2009, 2011a; McCullough and Rubin, this volume).

Scholars examining the contours of this dramatic, cultural shift over the last forty years emphasize the capacity of this imperative to health to stigmatize certain individuals and groups who are given responsibility for health on the one hand but have little power to affect actual change on the other (Lupton 1995; Petersen 1997, Petersen and Bunton 1997, Petersen and Lupton 1997; Saguy and Riley 2005; Peterson et al. 2010). They also highlight that the focus on individual responsibility renders invisible the very structural forces that limit people's choices and produce ill health and risk behaviors in the first instance, i.e., poverty, poor housing, racism, industrial pollution, etc. (Armstrong 2003: 213; Daykin and Naidoo 1995: 63).

It is within this context that the stigmatization of individual lifestyles has emerged as a way to combat chronic diseases such as diabetes, heart disease, and lung cancer (McNaughton 2013; see Rubin and Joseph and McCullough, this volume). Within these discourses, considerable emphasis is placed on promoting the risk factors associated with lifestyle (chronic) diseases. In recent years, overweight and obesity have almost overtaken their older comrades in harm, alcohol and tobacco, as the perceived leading risks for a number of lifestyle diseases, most notably T2DM (Bell et al. 2011a). In a series of annual reports from the WHO (1999, 2011) diabetes is referred to as a lifestyle disease that is now a leading cause of death globally. However, Michael Gard and Jan Wright (2005: 101–102), following Krieger (1994), have argued that "much of the rhetoric around the so-called 'obesity epidemic' is based on the spurious claim that obesity causes or is one of the important multiple causes of non-insulin dependent diabetes mellitus or ischemic heart disease" (see Becker and Yates-Doerr, this volume).

Thus although overweight and obesity are invariably held up as significant risk factors for T2DM, the relationship between them is actually very complex. While T2DM certainly does appear to be more prevalent among so-called obese people, individuals from a broad range of weights (including those considered healthy) can actually develop the disease. Furthermore, there are in fact, a number of risk factors for T2DM, including age, ethnicity, family history of the disease, previous gestational diabetes, nutrition, poverty, etc., and the interplay among them is still not well understood (Gard and Wright 2005; McNaughton 2013).

In recent years, however, the idea that fatness[1] is the central cause of T2DM has become increasingly prominent and thoroughly naturalized in the media, popular discourse, academic research, and public health campaigns (McNaughton 2013; see Rubin and Joseph, this volume). The larger-than-average body has come to signify not only poor health and poor self-control but also diabetes and, with that, disease. At the same time, diabetes (like obesity itself) is increasingly framed as self-inflicted: the result of wholly changeable and highly risky lifestyle factors such as overnutrition and physical inactivity, which are seen to be antithetical to a long and healthy life. At the same time, a person whose bodily form, lifestyle, or behaviors are read as evidencing that they are not heeding the call to health, or failing in their attempts to do so, is likely to experience some forms of stigma—social, political, economic, or medical (see Hardin, this volume).

As I have argued elsewhere (McNaughton 2103) the potency of overweight and obesity as a cultural signifier for diabetes and its iatrogenic consequences for those diagnosed with or deemed at risk for the disease has received little critical examination to date. In what follows, I set out to trace and unpack some of the contours of this relationship, exploring its potential impact on patient-provider interactions, health-seeking behavior, and its consequences for the timing of diagnosis and intervention. In short, the chapter also provides insights into the ethics and implications of stigmatizing lifestyle in an attempt to reduce chronic diseases like diabetes. Although there is no overarching theoretical framework in critical discourse analysis, by bringing together a variety of materials, media representations, and academic and public health research and conversations, I aim to show the ubiquity of certain discourses in which obesity has become entwined with and acts as a cultural signifier for diabetes, in particular T2DM.

From Globesity to Diabesity

Feminists were amongst the first to challenge biomedical models of weight and obesity, exposing the ongoing collusion between biomedical and cultural constructions of fatness (Orbach 1978, 1986; Millman 1980; Chernin 1981, 1986; Wolf 1990; Bordo 1993; Austin 1999; See Bell and McNaughton 2007 for a review). These works have also set the scene for more recent scholarship from a range of historical, queer, and feminist perspectives that examine the social constructions of fatness (Schwartz 1986; Stearns 1997; Gard and Wright, 2005: 160; Klein 1996; Sobal and Maurer 1999a, 1999b; Nichter 2000; Probyn 2000; Evans Braziel and LeBesco 2001; Stinson 2001; LeBesco 2004; Kulick and Meneley 2005; Gard 2010; Monaghan 2008 Bell et al. 2011a). While fatness is a mode of bodily trespass that has long been the focus of some social and moral scorn, during the last quarter of the twentieth century there was a seismic shift in its framing (Saguy and Riley 2005; Bell et al. 2011a). It has come to signify a person whose risky behavior and unhealthy lifestyle put them at risk for a range of health issues and diseases that range from cancer to diabetes (see McCullough, this volume; Bell et al. 2009). Even more than this, however, the overweight or obese body has come to represent an actual state of ill health (rather than merely the potential for sickness) and one that, I argue, is strongly identified with diabetes.

The reading of a bigger-than-average body as a sick body has been given much momentum via particular tropes from within obesity science as well as popular discourses on fat, weight, and risk (for further discussion on these, see Austin 1999; Campos 2004; Gard and Wright 2004; Campos et al. 2006; Murray 2008, Bell et al. 2009, 2011a; Petersen and Lupton 1997). The first is the idea that all fat is dangerous and that everyone is at risk—from the unborn fetus to our family pets (McNaughton 2011). Secondly, such discourses assume that we are getting fatter at an exponential rate and on a global scale, and thirdly, that overweight and obesity (like diabetes) are entirely preventable if individuals are vigilant and enact greater levels of self-control over their nutrition and physical activity. And finally, losing weight is seen to be a simple matter of reducing inputs (food) and increasing outputs (exercise)—grossly understating the complexity of issue (Gard and Wright 2004).

Critical examination of the evidence base for these assertions has led many commentators to question the existence, scale, and implications of the obesity epidemic (see for example: Campos 2004; Gard and Wright 2005; Campos et al. 2006; Campos 2008, Saguy and Riley 2005). Some have argued that the alleged obesity epidemic has all the hallmarks of what Cohen (1972) termed a "moral panic" (Campos 2004; Bell et al. 2009). Others have demonstrated that evidence for the health implications of weight is conflicted, contradictory, "replete with flawed and misleading assumptions," and has been consistently overstated (Gard and Wright 2005: 3; Lupton 1995; Campos 2004, 2006, 2008). For example, as Gard and Wright (2005) have shown, it is not clear that simple dietary intake causes many or most instances of overweight or obesity in adults or children. In a similar vein, Rolland-Cachera and Bellisle's (2002) analysis of the international literature found little evidence to suggest that overweight and obese children consumed more calories than did others. The exception was children experiencing the "highest indices of obesity," where a correlation was found between body weight and the amount of protein consumed.

A central conclusion that these and many other studies have drawn is that while being overweight or obese may have health consequences, the evidence is far from conclusive on how and to what extent these are caused by overweight or obesity. Indeed, it would seem that a wide range of healthy weights is clearly possible. Despite the conflicted and inconclusive state of the available evidence, overweight and obesity are invariably pronounced as dangerous threats to global health in medical and popular discourses—overstating both the current knowledge base and the risk. The wide-reaching and uncritical acceptance of a global obesity epidemic has resulted in a disproportionate response to the risks (See Galloway and Moffat, this volume). It has also provided many new opportunities for the monitoring and regulating of threatening, fat bodies, while simultaneously perpetuating certain medico-moral assumptions about individuals and the causes of fatness (Gard and Wright 2005; Bell and McNaughton 2007, McNaughton 2011).

More recently, broad acceptance within public health, government, and popular discourses that rates of overweight and obesity are skyrocketing globally has led a number of commentators to posit the onset of a diabetes epidemic (see Hardin, this volume). Obesity is often said to be the engine or driving force behind this emerging epidemic. A growing number of commentators are expressing grave concerns about these "escalating twin epidemics" of obesity and diabetes (Teixeira and Budd 2010: 527). For example, a senior commentator for the National Nutritionists Conference in Australia (May 2011) expressed this as follows:

> We are looking at an avalanche really, of people who are, who have become obese and are going to develop diabetes. It has very serious consequences for our health budget and for our community and for those individuals (Assoc. Prof. Jennifer Keogh, ABC News 2011).

The causative undertone of the "twin epidemics," i.e., that obesity leads to diabetes, is highly visible in this discourse, as these quotes suggests. However, in some quarters the independent identities of obesity and diabetes are merged into the so-called diabesity epidemic. One of the earliest uses of this term can be found in an Australian government report (Commonwealth of Australia 1999) titled "Diabesity & Associated Disorders in Australia—2000: The Accelerating Epidemic." In a similar vein, Kaufmann (2005a, 2005b), who is often attributed as having coined the term, also uses it to describe what she calls the "impending" "diabesity epidemic."

In this conflation, the order of the words—*dia* from diabetes and *besity* from obesity—do not necessarily suggest the order of things. Instead it is obesity that is presented or suggested as the central cause of the diabetes epidemic. For example, Professor Rob Moodie, head of Australia's National Preventative Health Taskforce, whose mission it is to turn around the obesity epidemic in Australia, described the situation as follows:

> It's going to require a massive effort to stop the increases in overweight and obesity…also that obviously has a major impact on levels of diabetes so there is a notion of a sort of "diabestiy" epidemic—the double epidemic of obesity and diabetes—[as] something that we have to take very seriously (ABC News 2008).

In commentaries like this from a leading spokesperson in the field of obesity, to media headlines such as "More than 50 per cent of Australian adults are overweight and there are an estimated 1.2 million people in Australia who suffer from Type 2 diabetes," we see firstly the (all too common) conflation of obesity and overweight and secondly the presentation of this convergence (overweight-obesity) as the cause of T2DM. As Gard and Wright (2005: 25) have argued, overweight and, in particular, obesity are commonly identified as the cause of diseases like T2DM, rather than as a symptom. However, overweight and obesity, like leanness or thinness, are not diseases or diagnosable illnesses but bodily conditions or states of being (Gard and Wright 2005: 25; McNaughton 2011).

Linking diabetes and overweight/obesity together in such politically charged ways serves to elevate the role of overweight and obesity as risk factors for diabetes. Indeed, the term "diabesity epidemic" implies (inaccurately) a single, all-pervasive cause for diabetes globally, namely obesity (overweight/obesity). Of course, this not only overstates the evidence, it also greatly underplays the complex relationships between the disease and body weight, while seriously understating both the existence and role of other risk factors and their interconnectedness (See Yates-Doerr, this volume). In addition, the character and effects of the structural forces that contribute to diabetes, overweight or obesity, such as poverty, migration experience, poor nutrition, etc., are also rendered invisible (see Becker, this volume).

Overweight and Obesity as Cultural Signifiers for Diabetes and an Unhealthy, Irresponsible, Diseased Body

In the 1980s and 1990s both Watson (1993: 248) and Crawford (1984: 70–71) found that those whose body weights were in the highest ranges were consistently assumed to be the persons most likely to be unhealthy. Drawing on Erving Goffman's (1963) early work and phrasing, these individuals were reckoned to have a "spoiled identity," because of their perceived inability to control their eating and weight (see McCullough, this volume). In another study Lupton and Chapman (1995: 488) note that "certain moral meanings associated with having a high blood cholesterol reading [were] related to cultural assumptions about the relationship between physical appearance, health states and self-control." Participants in this study commonly assumed a direct link between body shape and cholesterol: fatness, inactivity, and overnutrition equaled high cholesterol for many. One participant in the group interviews was assumed to have a high cholesterol simply because of his physical appearance: as one man expressed it, "I think you have got high cholesterol just looking at you" (Lupton and Chapman 1995: 488). In a similar vein, Davison et al.'s (1991) study into heart disease demonstrated that obese men and women were deemed the most likely contender for heart disease (see also Backett et al. 1994; Davison et al.1992). Similar framings, wherein body size or shape is taken to indicate disease or illness, are also central to and highly prevalent in, the discourses around weight and diabetes.

Clearly, overweight and obesity have come to act as powerful cultural signifiers for poor health and a range of diseases, including diabetes. In the idea of an obesity-diabetes epidemic we see several assumptions about the dangerousness of fat and the idea that poor health is simply the end result of changeable, risky behaviors, which in turn, have created the diabesity epidemic—potentially a much deadlier scourge. Overweight and obese people are imagined either as diabetic or as becoming diabetic. In this framing, the overweight or obese body/person signifies a diseased body/person or a body/person with high disease potential—both of which are self-inflicted through risky behavior. There is little room here for the idea of weight as a symptom of diabetes, for the notion that some overweight or obese people never develop the disease, that a range of healthy weights are possible, or that some people whose body weight is considered normal will be diagnosed with T2DM.

Overweight, Obesity, Diabetes, and Fat Prejudice

In Australia and elsewhere, fat prejudice is one of the last bastions of bigotry (Brewis et al. 2011). Although it does receive some public criticism in Australia, especially when directed at the young (Bell and McNaughton 2007), for the most part, anti-fat attitudes, unlike racism or sexism, are a "socially acceptable form[s] of prejudice" (Stunkard and Sorenson 1993: 1037). In such a context and at a time in which populations are said to be overflowing with corpulent citizens, it is not surprising to learn that the prevalence of weight stigma has increased in recent years (Puhl and Heuer 2009, 2010).

Although overweight and obesity are consistently proclaimed as dangerous national emergencies, fatness is also presented as the antithesis of the healthy body and the beautiful body. In Australia, the healthy body is the beautiful body: it is the fit, tight, trim, toned, and tanned body of the archetypal "bronzed Aussie" (Lupton and Chapman 1995). As LeBesco (2004: 1) has shown, because the fat person embodies both unhealthiness and unattractiveness, "fat people are widely represented in popular culture and interpersonal interactions as revolting—they are the agents of abhorrence and disgust."

In their analysis of Australian news stories on food risks over a fourteen-month period, Lupton and Chapman (1995) found that almost half (47 percent) reported specifically on the relationship between food intake and obesity: specifically overconsumption or an unbalanced diet. Many of these articles were features or front-page stories that presented the overweight body/person as reviled, as "grotesque, out of control, unhealthy and unAustralian"—as the opposite of the idealized tanned, fit, beautiful Aussie body (2004: 187). Overweight people were often depicted as headless or faceless and invariably consuming unhealthy foods, thus "presenting to the viewer both the type of body that is source of the anxiety and the very behaviors and lifestyles thought to create it" (Lupton and Chapman 1995:192). A third theme she identified was a focus on the purported rise in overweight and/or obesity and the role of lifestyle factors in this, which in turn was strongly linked to diets high in carbohydrates and to heart disease, insulin resistance, and diabetes (Lupton and Chapman 1995: 191, 194).

As Lupton and Chapman (1995) and many others have shown, the overweight person is commonly cast as stupid and deficient, their bodily forms reviled as grotesque and linked to moral categories such as laziness, irresponsibility, greed, and a lack of willpower or self-control (see for example Crawford 1984; Schwartz 1986; Bordo 1993; Saltonstall 1993; Lupton 1995; Cossrow et al. 2001; Puhl and Heuer 2009, 2010; Link and Phelan 2001; Schwartz and Brownwell 2004). If, as I have argued here, overweight and obesity are heavily stigmatized categories that also act as powerful cultural signifiers for diabetes, what are the implications of stigmatizing lifestyle as way to combat these? How might anti-fat attitudes affect patient-provider interactions, health-seeking behavior, and timing of diagnosis and intervention amongst those deemed to be at risk from diabetes, including those like my friend, who are not overweight and understand diabetes to be caused by fatness?

Fat Prejudice and the Medical Encounter

Unlike other stigmatized practices such as smoking, alcohol consumption, or drug use, fatness is highly visible and cannot be hidden from medical encounters or from daily social interactions (see McCullough, this volume; Bell et al. 2011b). In one survey of more than three thousand people, those with a BMI of 35 or greater were more likely to experience and report interpersonal discrimination, which for many occurred on a daily basis (Carr and Friedman 2005). A number of feminist scholars have argued that in fat-averse societies, the loathing of fatness is deeply gendered and a great deal of body scrutiny is directed toward women (Orbach 1978, 1986; Millman 1980; Chernin 1981, 1986; Lawrence 1984; Spitzack 1990; Wolf 1990; MacSween 1993; Bordo 1993). As I, and others, have argued elsewhere, this is also increasingly the case for men (Bell and McNaughton 2007; Monaghan 2008). Fat prejudice is a widespread social phenomenon, and health professionals are no less fixated on weight (particularly female weight) than are other members of society (Schwartz 1986; Bordo 1993; Sobal and Maurer 1999a, Puhl and Heuer 2009). Indeed, there is considerable evidence to suggest that health care providers hold negative and prejudicial attitudes toward people who are overweight (Oberriede et al. 1995; Teachman and Brownwll 2001; Ferraro and Holland 2002; Anderson and Wadden 2004).

For example, Ferraro and Holland's (2002) study indicated that doctors were more likely to evaluate their female patients as obese even when the women did not have a body mass index greater than 30. In Joanisse and Synnott's (1999) study of obesity and stigma, female interviewees were much more likely to have experienced abuse and bullying by health professionals than were their male counterparts. They also report that women attending medical appointments for issues quite unrelated to weight (e.g.: bladder infections, a broken arm, a nose bleed) were often lectured about their body size by doctors.

In this study, a number of women also described more subtle and insidious forms of stigma and judgment on the part of both male and female doctors in the form of callous jokes and comments about their weight. For example, one respondent was told by her doctor that "fat was unattractive to men"; another was asked how many chairs she had broken in the waiting room. And when one woman complained that her new medication made her vomit, her doctor responded that at least she would lose weight (Joanisse and Synnott 1999: 57).

As Cossrow et al. (2001) have argued, health care providers in all their variety can convey a lack of empathy toward overweight patients and this further contributes to the stigmatization of this population. Puhl and Heuer (2009) have argued that health care providers, who like other professionals in positions that are perceived as more powerful or authoritarian, may exert more of an influence on the lives of the stigmatized, and as a result their prejudices may have more of an impact. Teachman and Brownell's (2001) important study shows that there is a strong, implicit bias among health professionals, including those who work directly with overweight patients and do not consciously report negative feelings or assumptions. Although the internal and external obstacles to seeking health care have been well documented for diabetes (see, for example, Chin et al. 2001), Teixeira and Budd (2010: 529) note that little is known about the influence of obesity stigma. Their central concern is that fat prejudice among health professionals maybe acting as a barrier to diabetes management.

Diagnostically, the response to the onset of TD2M or indications that it may be developing is glycemic control, via diet, weight loss, exercise, medications, or insulin. However, as van der Does (1997: 34) notes, "[I]n Type 2 diabetes, definite conclusions about the role of long-term glycaemic control in preventing complications cannot be drawn yet." Nevertheless, weight management is often a central aim of glucose control. However, if patients are not losing weight or struggling to do so, health staff may lose patience or express a lack of empathy, shaming or further stigmatizing them (Cossrow et al. 2001; Teixeira and Budd 2010). Patients may also blame themselves for their alleged failure or be made to feel responsible for their diabetes in a way that is shaming or stigmatizing.

Conversations about weight, weight loss, diet, and exercise are commonplace in health care encounters around T2DM, and several studies suggest that experiencing or expecting weight discrimination may be causing people to evade or delay health care or treatment. Teixeira and Budd (2010) suggest that the shame of not having lost weight and the fear of being reprimanded are key factors in T2DM patients postponing or avoiding follow-up visits. Peyrot et al.'s (2005) study into possible psychological barriers to diabetes care also found that many participants with T2DM felt very anxious about their weight.

Relatedly, a survey undertaken in Aotearoa-New Zealand by Simmons et al. (2007) indicated that obesity was an obstacle to patients seeking diabetes support, along with other health conditions and economic barriers. Another study by Drury and Louis (2002) indicates a direct correlation between avoidance or delay of health care with women's perceptions of weight and stigma. Although this study did not consider men's experiences, broader arguments about men, service use, and weight stigma would suggest that they, too, may be avoiding health care (Bell and McNaughton 2007; Monaghan 2008).

Teixeira and Budd (2010) argue that obesity stigma is a likely barrier to ongoing diabetes management and that health providers need to improve their sensitivity, devote more time to interactions with overweight patients, and reflect more self-critically on their own assumptions about weight and how these are being communicated to clients. They also call for health staff to employ particular counseling strategies with their obese T2DM patients that will improve disease management and reduce patients' experience of weight stigma. Of course, the assumption here is that most diabetics are overweight, and this is the focus of most studies, overlooking those who may not be overweight but are still at risk for the disease.

Conclusion: The Consequences of Stigmatizing Lifestyle

The central aim of this chapter is to demonstrate some of the ways in which a larger than average body size has come to act as a powerful cultural signifier not only of a diseased or unhealthy body, but of a diabetic body—or a body soon to be diabetic. I have argued that this is due in part to the ways in which overweight and obesity have been imagined in recent years as the central cause of T2DM— an assumption I argue that has become thoroughly naturalized in the media, academic research, popular culture, and public health campaigns. The questions then posed are what are the iatrogenic consequences of overweight and obesity as a cultural signifier for those diagnosed or deemed at risk from T2DM—something that has received very little critical examination in the extant literature.

I began by reviewing the growing body of literature demonstrating that a fat body/person provokes a range of moralistic and prejudicial attitudes from the person themselves, their families, peers, and their health care providers. I demonstrated that the fat person is framed as lacking in beauty, desirability, willpower, responsibility, discipline, and health: they are irresponsible, bad citizens, morally inferior, grotesque, and out of control (Bell et al. 2011a). Although some people may resist these messages or counter these evaluations of their persons, they are nevertheless surrounded by messages that speak to their "lifestyles," their bodies, and their selves as irresponsible failures.

As I, and others, have argued elsewhere (Bell et al. 2011a), the greatest risks to health tend to coalesce around specific (often poor) populations and particular substances and practices, notably: tobacco, alcohol, overnutrition, and illicit drugs. Said to present the greatest risks to personal health, these substances and practices are also presented as wholly preventable if individuals simply take charge of their health and their bad lifestyles and avoid smoking, drinking, drugs, and overeating (Bell et al. 2011a, 2011b).

However, this focus on lifestyle-induced risk factors can produce disturbing alignments or mergers like diabesity and the "overweight or obesity causes diabetes" linkage examined here. This turns a symptom (weight) into a causal disease agent (see Yates-Doerr, this volume). In doing so, it downplays or renders invisible the role of age and genetics, and diabetes, like overweight and obesity, comes to be seen as the result of factors within the realms of personal control (see also Burris 2008). Diabetes, like weight, is thus (re)framed as self-inflicted, as the result of risky and utterly changeable lifestyles, antithetical to a long life and to good, responsible citizenship. This reframing also places responsibility for health directly onto the individual while rendering invisible the very structural forces that create ill health in the first place. Given that T2DM can emerge in people from range of weight ranges—including those considered healthy—merging weight and diabetes in these ways will likely have ethical implications for their experience and interpretation of the symptoms of the disease as well as its prevention and diagnosis.

Although we know that diabetes occurs in people from a broad array of weight ranges, there is little research to indicate how those with or at risk from T2DM might be responding to the stigma associated with diabesity. Studies into the stigmatizing of drug users strongly indicates that stigmatizing and marginalizing people in these ways is likely to leave them alienated, anxious, and removed from the kinds of services that they might need and potentially with poor mental and physical health as a result (Krieger 2000; Mason 2001; Kvernmo and Heyerdahl 2003; Todd and Fisher 1993). It also shows that the more insidious, subtle daily expressions of discrimination provide a powerful baseline from which patients evaluate their health care experiences (Johnson et al. 2004; Browne 2003) and may discourage people from seeking support or attending follow-up visits. Many researchers have, as a result, highlighted the need to address fat prejudice as an important component to addressing barriers to care. I argue here for the need to expand this to include assumptions and readings of larger than average bodies as diseased bodies—notably as "diabese" bodies.

Notes

1. Although some authors do not use the word *fat* because of its disparaging connotations, others have argued that it needs be reclaimed, re-politicized, and revalued, and this is way it is used here.

References

ABC News. 2008. "Taskforce Chair Warns of 'Diabesity' Epidemic." Available at http://www .abc.net.au/news/stories/2008/05/28/2258241.htm, accessed May 29, 2011.

———. 2011. "Healthy Foods often Salty." Available at http://www.abc.net.au/news/video/ 2011/05/28/3229757.htm, accessed May 29, 2011.

Anderson, D.A., and T.A. Wadden. 2004. "Bariatric surgery patients' views of their physicians; weight-related attitudes and practices." *Obesity Research,* 12 (10),1587–1595.

Austin, S. B. 1999. "Fat, Loathing and Public Health: The Complicity of Science in a Culture of Disordered Eating." *Culture, Medicine and Psychiatry* 23: 245–268.

Armstrong, E. M. 2003. *Conceiving Risk, Bearing Responsibility: Fetal Alcohol Syndrome and the Diagnosis of Moral Disorder.* Baltimore: The John Hopkins University Press.

Backett, K., C. Davison, and K. Mullen. 1994. "Lay Evaluation of Health and Healthy Life-styles: Evidence from Three Studies." *British Journal of General Practice* 44: 277–280.

Bell, K., and D. McNaughton. 2007. "Feminism and the Invisible Fat Man." *Body and Society* 13, no. 1: 108–132.

Bell, K., D. McNaughton, and A. Salmon. 2009. "Medicine, Morality and Mothering: Public Health Discourses on Alcohol Exposure, Smoking around Children and Childhood Over-nutrition." *Critical Public Heath* 19, no. 2): 155–170.

———., eds. 2011a. *Alcohol, Tobacco and Obesity: Morality, Mortality and the New Public Health.* Routledge: United Kingdom.

———. 2011b. "Introduction." In *Alcohol, Tobacco and Obesity: Morality, Mortality and the New Public Health.* Routledge: United Kingdom.

Bordo, S. 1993. *Unbearable Weight: Feminism, Western Culture, and the Body.* Berkeley, Los Angeles, and London: University of California.

Brandt, A., and P. Rozin. 1997. *Morality and Health.* New York: Routledge.

Brewis, A., A. Wutich, A. Falletta-Cowden, and I. Rodriguez-Soto. 2011. "Body Norms and Fat Stigma in Global Perspective." *Current Anthropology* 52, no. 2: 269–276.

Browne, A. J. 2003. *First Nations Women and Health Care Services: The Sociopolitical Context of Encounters with Nurses.* Unpublished doctoral dissertation, University of British Columbia.

Burris, S. 2008. "Stigma, Ethics and Policy: A Commentary on Bayer's 'Stigma and the Ethics of Public Health: Not Can We But Should We.'" *Social Science and Medicine* 67: 473–475.

Campos, P. 2004. *The Obesity Myth: Why Our Obsession with Weight is Hazardous to Our Health.* London: Penguin.

————. 2008. "A 10,000 Obesity Challenge." *Rocky Mountain News,* available at http://www .rockymountainnews.com/news/2008/may/20/campos-a-10000-obesity-challenge/, accessed July 24, 2008.

Campos, P., A. Saguy, P. Ernsberger, E. Oliver, and G. Gaesser. 2006. "The Epidemiology of Overweight and Obesity: Public Health Crisis or Moral Panic?" *International Journal of Epidemiology* 35: 55–60.

Carr, D., and M. Friedman. 2005. "Is Obesity Stigmatizing? Body Weight, Perceived Discrimination, and Psychological Well-being in the United States." *Journal of Health and Social Behavior* 46: 244–259.

Chernin, K. 1981. *The Obsession: Reflections on the Tyranny of Slenderness.* New York: Harper.

————. 1986. *The Hungry Self: Women, Eating and Identity.* New York: Random House.

Chin, M. H., S. Cook, L. Jin, M. L. Drum, J. F. Harrison, and J. Koppert. 2001. "Barriers to Providing Diabetes Care in Community Health Centers." *Diabetes Care* 24, no. 2: 268–274.

Cohen, S. 1972. *Folk Devils and Moral Panics.* London: Routledge.

Commonwealth of Australia. 1999. "Diabesity & Associated Disorders in Australia—2000: The Accelerating Epidemic." In *National Diabetes Strategy 2000–2004,* Canberra: Commonwealth Department of Health and Aged Care.

Cossrow, N. H., R. W. Jeffery, and M. T. McQuire. 2001. "Understanding Weight Stigmatization: A Focus Group Study." *Journal of Nutrition Education* 33, no. 4: 208–214.

Crawford, R. 1984. "A Cultural Account of 'Health': Control, Release, and the Social Body." In *Issues in the Political Economy of Health Care,* ed. J. B. McKinlay. New York: Tavistock, 60–103.

————. 1994. "The Boundaries of the Self and the Unhealthy Other: Reflections on Health, Culture and AIDS." *Social Science and Medicine* 10: 1347–1365.

Daykin, N., and J. Naidoo. 1995. "Feminist Critiques of Health Promotion." In *The Sociology of Health Promotion: Critical Analyses of Consumption, Lifestyle and Risk,* ed. R. Bunton, S. Nettleton, and S. Burrows. London: Routledge, 59–69.

Davison, C., G. Davey Smith, and S. Frankel. 1991. "Lay Epidemiology and the Prevention Paradox: The Implications of Coronary Candidacy for Health Education." *Sociology of Health and Illness* 13: 1–19.

Davison, C., S. Frankel, and G. Davey Smith. 1992. "The Limits of Lifestyle: Re-assessing 'Fatalism' in the Popular Culture of Illness Prevention." *Social Science and Medicine* 34: 675–685.

Drury, C. A., and M. Louis. 2002. "Exploring the Association between Bodyweight, Stigma of Obesity, and Health Care Avoidance." *Journal of the American Academy of Nurse Practitioners* 14, no. 12: 554–561.

Evans Braziel, J., and K. LeBesco, eds. 2001. *Bodies Out of Bounds: Fatness and Transgression.* Berkeley: University of California Press.

Ferraro, K. F., and K. B. Holland. 2002. "Physician Evaluation of Obesity in Health Surveys: 'Who Are You Calling Fat?'" *Social Science and Medicine* 55: 1401–1413.

Gard, M. 2010. *The End of the Obesity Epidemic.* London: Routledge.

Gard, M., and J. Wright. 2004. *The Obesity Epidemic: Science, Morality and Ideology.* London: Routledge.

Goffman, E. 1963. *Stigma: Notes on the Management of Spoiled Identity.* Englewood Cliffs, NJ: Prentice-Hall.

Joanisse, L., and A. Synnott. 1999. "Fighting Back: Reactions and Resistance to the Stigma of Obesity." In *Interpreting Weight: The Social Management of Fatness and Thinness*, ed. J. Sobal and D. Maurer. New York: Aldine de Gruyter, 49–72.

Johnson, J. L., J. L. Bottorff, A. J. Browne, et al. 2004. "Othering and Being Othered in the Context of Health Care Services." *Health Communication* 16, no. 2: 255–271.

Kaufmann, F. R. 2005a. *Diabesity: A Doctor and Her Patients on the Front Lines of the Obesity-Diabetes Epidemic*. New York: Bantam.

———. 2005b. *Diabesity: The Obesity-Diabetes Epidemic that Threatens America–and What We Must Do to Stop It*. New York: Bantam.

Klein, R. 1996. *Eat Fat*. New York: Pantheon.

Krieger, N. 1994. "Epidemiology and the Web of Causation: Has Anyone Seen the Spider?" *Social Science and Medicine* 39, no. 7, 887–903.

———. 2000. "Refiguring 'Race': Epidemiology, Racialized Biology, and Biological Expressions of Race Relations." *International Journal of Health Services* 30, no. 1: 211–215.

Kulick, D., and A. Meneley, eds. 2005. *Fat: The Anthropology of an Obsession*. New York: Jeremy P. Tarcher/Penguin.

Kvernmo, S., and S. Heyerdahl. 2003. "Acculturation Strategies and Ethnic Identity as Predictors of Behavior Problems in Arctic Minority Adolescents." *Journal of the American Academy of Child and Adolescent Psychiatry* 42, no. 1: 57–65.

Lawrence, M. 1984. *The Anorexic Experience*. London: Woman's Press.

LeBesco, K. 2004. *Revolting Bodies? The Struggle to Redefine Fat Identity*. Amherst, Boston: University of Massachusetts Press.

Libman, K., and N. Freudenberg. 2007. *Reversing the Diabetes and Obesity Epidemics in New York City: A Call to Action to Confront a Public Health, Economic and Moral Threat to New York City's Future*. City University of New York Campaign Against Diabetes.

Link, B. G., and J. C. Phelan. 2001. "Conceptualizing Stigma." *Annual Review of Sociology* 27: 363–385.

Lupton, D. 1995. *The Imperative of Health: Public Health and the Regulated Body*. United Kingdom: Sage Publications.

———. 2004. "'A Grim Health Future': Food Risks in the Sydney Press." *Health, Risk, and Society* 6, no. 2: 187–200.

Lupton, D., and S. Chapman. 1995. "'A Healthy Lifestyle Might be the Death of You': Discourses on Diet, Cholesterol Control and Heart Disease in the Press and among the Lay Public." *Sociology of Health and Illness* 17: 477–494.

MacSween, M. 1993. *Anorexic Bodies: A Feminist and Sociological Perspective on Anorexia Nervosa*. London: Routledge.

Mason, T., ed. 2001. *Stigma and Social Exclusion in Healthcare*. London: Routledge.

McNaughton, D. (2013) 'Diabesity' Down Under: Overweight and obesity as cultural signifiers for Type 2 Diabetes Mellitus, Critical Public Health (10.1080/09581596.2013.766671)

McNaughton, D. 2011. "From the Womb to the Tomb: Obesity and Maternal Responsibility." *Critical Public Health* 21, no. 2: 179–190.

Millman, M. 1980. *Such a Pretty Face: Being Fat in America*. New York: W.W. Norton.

Monaghan, L. 2008. *Men and the War on Obesity: A Sociological Study*. London: Routledge.

Murray, S. 2008. Pathologising 'fatness': Medical authority and popular culture. *Sociology of Sport Journal*, 1: 7–21.

Nichter, M. 2000. *Fat Talk: What Girls and their Parents Say about Dieting.* Cambridge, MA: Harvard University Press.

Oberrieder, J., R. Walker, D. Monroe, and M. Adeyanju. 1995. "Attitude of Dietetics Students and Registered Dietitians toward Obesity." *Journal of the American Dietetic Association* 95, no. 8: 914–916.

Orbach, S. 1978. *Fat is a Feminist Issue.* New York: Berkeley.

———. 1986. *Hunger Strike.* London: Faber and Faber.

Petersen, A. 1997. "Risk, Governance, and the New Public Health." In *Foucault, Health and Medicine,* ed. A. Petersen and R. Bunton. London: Routledge, 189–206.

Petersen, A., and R. Bunton, eds. 1997. *Foucault, Health and Medicine.* London: Routledge.

Petersen, A., and D. Lupton. 1997. *The New Public Health: Health and Self in the Age of Risk.* United Kingdom: Sage Publications.

Petersen, A., M. Davis, S. Frazer, and J. Lindsay. 2010. "Healthy Living and Citizenship: An Overview." *Critical Public Health* 20, no. 4: 391–400.

Peyrot, M., J. F. McMurry Jr., and D. F. Kruger. 1999. A Biopsychosocial Model of Glycemic Control in Diabetes: Stress, Coping and Regimen Adherence. *Journal of Health and Social Behavior,* 40 (2), 141–158.

Probyn, E. 2000. *Carnal Appetites: FoodSexIdentities.* London: Routledge.

Puhl, R. M., and C. A. Heuer. 2009. "The Stigma of Obesity: A Review and Update." *Obesity* 17, no. 5: 941–946.

———. 2010. "Obesity Stigma: Important Considerations for Public Health." *American Journal of Public Health* 100, no. 6: 1019–1028.

Rolland-Cachera, M. F., and F. Bellisle. 2002. "Nutrition." In *Child and Adolescent Obesity: Causes and Consequences, Prevention and Management.* ed. W. Burniat et al. Cambridge: Cambridge University Press, 69–86.

Saguy, A. C., and K. W. Riley. 2005. "Weighing Both Sides: Morality, Mortality, and Framing Contests over Obesity." *Journal of Health Politics* 5: 869–921.

Saltonstall, R. 1993. "Healthy Bodies, Social Bodies: Men's and Women's Concepts and Practices of Health in Everyday Life." *Social Science and Medicine* 36: 7–14.

Schwartz, H. 1986. *Never Satisfied: A Cultural History of Diets, Fantasies and Fat.* New York: Doubleday.

Schwartz, M. B., and K. D. Brownell. 2004. "Obesity and Body Image." *Body Image* 1, no. 1: 43–56.

Simmons, D., S. Lillis, J. Swan, and J. Haar. 2007. "Discordance in Perceptions of Barriers to Diabetes Care between Patients and Primary Care and Secondary Care." *Diabetes Care* 30, no. 3: 490–495.

Sobal, J., and D. Maurer, eds. 1999a. *Weighty Issues: Fatness and Thinness as Social Problems.* New York: Aldine De Gruyter.

———. 1999b. *Interpreting Weight: The Social Management of Fatness and Thinness.* New York: Aldine De Gruyter.

Spitzack, C. 1990. *Confessing Excess: Women and the Politics of Body Reduction.* New York: State University of New York Press.

Stearns, P. 1997. *Fat History: Bodies and Beauty in the Modern West.* New York: NYU Press.

Stinson, K. 2001. *Women and Dieting Culture: Inside a Commercial Weight Loss Group.* New Brunswick, NJ: Rutgers University Press.

Stunkard, A. J., and T. I. Sorensen. 1993. "Obesity and Socioeconomic Status—A Complex Relation." *New England Journal of Medicine* 329, no. 14: 1036–1037.

Teachman, B. A., and K. D. Brownell. 2001. "Implicit Anti-fat Bias among Health Professionals: Is Anyone Immune?" *International Journal of Obesity* 25: 1525–1531.

Teixeira, M. E, and G. M. Budd. 2010. "Obesity Stigma: A Newly Recognized Barrier to Comprehensive and Effective Type 2 Diabetes Management." *Journal of the American Academy of Nurse Practitioners* 22: 527–533.

Todd, A. D., and S. Fisher, eds. 1993. *The Social Organization of Doctor-Patient Communication*. Norwood, NJ: Ablex Publishers.

Van der Does, J. 1997. *Influence of Glycaemic Control on Well-Being and Cardiovascular Risk Indicators in Type 2 Diabetes: A Randomized Trial in General Practice*. Vrije Universiteit: Netherlands.

Watson, J. M. 1993. "Male Body Image and Health Beliefs: A Qualitative Study and Implications for Health Promotion Practice." *Health Education Journal* 52: 246–252.

WHO (World Health Organization). 1999 *Definition, Diagnosis and Classification of Diabetes Mellitus and its Complication, Report of a WHO Consultation, Part 1: Diagnosis and Classification of Diabetes Mellitus*. Department of Noncommunicable Disease Surveillances. Geneva: World Health Organization.

———. 2011. The Global Status Report on Noncommunicable Diseases 2010: Description of the global burden of NCDs, their risk factors and determinants. Geneva: World Health Organization.

Wolf, N. 1990. *The Beauty Myth: How Images of Beauty are Used against Women*. London: Vintage.

✛ ✛ ✛

PART

II

Large Embodiment and Histories of Fat

CHAPTER 4

Obesity in Cuba

Memories of the Special Period and Approaches to Weight Loss Today

Hanna Garth

✛ ✛ ✛

In this chapter I analyze the role of memories of food scarcity and the psycho-social effects of nationalized food provisioning, which includes food rationing and state-subsidized food sales, on present day efforts to reduce obesity through dieting. My objective is to consider the impact of memories of food scarcity during Cuba's Special Period, a period of economic hardship that I elaborate further below, on the rising rates of obesity in Cuba as well as current efforts to control body weight. My analytic focus is on the role that memories of earlier crises play in coping with difficult situations in the present (Bruner 1990; Garro 2000; Sutton 2001), specifically the ways in which memories of food scarcity affect dieting during periods of abundance after scarcity ends (cf. Franco et al. 2007). Research has shown that the psychological effects of chronic restriction can dramatically affect consumption behavior even when restrictions, whether cognitive or economic, are lifted (cf. Birch and Davidson 2005; Fisher and Birch 1999; Polivy 1996).

The data analyzed here are part of a larger project based on sixteen months of fieldwork conducted between 2008 and 2011, which includes over 100 interviews with people living in Santiago de Cuba ranging in age from nineteen to ninety-five years old. In the larger project, I examined how household members use the current food system and, in turn, how the tactics employed to acquire food strain, shift, and strengthen social relationships, thus affecting household and community social dynamics. As a part of this broader research project, data were systematically collected on memories and perceptions of Santiago's changing food system. For this chapter I draw on eight interviews with individuals ranging in age from twenty-seven to sixty-two years old, which are representative of general themes related to food consumption, dieting, and exercise in Santiago today.

These data indicate that despite the difficulties of food acquisition, obesity linked to food consumption and sedentarism has been a national concern for several decades. Obesity reduction today is complicated by the current food rationing system and memories of food scarcity that lead Santiagueros (people living in the city of Santiago de Cuba) to take advantage of the presence of sweets and high-fat foods to vary their food consumption and please the palate. In contrast to dieting, exercise is associated with healthy living practices and stress reduction and does not appear to have a strong connection to memories of the Special Period when increased physical activity was obligatory due to decreased availability of transportation.

This work focuses on Cuba's second-largest city, Santiago, which is located in the southeastern part of the island. Though Santiago de Cuba is an urban center with a population of approximately 500,000 people, Santiagueros often self-identify as *guajiros,* or peasants. In this chapter, specific attention is given to participants whose reflections on food memories, exercise, and the body are particularly useful for understanding local concepts of obesity and weight loss (see Trainer and Hardin, this volume). My analysis deepens an earlier work on food scarcity and memory in Santiago de Cuba (Garth 2009). The ways in which people remember and express memories of the past can reveal important aspects of their social lives. The analysis of salient memories reveals significant emotions about what might be taken for granted as everyday banal food consumption practices. The eating associated with previous periods of scarcity may be characterized as a form of binge eating tied up with emotional, personal, and socially relevant issues (see Becker, this volume).

The Cuban Food System

To analyze the interrelationship between obesity and diet in Cuba today, it is important first to understand the local food system. Cuba's food rationing system was officially established on March 12, 1962; it is referred to locally as *la libreta,* a reference to the ration cards administered to all Cubans for the purchase of basic food items. In the early 1960s, the need for the rationing system emerged because of an increase in demand for food due to increased purchasing power and decreases in domestic food production resulting from the shift toward state ownership of farmland and food production enterprises (Alvarez 2004).[1] The rations were initiated during Cuba's transition to socialism to ensure that the population had access to basic food staples at affordable prices. As its long history of rationing illustrates, Cuba's current food system was borne of a complex history of strained economic periods and the need to innovate solutions in the face of deficient international trade relationships.

The foods provided in the ration have changed over time as the needs of the population have changed. Prices are still very heavily subsidized, but households must still pay a small amount for the rationed food. The rations are distributed at what Cubans call *bodegas, placitas/puestos,* and *carnicerias.*[2] During the course of my research in Santiago the items available in the ration slowly changed. The monthly ration per person included: 5 pounds of white rice, 10 ounces of beans, 3 pounds refined sugar, 1 pound raw sugar, 1 kg of salt, 4 ounces of coffee, 250 ml of oil, and a roll of bread per day.[3] Meat products include 6 ounces of chicken, 11 ounces of fish, 10 eggs, and 8 ounces of ground meat mixed with soy.[4] If there is a national shortage at any given time, some of these meat products are substituted with pork-based sausages and processed meats or extra chicken. All of these items together cost about 25 national pesos a month, or about $1.00 (U.S.).

This ration is essential for making ends meet in most Santiago households, yet complaints about insufficient food in the monthly ration are widespread in Cuba (Gjelten 2008). Although the rations are the most common and important way that Santiagueros acquire food, all of the people I interviewed within the larger sample claimed that no one would be able to survive on rations alone. Most participants stated that the food provided in the ration only lasted from one to two weeks rather than the full month. Santiagueros supplement their monthly food rations in several other ways, listed here in order of importance: peso purchases, CUC shoppin,[5] black market purchases, informal trades, self-production, and gifts.

Despite this daily struggle to acquire food, obesity linked to food consumption and sedentarism has been a national concern for several decades (Garth 2009). Historically, Cubans have maintained high caloric diets based heavily on high-fat and high-sugar foods. Already in the mid 1980s, "Cuba's preventive attention [was] increasingly concentrated on heart disease, cancer, and stroke. Risk factors related to diet, smoking, obesity, sedentarism, and occupational accidents contributed to Cuba's 'double burden of health risks': those related to underdevelopment in rural areas and those associated with development in urban areas" (Guttmacher 1987: 179).[6] As Sarah Trainer discusses in this volume, similar trends are occurring across the globe.

Through Cuba's Medicine in the Community Program implemented in 1976, national campaigns promoted healthy lifestyles and "included community participation as a cornerstone of the health system's strategy to combat problems such as sedentarism, obesity, and smoking" (Barberia and Castro 2003: A23). Citizen participation in maintaining a healthy lifestyle was encouraged by state institutions and public service announcements. Organizations like the Casas de Abuelos (Seniors Day Care) initiated campaigns against sedentarism, smoking,[7] and obesity (Barberia and Castro 2003). McCullough's discussion (see McCullough, this volume) that draws on Saguy and Alemling (2008) focuses on the individualization of a social problem resulting in blaming the individual. In contrast, much of the literature on Cuba focuses on the role of the state, which has made strong efforts to look at systemic causes and developed subsequent prevention programs at the national level. Between 1972 and 1993, the prevalence of chronic malnutrition fell to 32.6 percent, acute malnutrition was reduced by 69.2 percent; malnutrition of all types decreased by 44.4 percent; and overweight fell 48.5 percent (Esquivel et al. 1997).[8] That is, whereas obesity has historically been a problem in Cuba throughout the 1970s and 1980s, due to both economic factors and state prevention efforts, overweight prevalence was cut in half from the early 1970s to the early 1990s. After the economic crisis of the 1990s after the collapse of the Soviet Union, obesity and overweight have reemerged as significant public health and social problems in Cuba. Along with government programs to combat obesity, social constructions perpetuated by audiovisual and print media used both for public health campaigns and for entertainment designate lean bodies as preferential in Cuba today (see Rubin and Joseph, this volume).

As Campos et al. (2006) illustrate, social constructs and medical discourses frame overweight or obese bodies as unhealthy and undesirable. At the same time, extremely thin bodies are not favored either; in Cuba as in other parts of the world, thin bodies are seen as aesthetically displeasing, potentially diseased, and indicative of weak social networks or family problems (cf. Becker 1995; Pollock 1995). Visible attributes of the physical body are often seen as a representation of control conflated with morality, responsibility, and respectability (Crawford 1984). Fit or thin bodies are usually associated with control; the assumption is that individuals with slim bodies are aware and in control of what they take into their bodies. Eating therefore becomes a deliberate action with the result of a slim, under-control body (see McCullough, this volume). As such, in many parts of the world overweight and obese bodies are often linked to a lack of control (Lester 1997; Sobo 2000). However, as I will elaborate below in the case of Cuba today after a decade of food scarcity the link between obesity, concepts of healthy bodies, and how one maintains control over the body must be problematized; indeed for some Cubans maintaining extra body fat is seen as a form of control and a physical protection against potential future food insecurity. In Santiago, memories of food scarcity position ideal body size within the margins of too fat and too thin, or as one participant put it, "Not fat but wrapped in meat" (*No gorda pero envuelta en carne*).

The Special Period

Following the collapse of the Soviet Union beginning in the late 1980s, Cuba suffered its most recent period of acute economic hardship, known as the Special Period in Time of Peace. The Soviet collapse was so devastating for Cuba not only due to heavy reliance upon the USSR as a trade partner, but also due to the subsidized price for petroleum, free armaments, and low-interest development loans that Soviet support for Cuba entailed (Dominguez 2005: 12). During the period of Soviet financial and material aid, there was an abundance of cheap imported food products and other goods that were accessible even to poor Cubans. The Special Period brought an end to these cheap imports and triggered food scarcity. From 1989 to 1992, imports were cut by 73 percent from $8.1 billion to $2.2 billion (Preeg 1993; Roca 1977). With the drastic reduction of oil, fertilizer, and pesticide imports from the Soviet Union, the agricultural crisis gave rise to a food emergency. For instance, the bread ration was cut by 20 percent in Havana to 3 ounces daily and the bread price was raised by 30 percent outside of Havana (Chaplowe 1996).

In the 1990s, "caloric intake fell by 27 percent between 1990 and 1996" (Dominguez 2005: 14). In late 1993 the average daily caloric intake[9] dropped from 2,865 calories to 1,863 (Languepin 1999).[10] During these years many food products became scarce and those that were available were difficult for average Cubans to access due to their increased prices.[11] Due to these scarcities of the early 1990s and the creation of the dual-currency system,[12] "12 percent of urban Cubans earned less than 100 pesos per month (less than $5 per month at the prevailing exchange rate), had no access to dollars, grew no food and received no food subsidies" (Dominguez 2005: 15).[13] Nevertheless, during the worst of the Special Period in 1993, overweight was still the most common type of malnutrition in Cuba, with a prevalence of 5.2 percent (Esquivel et al. 1997). Although food access became more difficult, even during a period of economic crisis, rates of hunger and protein-energy malnutrition did not surpass rates of obesity. Nonetheless, experiences of food scarcity and difficulty accessing food during Cuba's Special Period influence present day approaches to weight loss through dieting and exercise.

After the Special Period

It has been nineteen years since the worst of the Special Period, and over time food accessibility has improved throughout the island (cf. Chaplowe 1996; Dominguez 2005; Isreal 2008; Koont 2004; Murphy 1999; Premat 1998; Stricker 2007). With the legalization of the dollar and the subsequent creation of hard currently, the Convertible Cuban peso (CUC), the opening of Cuba to tourism, increasing joint ventures with foreign companies, and the opening of small-scale enterprise, the shortages of the Special Period slowly faded. As such, especially from the perspective of people in their twenties, who do not remember Cuba before the 1990s, the availability of food items and other material goods has slowly increased across the island.[14]

For those who do remember Cuba before the 1990s, previous restrictions in food supply have several long-term consequences. Long periods of food restrictions can dramatically affect consumption practices when foods become more available. In developed and underdeveloped countries alike, some of the noted psychological consequences of deprivation included obsessions with food, preoccupation with eating for longer periods of time, binge eating, and significant increases in introversion, irritability, anxiety, anger, and depression (Alaimo 2005). Nutrition studies suggest that food deprivation in childhood has the potential to induce binge eating behavior and overweightness when food is readily available later in life (Fisher and Birch 1999). Overweightness has been shown to occur in response to mild or moderate levels of food insecurity even when past food restriction was only temporary (Frongillo et al. 2007). Such factors impact present day food consumption and weight loss practices in Santiago, both for younger generations and for those who remember before the Special Period but live with memories of food scarcity.

Memories of Food Scarcity

Memories of food scarcity during Cuba's Special Period still haunt many Santiagueros today. In my fieldwork, people in Santiago de Cuba have diverse ways of explicitly linking their own food consumption behaviors with their memories of the Special Period. For example, toward the end of an hour-long interview forty-year-old Mickey[15] explained to me that[16]:

> In those years [before the 1990s] the people were, they were…were… it's like— in Cuba, there is this saying: God was in the land, in the Cuban soil. Before, people had better hearts, they were more human … the Special Period started to change the character of the Cuban people, a change of disposition. Many people transformed and started to do things, things I don't view as right, like stealing or not sharing food with their own family members. And, well, really the mind of the Cuban has suffered a lot over these things, because of the scarcities. Yes, so the Cuban way of being changed a lot because of the shortages of goods, things became scarce until everything was gone, everything, to the point where even a leaf from a tree had a value. Like the other day we were talking about, that many people shrunk—they got smaller—their body size. I am talking about a lot of people who came to lose like 30, 40 pounds—40 pounds without any money, without anything. It was a very critical situation, it was seriously severe.

"So," he said, turning to the huge plate of rice and beans in front of him, "that is why I need to eat so much right now. I am working on having a big belly, so that in case there is another Special Period I will have an extra 40 pounds to lose," and he laughed as he began to shovel food into his mouth. Enacting the very practices that he had just reflected on in the interview, Mickey engaged in a controlled attempt to overeat.

Mickey's decision to overeat in an attempt to gain weight shows that over-weightness is not just a matter of out-of-control eating, but rather requires important considerations of economic decision making, historical conditions, and psychosocial stress. Mickey is a self-identified black[17] man from in Santiago de Cuba, and in this powerful statement he references his own memories of Cuba's Special Period and the effects of those memories on his present day actions. Mickey not only relates Cuban food to his identity, but he also makes explicit reference to the relationship between the food he eats and his own body. In particular, he states his awareness of using food and his own agency over it to control his body size, a response to his memories of a time when people were even more powerless with respect to food access. Mickey's memories of the past instill in him a sense of fear or insecurity about the future, which he responds to by vigilantly controlling his food intake to gain weight. His jovial demeanor and humorous response to his interview on this topic illuminate both his joy in succeeding to overeat and that he feels that it is somewhat strange to be trying to gain weight in this way. As Jessica Hardin discusses in the case of Samoa (this volume), food consumption and obesity today is seen by some as a sign of power and control over the body, social connectedness, and financial success. In the Cuban case, rather than linking obesity to the morality of individuals, obesity and the diseased body are usually considered a problem of national political economy. Indeed, as I show later in this chapter, some Santiagueros view obesity and excess consumption as a sign of lack of access to food in abundance that forces them to "take advantage" (*aprovechar*) of whatever foods "appear" (*lo que aparece*), whether they are healthy foods or not.

In contrast to Mickey, Tomas, a sixty-two-year-old white university professor from Santiago de Cuba, connects his current thin frame and what he considers poor eating habits with the practices he developed in the 1990s. After several months of observing how little he eats, one day I explicitly asked Tomas about his daily food intake. He paused and responded with a memory of the Special Period:

> I remember one day my sons—they were eight and eleven—came home from school hungry for lunch and there was absolutely nothing to give them. Nothing. So we went to the corner where they were selling shaved ice with syrup and that was what we all had for lunch. Nothing more than sugar water. The Special Period was hard, very hard. [...] After living through those years we just stopped really eating. For example, we used to sit down to lunch in my family, I mean in the 1970s and 1980s, we actually ate like you are supposed to. Now we have lost that. I basically just drink soft drinks and eat little sandwiches and

sweets, and my wife and son are the same way. I know I am unhealthy and too thin. I am probably malnourished and my eating habits are probably the cause of my gallbladder problems. But after those years we just never returned to the table. It's like we are afraid to go back because it might disappear again.

Tomas' understanding of how past food scarcities changed his present day food habits are based in what he views as the loss of the tradition of eating a proper meal seated at a table as a family—what he refers to as "really eating." Unlike Mickey, Tomas is more relaxed about his ability to control his body through his eating. Although he believes that his poor eating habits may be the cause of illness, he does not change because of a latent fear that if he returns to his old eating practices he may again suffer the trauma of food scarcity. Although it is certainly true that a number of sociocultural, political, and economic factors influence changes in food consumption practices, it is important that for both of these participants the years of food scarcity of the 1990s were a critical turning point in their food consumption practices. These interviews indicate that despite their class and skin color differences, Mickey and Tomas appear to have had similar experiences of food scarcity during the Special Period, similar increased access to food today, and similar feelings of fear and insecurity about the future. Although Tomas's case does not concern issues related to obesity and dieting, these two cases illustrate that individuals react differently to memories of food scarcity; it is not clear or predictable how people will cope with memories of food scarcity once access increases again.

Dieting in the Shadow of the Special Period

The Special Period in Cuba was extremely difficult for many families across the island, especially with respect to food. Individuals react differently to memories of food scarcity. The restriction of food intake is complicated by the fact that many people are uncertain that certain food items will remain available given past shortages. For example, during an interview in 2011, Yaicel, a twenty-seven-year-old black-identified Santiaguera, explained to me her approach to weight loss.

> Hanna: I heard you mention that you want to lose weight…
>
> Yaicel: Look, let me tell you, I am a dancer. If I want to be treated seriously and to one day be part of a professional group I have to maintain my body. You know that, as a dancer, I have to train every day. I dance for two or three hours a day, which you know is exercise and it's not easy; it's hard work. I am there sweating and panting for two or three hours a day. But I don't lose weight, since I had the second baby I just can't seem to lose weight. It's here [grabs her stomach] that has me crazy, I want to lose this belly.

Hanna: Apart from the dancing have you tried changing what you eat?

Yaicel: Well, this is complicated. I have to eat and there are certain things like sometimes there is not enough rice so we have to eat pasta and you know that pasta makes you fat. But if there is nothing else we have to eat it. And for example when the chicken arrives at the ration station we have to eat it because you don't know if chicken will arrive again.

Hanna: What about things like sweets and ice cream?

Yaicel: Ice Cream! Why wouldn't I eat ice cream? It has calcium and vitamins that I need. It's like with sweets you have to eat them when they are around because you don't know if there will be more later. Like a few summers ago there was no ice cream, there was some problem and there was no ice cream in the city. I have to take advantage of it when it's here because you never know when it will disappear.

Yaicel is explicit about the complications of food restriction under Cuba's food rationing system, using chicken as an example she notes that she has to take advantage of the food that is offered in the ration both because of its low cost and her uncertainty of when it will arrive again. Like Yaicel, Maria Julia, a forty-five-year-old white women who is relatively well off and lives in the city center, practices her own form of dieting that involves taking advantage of what "appears," but unlike Yaicel, Maria Julia later cuts her calories.

Hanna: Why did you start dieting?

Maria Julia: Well it's a long story but basically I got really fat after my divorce because I started drinking and overeating. One day I was crying and feeling awful about my divorce and I just realized that I had to stop, that I was still young and I could find another man and be happy. So [my current boyfriend] was already expressing interest in me but I didn't pay attention to him. First I stopped drinking and I lost about 3 k [6.6 pounds] but I still had a big belly so I started to think more about what I was eating. I basically stopped eating for the sake of eating. Like if there was nothing interesting to eat if it was just rice and beans I wouldn't eat, but if there was something good like chicken or beef or some sweets I would eat and then later not eat. I would take advantage of what appeared but then not continue eating what was just always around. Until today, after I lost the weight, now I eat whatever I want all day long—sweets, soda, pasta—whatever appears, but I don't eat anything at night. Maybe I will have a bit of salad or a boiled egg, but more than that never. And like this I have maintained a lower weight and I have my boyfriend. I am happy again.

Carlos, a sixty-five-year-old Mestizo-identified Santiaguero who lives in the city center and works as a Spiritual consultant, started to lose weight through dieting when he was diagnosed with diabetes in late 2009. When he was first diagnosed he weighed 230 pounds, and over the course of a year and a half he has reduced his weight to 180 pounds. Carlos has always exercised; he takes exercise classes three days a week, and walks approximately 3 miles a day because his work requires that he go to his clients' homes. He believes that he lost most of his weight not from exercise but from modifications in his diet.

> When I was diagnosed with diabetes I had to stop eating whatever I wanted and start having control over my diet. I used to just eat whatever I wanted, like I would stop and eat a pizza or a sandwich from the food carts whenever I wanted. Then I would go to my clients' houses and they would offer me cakes or sandwiches or whatever and I would eat it—why not!? It was part of my payment, really, for my work. But I had to stop; now I explain that I am diabetic and it's very serious. I could get a leg amputated or go blind if I don't take control, so I have to tell them no. And it has worked I have lost 50 pounds just from controlling what I eat. I eat breakfast, lunch, and a small dinner at home and never at someone else's house, and I have lost weight because I know what I am eating.

As the examples of Yaicel and Maria Julia demonstrate, memories of food scarcity lead people to "take advantage of" (aprovechar) the availability of whatever foods "appear" (lo que aparece) because they are uncertain that these items will remain available given past shortages. For Yaicel, it is important to both take advantage of what appears, like in the case of ice cream and other sweets, and to conform her tastes to what is available, as in the case of the chicken ration. "Taking advantage" (*aprovechando*) and conforming to what is available were very important during the Special Period. Given the increasing availability of nutrients and calories, this practice of "taking advantage" (aprovechando) of what is now available is one factor among many that has led to increasing levels of obesity on the island. The resulting weight gain in turn leads to dissatisfaction with body shape and size. People turn to various types of practices to rectify the situation, to change the shapes of their bodies through diet, exercise, or some combination of practices; however, as I elaborate further below, there are certain foods that many people are not willing to give up for the sake of weight loss despite body dissatisfaction.

I found that among my research participants who expressed a desire to lose weight, many shared with Yaicel and Maria Julia views that there were certain high-fat or high-sugar foods that they simply could not give up as part of their efforts to lose weight. I believe that their desires to continue consuming such foods is deeply tied to their memories of food scarcity and fears of future food scarcities that might prevent their access to such foods. Sometimes efforts to reduce the quantity of food consumed were pursued; if this was the case it was often in a manner similar to how Maria Julia approaches caloric restriction during the evening meal. Others would try to reduce proportions of food throughout the day. As Yaicel and Maria Julia express, the possibility of food scarcity and clear memories of the experience of deprivation lead such dieters to continue eating foods that they feel they must take advantage of despite high caloric content. Very few research participants shared memories of hunger or malnutrition; rather, they focused on the scarcity of particular foods and the difficulty of acquiring the foods that they wanted during the years of the Special Period.

Carlos, in contrast, has been able to reduce his consumption of sweets and high-fat foods. Carlos's diabetes diagnosis helps motivate him to resist the temptations to eat whatever he wants and to respectfully decline snacks he is offered when he visits his clients' homes. I interpret Carlos's dietary practices as a shift from living to eat, to eating to live. Like Mickey he asserts his own agency over his food consumption by no longer eating whatever seems appetizing in the moment, but by maintaining a rigid balanced eating plan, preparing all of his own meals, and eating them at home so that he knows exactly what goes into the food that he consumes.

Raulnelis is a forty-one-year-old Santiaguero who ethnically identifies as *Chino*.[18] My conversation with Raulnelis eventually led to the topic of gender, and he shared that from his perspective the obesity problem in Cuba was more concentrated in women. I asked him to explain further:

> Raulnelis: Well obesity [in Cuba] seems to be concentrated in women over thirty, or better said women who have already had their children. Why exactly I don't really know, but I suspect that it's both biological and social. Women's metabolism changes at this age, but also since most women in Cuba dedicate themselves to their children and running their households once the kids go to school they become more sedentary. After they make the meals and clean the house they relax, watch novellas, talk to each other and that is when they start to gain weight [*aumentar grasa*].
>
> Hanna: Why aren't men gaining weight?
>
> Raulnelis: Because they are out in the street working.
>
> Hanna: And if they are out of work like yourself?
>
> Raulnelis: Well, really most men in Cuba are never without work. They might have lost their jobs but then they go out in the street and invent something. They have to earn money. They might sell things or hustle something or they are at the employment office waiting in line, but they aren't sitting around watching novellas.

Raulnelis introduces an important perspective on the gendered aspects of obesity and weight loss. As noted above, rates of obesity and overweight appear to be relatively equal in men and women in Cuba. As Raulnelis points out, the gendered division of labor in Cuba is such that women are more likely to attend to household needs and child rearing, whereas men are more likely to work outside the home (cf. Garth 2010; Pertierra 2008). Similar to what Galloway and Moffet discuss in this volume, drawing on Counihan (1992), Raulnelis here reifies gendered notions of labor and consumption, with an underlying ideological position that values thinness and self-control as well as labor outside the home.

Conclusions

Although none of the research participants explicitly mentioned it, Cuba's food rationing system has been central in defining Cubans' relationships with food and is particularly important to understanding obesity and food consumption in Cuba. For nearly half a century the majority of Cubans have mainly had access to the basic foods provided in ration, nearly everyone eats the same foods, and cuisine varies little from week to week. Based on my observations, the lack of variety in everyday food is one factor that leads Santiagueros to seek variety through snacking and eating street foods. Consistent with this hypothesis, most of the research participants presented in this chapter expressed that they did not limit consumption of sweets and high-fat foods as part of weight loss efforts. Indeed they feel that they need to take "advantage of them" when they were around for dietary variety and for fear of food scarcities. The food rationing system and memories of food scarcity are factors that lead Santiagueros to take advantage of sweets and high-fat foods to vary their food consumption and please the palate.

As the interviews with Tomas and Mickey illustrate, individuals react differently to memories of food scarcity; it is not clear how people will cope with memories of food scarcity once access improves. However, several of the cases in this chapter reveal that memories of food scarcity lead people to "take advantage of" the availability of whatever foods "appear" because they are uncertain that these items will remain available given past shortages. Many participants share similar perspectives to those of Yaicel and Maria Julia presented above; there were certain high-fat or high-sugar foods that they simply could not give up as part of their efforts to lose weight. Sometimes efforts to reduce the quantity of food consumed each way were pursued; if so, it was often similar to Maria Julia's approach to caloric restriction during the evening meal. Others reduce proportions of food throughout the day. Haunted by memories of food scarcity and fears of future scarcities dieters continue eating foods that they feel they must take advantage of despite high caloric content. Given the increasing availability of nutrients and calories, this approach to food consumption is one factor among many that has led to increasing levels of obesity on the island.

This chapter indicates the importance of ethnographic research for understanding the relationship between memories of past food scarcity and present day weight loss efforts to create effective weight loss programming and public health policy. The data presented here indicate that obesity and overweight "epidemics" are particular to time, place, and sociocultural meaning making (see also Hardin, this volume). These data show that memories of the food scarcities of the 1990s still haunt Santiagueros. Their behaviors and choices today are shaped by their memories of the past and have a specific impact on dieting practices as a part of weight loss efforts today. Although body size and weight serve for proxy of health status in Cuba (see Becker and Yates-Doerr, this volume), the trauma from past food scarcities interferes with individual desires to maintain low body weight. Santigueros express the need to "take advantage of" (aprovechar) certain foods while they are available because they are uncertain of future access. These ideas directly affect their eating practices and dieting efforts.

Notes

1. Cuba's postrevolutionary government implemented agrarian reforms in 1959 and 1962, which eliminated a land ownership system through redistribution and nationalization of the land and encouraged the development of cooperatives on large estates. In an effort to improve food access, the postrevolutionary government encouraged the cultivation of easily grown, highly nutritive crops such as viandas (a category that includes tubers such as yuca, malanga' sweet potato, and yam, as well as plantains). However, the agricultural transition has not resulted in sufficient food production to feed the population. Today more than 80 percent of Cuba's food is imported (USDA 2010).
2. The original ration booklet optimistically included ham, cheese, pepperoni, sausage, beef, pork, lamb, goat, fish, seafood, fruits, and vegetables. However, many of these items were never actually available in the ration.
3. As of March 2011.
4. People with certain chronic conditions, such as high cholesterol, diabetes, cancer, renal problems, etc., are able to purchase additional or different food items.
5. Cuba has a dual-currency economy. At the time of this research, the convertible peso or CUC was a close equivalent to the Euro, and the national peso is worth about four cents. Cubans get paid in the national peso. One CUC can be purchased for twenty-five national pesos. When making purchases in CUC, Santiagueros use the word shoppin from the English word "shopping" as both a verb to describe the act of making CUC purchases and as a noun to describe the location in which the purchases are made. Statements such as "I am going shoppin," and "I am going to the shoppin" are used interchangeably to denote the act of making CUC purchases. Despite the discursive distinction between CUC shoppin and other types of purchases, currently shoppin in the CUC stores is the only way to acquire many of the products Cubans feel are necessary, including additional cooking oil, imported spices, and personal hygiene products such as deodorant.
6. In a study of Cubans who migrated to Florida in the 1980s, "obesity was found in 17 percent of women, 25 percent of adults had significantly low adipose tissue stores, and

lean body mass was estimated by anthropometry and found to be adequate in 88 percent of adults" (Gordon 1982). The foods most frequently consumed in Cuba were bread, eggs, rice, and garbanzo beans. In interviews they found that fruits and vegetables were not commonly consumed in Cuba daily (Gordon 1982: 582). The Cuban diet was then, as it is now, high in fat and sugar.

7. "Fidel Castro himself contributed to the anti-smoking campaign when he stopped smoking in public in 1985, and announced he had quit in 1986, thereby promoting himself as a role model" (Barberia and Castro 2003).

8. Additionally, according to Rodríguez-Ojea and Jiménez Acosta, "The largest survey on the nutritional status in adult population conducted in Cuba assessed a sample of 30063 adults 20–59 years (62.2 percent females) selected both, in urban and rural areas in 1985. BMI ≥ 30 kg/m2 was measured in 5.1 percent males and 12.2 percent females. Overweight, (BMI≥ 25–29.9 kg/m2) was 26.4 percent in males and 27.2 percent females. Overweight and obesity prevalence were higher in urban as compared to rural areas for both genders (Berdasco and Romero 1992). Shortly after the early nineties Cuba's economy underwent serious constraints, and prevalence of obesity decreased sharply. The percentage of adult population with chronic energy deficiency (BMI ≤ 18.5 kg/m2) more than doubled in women and increased 88 percent in men in Havana City; whereas overweight and obesity prevalence rates significantly decreased, both in men and women in urban population above 19 years (n=22851) in both genders."

9. The United Nation's Food and Agriculture Organization (FAO) has set the minimum daily nutritional requirements for Cuba at 2,400 calories, 75g of fat, and 72g protein (2009).

10. Others argue that there was a greater drop in caloric intake from 3,100 calories in 1989 to less than 1,800 in 1993 (PAHO 1999; see also Chomsky 2000).

11. Additionally, school cafeterias, day care centers, and government job sites provided fewer and lower-quality foods than they had before.

12. In 1993, the government began to allow Cubans to use foreign currency legally; previously the possession of hard currency was a punishable crime. Cuba operated on a dual U.S. dollar–Cuban peso economy until 2004 when dollars ceased to be accepted and the convertible Cuban peso (CUC, or chavitos) came into circulation. At the time of my research the CUC was equivalent to $1.08. However, Cubans do not get paid in CUC; Cuba's second currency, the Cuban national peso, is the currency that most Cubans are paid in. There are 25 national pesos per CUC. Whereas there used to be many stores that accepted the national peso, these stores are increasingly converting to CUC, thus forcing Cubans to convert their Cuban national pesos into CUC to make their purchases (Centero and Font 1997; De La Fuente and Glasco 1997; Phillips 2009). Note that after converting to CUC, a Cuban worker who receives 300 national pesos a month in salary has only 12 CUC a month.

13. Carmelo Mesa-Lago argues that decreasing wages, decreasing purchasing power, and exceedingly high prices for essential goods coupled with the reduction in food rations from one month's supply to only about ten days' supply, caused a significant decline in the Cuban standard of living (Mesa-Lago and Perez Lopez 2005).

14. In Santiago de Cuba, availability and accessibility of various food items has increased greatly with the appointment of Lázaro Éxposito as Santiago's new provincial first secretary

of the Cuban communist party (PCC) in 2010. After decades of neglect, Santiago and Guantánamo had acquired reputations within and beyond Cuba as the most resource-poor and least functional provinces on the island, especially in comparison to the city of Havana. Éxposito, formerly first secretary of Granma province, was received in Santiago with great anticipation following his success in revitalizing Granma and its capital, Bayamo. In his short time in Santiago, Éxposito has already completed several projects, including road improvements, the installation of streetlights, water pipes, and telephone connections throughout the city of Santiago. In addition to these pressing infrastructural improvements, Éxposito has expanded food availability through the opening of new seafood restaurants, juice bars, ice cream and pizza parlors, bakeries, dairies, and street food carts. Established markets have been painted, new signs have been posted, and repairs have been made to once crumbling structures.

15. All names and some identifying details of research participants have been changed throughout this chapter.
16. All of the interviews were conducted in Spanish and transcribed by the author.
17. In this chapter I include participants self-identified skin color and/or ethnicity to illuminate any differences in weight-loss practices or experiences of the special period across skin color lines. Furthermore, the global literature on obesity and weight-loss indicates differentiated experiences and practices based on race, ethnicity, or skin color (cf. Bramble et al. 2009; Caldwell et al. 1997; Kumanyika 1987; Rucker and Cash 1992; Williamson et al. 1991).
18. His ethnic identification as "chino" is based on his understanding that his ancestors were Chinese migrants who came to Cuba to work on the railroads during the nineteenth century. Although he acknowledges that his skin color is locally interpreted as mestizo, he makes an effort to distinguish himself from other Cuban mestizos.

References

Alaimo, K. 2005. "Food Insecurity in the United States: An Overview." *Topics in Clinical Nutrition* 20: 281–298.

Altieri, M. A., N. Companioni, K. Caniezares, C. Murphy, P. Rosset, M. Bourque, and C. Clara Nicholls. 1999. "The Greening of Barrios: Urban Agriculture for Food Security in Cuba." *Agriculture and Human Values* 16: 131–140.

Alvarez, J. 2004. *Cuba's Agricultural Sector,* Gainesville: University Press.

Barberia, L., and A. Castro. 2003. "Seminar on Cuban Health System: Its Evolution, Accomplishments and Challenges." *David Rockefeller Center for Latin American Studies Working Papers in Latin America,* Paper No. 2/3-4.

Barchfield, J. 2011. "Vegetarians Push Soy, but Cubans Prefer Pork." *Associated Press,* available at http://www.washingtonpost.com/wpdyn/content/article/2011/02/17/AR2011021701 067pf.html, accessed February 17, 2011.

Becker, A. E. 1995. *Body, Self and Society: The View from Fiji.* Philadelphia: University of Pennsylvania Press.

Birch, L. L., and K. K. Davison. 2005. "Family Environmental Factors Influencing the Developing Behavioral Controls of Food Intake and Childhood Overweight." *Pediatric Clinics of North America* 48: 893–907.

Bramble, J., L. J. Cornelius, and G. Simpson. 2009. "Eating as a Cultural Expression of Caring among Afro-Caribbean and African American Women: Understanding the Cultural Dimensions of Obesity." *Journal of Health Care for the Poor and Underserved* 20: 53–68.

Bruner, J. 1990. *Acts of Meaning.* Cambridge, MA: Harvard University Press.

Caldwell, M. B., K. D. Brownell, and D. E. Wilfley. 1997. "Relationship of Weight, Body Dissatisfaction, and Self-esteem in African American and White Female Dieters." *International Journal of Eating Disorders* 22: 127–130.

Campos, P., A. Saguy, P. Ernsberger, E. Oliver, and G. Gaesser. 2006. "The Epidemiology of Overweight and Obesity: Public Health Crisis or Moral Panic?" *International Journal of Epidemiology* 35: 55–60.

Centero, M. A., and M. Font, eds. 1997. *Toward a New Cuba? Legacies of a Revolution.* Boulder, CO: Lynne Rienner Publishers.

Chaplowe, S. G. 1996. "Havana's Popular Gardens: Sustainable Urban Agriculture." *World Sustainable Agriculture Association Newsletter* 5: 22.

Chomsky, A. 2000. "The Threat of a Good Example: Health and Revolution in Cuba." In *Dying for Growth: Global Inequality and the Health of the Poor,* ed. J. Y. Kim. Monroe: Common Courage, 331–357.

Conover, S., S. Donovan, and E. Susser. 2001. "Reflections on Health Care in Cuba." *Lancet* 2, no. 8201: 958–960.

Counihan, C. M. 1992. "Food Rules in the United States: Individualism, Control and Hierarchy." *Anthropological Quarterly* 65, no. 2: 55–66.

Crawford, R. 1984. "A Cultural Account of 'Health': Control, Release, and the Social Body." In *Issues in the Political Economy of Health Care,* ed. J. McKinlay. New York: Tavistock Publications, 60–103.

———. 1994. "The Boundaries of the Self and the Unhealthy Other: Reflections on Health, Culture, and AIDS." *Social Science and Medicine* 38: 1347–1365.

De La Fuente, A., and L. Glasco. 1997. "Are Blacks 'Getting Out of Control'? Racial Attitudes, Revolution, and Political Transition in Cuba." In *Toward A New Cuba? Legacies of a Revolution,* ed. M. A. Centero and M. Font. Boulder, CO: Lynne Rienner Publishers, 53–72.

Deere, C. D., N. Perez, and E. Gonzales. 1994. "The View from Below: Cuban Agriculture in the 'Special Period in Peacetime.'" *Journal of Peasant Studies* 21, no. 2: 194–234.

Dominguez, J. I. 2005. "Cuba's Economic Transition: Successes, Deficiencies and Challenges." In *Transforming Socialist Economies: Lessons for Cuba and Beyond,* ed. S. J. Burki and D. P. Erikson. New York: Palgrave.

Esquivel, M., J. M. Romero, A. Berdasco, J. A. Gutiérrez, J. M. Jiménez, E. Posada, and M. Ruben. 1997. "Nutritional Status of Preschool Children in Ciudad de La Habana from 1972 to 1993." *Revista Panamaericana de Salud Publica* 1, no. 5: 349–354.

Fisher, J. O., and L. L. Birch. 1999. "Restricting Access to Food and Children's Eating." *Appetite* 32, no. 3: 405–419.

Food and Agriculture Organization of the United Nations. 2009. "FAO and Emergencies: Cuba." Available at www.fao.org/emergencies/country_information/list/latinamerica/cuba/en/, accessed July 22, 2009.

Franco, M., P. Ordúñez, B. Caballero, J. A. Tapia, M. Lazo, J. L. Bernal, E. Guallar, and R. Cooper. 2007. "Impact of energy intake, physical activity and population-wide weight loss on cardiovascular disease and diabetes mortality in Cuba, 1980–2005." *American Journal of Epidemiology* 166, no. 12, 1374–1380.

Frongillo, E. A., B. S. Rauschenbach, C. M. Olson, A. Kendall, and A. G. Colmenares. 2007. "Questionnaire-based Measures are Valid for the Identification of Rural Households with Hunger and Food Insecurity." *Journal of Nutrition* 127: 699–705.

Garro, L. C. 2000. "Cultural Knowledge as Resource in Illness Narrative: Remembering through Accounts of Illness." In *Narrative and the Cultural Construction of Illness and Healing,* ed. C. Mattingly and L. C. Garro. Berkeley and Los Angeles: University of California Press, 70–87.

Garth, H. 2009. "Things Became Scarce: Food Availability and Accessibility in Santiago de Cuba Then and Now." *NAPA Bulletin* 34: 178–182.

———. 2010. "Toward Being a Complete Woman: Reflections on Mothering in Santiago de Cuba." *Center for Study of Women Newsletter,* December. University of California Los Angeles.

Gjelten, T. 2008. "Raul Castro's Reforms Raise Expectations in Cuba." *All Things Considered,* National Public Radio, May 9.

Gordon, A. M., Jr. 1982. "Nutritional Status of Cuban Refugees: A Field Study on the Health and Nutrition of Refugees Processed at Opa Locka, Florida." *American Journal of Clinical Nutrition* 35, no. 3: 582–590.

Guttmacher, S. 1987. "The Prevention of Health Risks in Cuba." *International Journal of Health Service* 17, no. 1: 179–189.

Heinberg, L. J., J. K. Thompson, and J. L. Matzon. 2001. "Body Image Dissatisfaction as a Motivator for Healthy Lifestyle Change: Is Some Distress Beneficial?" In *Eating Disorders: Innovative Directions in Research and Practice,* ed. R. H. Striegel-Moore and L. Smolak. Washington, DC: American Psychological Association, 215–232.

Ibarra Cuesta, J. 1995. "Cuba: 1898–1958 Estructura y Procesos Sociales." *Editorial de Ciencias Sociales,* La Habana, Cuba.

Israel, E. 2008. "In 'Eat Local' Movement, Cuba is Years Ahead." *Reuters,* December 15.

Kumanyika, S. 1987. "Obesity in Black Women." *Epidemiologic Reviews* 9: 31–50.

Koont, S. 2004. "Food Security in Cuba." *Monthly Review* 55, no. 8: 11–20.

Languepin, O. 1999. *Cuba: La Faillite d'une Utopie.* Paris: Gallimard.

Lester, R. 1997. "The (Dis)embodied Self in Anorexia Nervosa." *Social Science and Medicine* 44, no. 4: 479–489.

Mesa-Lago, C. and J. Perez-Lopez. 2005. *Cuba's Aborted Reform: Socioeconomic Effects, International Comparisons, and Transition Policies.* Gainesville: University of Florida Press.

Murphy, C. 1999. "Cultivating Havana Urban Agriculture and Food Security in the Years of Crisis." *Development Report #12,* Oakland, CA: Food First—Institute for Food and Development Policy.

Pan American Health Organization (PAHO). 1999. *Cuba: Profile of the Health Services System.* Washington: Pan American Health Organization.

Pertierra, A. C. 2008. "En Casa: Women and Households in Post-Soviet Cuba." *Journal of Latin American Studies* 40: 743–767.

Phillips, E. 2009. "Dollarization, Distortion, and the Transformation of Work." Paper presented at A Changing Cuba in a Changing World Conference, New York, March 12.

Pilcher, J. 1998. *¡Que vivan los tamales! Food and the Making of Mexican Identity.* Albuquerque: University of New Mexico Press.

Polivy, J. 1996. "Psychological Consequences of Food Restriction." *Journal of the American Dietetic Association* 96: 589–592.

Pollock, N. J. 1995. "Social Fattening Patterns in the Pacific—The Positive Side of Obesity: Naru Case Study." In *Social Aspects of Obesity*, ed. I. de Garine and N. J. Pollock. Amsterdam: Gordon and Breach, 87–106.

Prager, J. 1998. *Presenting the Past: Psychoanalysis and the Sociology of Misremembering.* Cambridge, MA: Harvard University Press.

Preeg, E. 1993. *Cuba and the New Caribbean Order.* Washington, DC: Center for Strategic and International Studies.

Premat, A. 1998. "Feeding the Self and Cultivation of Identities in Havana Cuba." Ph.D. dissertation, York University.

Roca, S. G. 1977. "Cuban Economic Polity in the 1970s: The Trodden Paths." In *Cuban Communism.* I.L. Horowitz, ed. New Brunswick: Transaction Books.

Roca, S. G. 1998. "Cuban Economic Polity in the 1970s: The Trodden Paths." In *Cuban Communism*, ed. I. L. Horowitz. New Brunswick: Transaction Books, 338–371.

Rodríguez-Ojea Menéndez, A., and S. J. Acosta. 2005. "Is Obesity a Health Problem in Cuba?" *Human Ecology* 13: 103–108.

Rucker, C. E., and T. F. Cash. 1992. "Body Images, Body-size Perceptions, and Eating Behaviors among African American and White College Women." *International Journal of Eating Disorders* 12: 291–299.

Saguy, A., and K. Riley. 2005. "Weighing Both Sides: Morality, Mortality and Framing Contests over Obesity." *Journal of Health Politics, Policy and Law* 30, no. 5: 869–921.

Stricker, P. 2007. *Toward a Culture of Nature: Environmental Policy and Sustainable Development in Cuba.* New York: Lexington Books.

Sobo, E .J. 2000. "The Sweetness of Fat: Health, Procreation, and Sociability in Rural Jamaica." In *The Visible Self: Global Perspectives on Dress, Culture and Society, 2nd ed.*, ed. J. B. Eicher and H. A. Lutz. New York: Fairchild Eiche, 384–388.

Sutton, D. 2001. *Remembrance of Repasts: An Anthropology of Food and Memory.* Oxford: Berg Publishers.

USDA. 2010. "Agricultural Baseline Projections." Available at http://www.ers.usda.gov/Briefing/Baseline/, accessed February 10, 2010.

Williamson, D. E., H. S. Kahn, and T. Byers. 1991. "The 10 Year Incidence of Obesity and Major Weight Gain in Black and White US Women Aged 30–55." *American Journal of Clinical Nutrition* 53: 1515s–1518s.

Acknowledgments

I would like to acknowledge my friends in Santiago who have made this project by sharing their stories with me. In particular I thank the Casa del Caribe for supporting my work along with my doctoral committee members: Carole Browner, Robin Derby, Linda Garro, Akhil Gupta, and Jason Throop. I am grateful to Netta Avineri, Hadi N. Deeb, and Mara Buchbinder for comments on an earlier draft. I would also like to thank the editors, Jessica Hardin and Megan McCullough, and anonymous reviewers for their comments, which greatly improved this chapter. This project was funded in part by the following organizations: UC Diversity Initiative for Graduate Study in the Social Sciences, UC Cuba Initiative Travel Grant, National Science Foundation, Social Science Research Council, UCLA Latin American Institute, UCLA Center for Study of Women, and UCLA's Department of Anthropology.

CHAPTER 5

Fasting for Health, Fasting for God

Samoan Evangelical Christian Responses to Obesity and Chronic Disease

Jessica A. Hardin

✛ ✛ ✛

O fanau a tagata e fafaga i upu a o fanau a manu e fafaga i fugalaau.
People nourish their young with words, while birds nourish their young with seeds.

— Samoan Proverb

The motivation to write this paper was sparked during conversations with public health practitioners and Pacific scholars after returning from preliminary field-work trips over the course of three years.[1] Whenever I would mention to Pacific scholars working in the United States or public health practitioners working with Pacific Islanders that I was doing research on fasting, the response was generally: "Samoan people fast?" This motivated me to explore why the Samoan practice of fasting seems like such a contradictory idea.

The first part of this puzzle is that anthropologists often associate Samoans with lavish food presentations as a key dimension of exchange relationships; this association informs not only social relationships but also bodily idioms and sub-jectivity. For many public health practitioners, Samoa elicits an image of fast foods, fatty meats, obesity, and attendant diseases. The question arises, then, how and why is the practice of fasting a common topic of discussion among Samoan Christians when it seems, at least on the surface, to contradict Samoan food ideologies and anthropological understanding of the connection between con-sumption, body size, and abundance? How is fasting appropriated into a food ideology that values large body sizes and views eating as a central dimension of sociality? Can fasting be considered a Samoan way to address pressing epidemiological issues in Christian terms? Concordantly, what can we learn about obesity prevention and local understandings of chronic illness by exploring not only diet and exercise but also expanding the scope of medical anthropology research to include religious motivations for abstaining from eating? How might obesity and chronic disease interventions be designed to incorporate socially productive and culturally embodied modes of food abstinence? To best understand the epidemiological context of Samoa, as these questions suggest, it is important to couple health and religion and look beyond more strictly defined medical or wellness contexts to understand how health can be socially mobilized.

The puzzle for researchers is that fasting seems like a counterintuitive practice given that so much of Samoan social life focuses on food; however, the very act of fasting, which focuses on spiritual "food," explains why fasting is increasingly popular among evangelical Christians.[2] Fasting is meaningful within a context in which eating and sharing food are powerful ways to concretize social relationships; fasting is conceptualized as not simply abstaining from eating but feeding on spiritual materials, like the Word of God or the Holy Spirit. Abstaining, like eating, becomes socially productive and spiritually valuable, as opposed to dieting, which does not accomplish valuable social work. Dieting restricts one's ability to relate socially, whereas fasting expands opportunities to build social and spiritual relationships in new ways. In a time when the meaning of eating and food is changing because of increased chronic diseases and lifestyle-focused health interventions, fasting permits Samoan food ideology to prosper while also fashioning a local response to epidemiological change.

In this chapter, I explore multiple dimensions of fasting that make this Samoan practice a meaningful response to the everyday dilemmas posed by the experiences of chronic illness. Food ideology, the morality of hunger, and the acquisition of knowledge all play a part in constituting fasting as a Christian response to epidemiological and social change. To understand fasting, first it is important to understand that there are profound changes occurring across the Samoan islands. These changes include: (1) amplified dependence on imported and high fat content foods, (2) the efflorescence and diversification of Christian denominations that often challenge kin-based village organization, and (3) the rapid increase in chronic diseases, including type 2 diabetes, cardiovascular disease, and hypertension since the 1970s.

In this context, public health organizations and evangelical churches alike often link rates of chronic disease with traditional food practices, deeming them immoral and greedy (Hardin under review). In particular, *fa'alavelave*, "life-crisis," or ritual exchange events, with lavish food presentations, provide ample semiotic grounds to link chronic disease, embodied as evidence, to immoral social and financial practices. As elsewhere in the world (see McCullough, this volume), the obese and chronic diseased body can become evidence of corrupt morality.

Samoan food ideology centers on eating as a way to create and sustain social relationships. Discussions of food, eating together, and sharing food are fundamental ways of relating and a mode of being in the world for Samoans in the islands and the diaspora. Fasting brings God into this equation and challenges the foundation for how kin relate and constitute affective, economic, and political networks (cf. Besnier 1995). Fasting is embedded in this food ideology and frames eating in spiritual terms as a way to create and sustain a relationship with God. In my interviews, fasting is discussed as a moral solution to the problems of material and kin-based relationships. Disease is often taken as the embodied evidence of immoral worldly relationships. This in turn reframes what is considered a disease crisis in moral and Christian terms, both explaining the problem and offering solutions.

According to Samoan epistemology, food connects people in the social world through consumption, labor, commensality, and the experience of heaviness in the body. From the proverb that frames this paper, "People nourish their young with words, while birds nourish their young with seeds," we see that even before Christian idioms of consumption, Samoans analogically linked eating with learning or coming to know things about the world. Food acts to connect people socially but also as a mode of nourishing knowledge and understanding. Today, however, for many Samoan evangelical Christians, food also disconnects individuals spiritually.

This disconnection rests in the idea that the body is often perceived to be consumed with the commitments of social relationships. The implicit message is that individuals are overextended and too deeply connected to social networks and the effort of giving and providing to others at the expense of feeding the spirit. The role of food is thus contested as a central dimension of social organization where somatic experiences of *fa'aaloalo*, "respect," and *alofa*, "love," are questioned. Respect and love manifest by making the body feel *mamafa*, "heavy"; these concepts are often reflected upon after eating staple Samoans foods, including taro and breadfruit. This somatic experience is contrasted to the lightness of the body experienced while fasting; heaviness and lightness not only reflect states of hunger or satiation, but also, at times, the weightedness of the body in relation to social connections (cf. Yates-Doerr 2012). In this chapter, I examine how fasting is a mode of attention through which the burden of disease is placed on individual moral actors and not considered a problem of global political economy. This in turn combats stereotypes of obese Samoans while rendering invisible global economic shifts that have changed food and labor patterns for Samoans in the islands and in the diaspora.

Methods

The data for this paper are selected from three preliminary research trips to Hawaii, American Samoa, and Samoa, where I conducted twenty interviews on fasting. Other methods included participant observation and focus groups on fasting. I conducted participant observation in three evangelical churches in Hawaii and Samoa, and while in American Samoa I conducted participant observation in mainline churches, including Congregational, Methodist, and Catholic denominations. I participated in daily worship activities, including prayer and Bible study, communal and household meals, and church fundraising activities. I also interviewed health practitioners at hospitals, clinics, and health oriented NGOs. I conducted interviews in Samoan, English, or both depending on the preferences of the interviewee. I recorded interviews and transcribed and translated these interviews with assistance from University of Hawaii Samoan Studies faculty. I analyzed transcripts for themes and also included informal interviewing data from my field notes. My interlocutors include a wide range of individuals who are diverse in rank, Christian denomination, age, and identified homeland. Despite the diversity of my interlocutors, each interlocutor articulated to some degree the themes presented below.

Two Perspectives on Obesity in Oceania

In the following section I explore two overlapping approaches to culture and biology in the study of obesity in Oceania: cultural preferences for large body size (Becker 1995; Firth 1940; Pollock 1992, 1995; Shore 1989) and the thrifty-gene hypothesis (McGarvey 1995; Neel 1962; Zimmet et al. 1997).

The Meaning of Body Size

Anthropological investigations of body size in Oceania are often taken as "classic" examples of the culturally relative values placed on body size. Famously, studies of mana contribute to an understanding of the relationship between local theories of power and body size. Raymond Firth (1940) is one of the first to recognize that anthropological theory in the case of mana was built at the conceptual level through cross-cultural comparisons of mana as supernatural force (Codrington 1915), religious force (Durkheim 2001), truth (Hocart 1922), or prestige (Tregear 1904). Bradd Shore describes mana in relation to a general Polynesian epistemological bias toward knowing things in their specific context and through their perceptual effects in the world rather than in terms of essential or intrinsic features (1989: 138).

Shore challenges a monolithic and static understanding of mana as power and instead explains mana as fickle, cultivated, and fluctuating in relation to an individual's success. Mana then, is not power per se, but generative potency, where large body size is seen as evidence of the gods' presence in the life of the individual and the family. Shore writes: "The divine mana of chiefs is manifest in their brilliance, their shining. This, as much as corpulence, was the 'beauty' that marked chiefly status" (Sahlins 1981 quoted in Shore 1989: 139). From Shore, we see the complex ways that large body size signifies transcendent connection with the gods, reproductive potency, and sexuality.

Anne Becker's work in Fiji (1995) has shaped how anthropologists think about the morality of body morphology. Becker argues that body size cannot be read as a sign of wealth but as a sign of dense social networks, nurturance, and care on the part of the family. Conversely, obesity is considered morally problematic because overly large bodies are perceived to be incapable of labor and suggests an inability to provide care for others. Becker enriches anthropological understandings of the sensory, symbolic, and somatic explanations for large body size preference. By drawing attention to how body morphology can be used as an idiom for nurturance and care, Becker explains how exchange activities and practices are fundamental to body cultivation and ideology. Thus, the sharing of food is an act of expanding one's social universe and highlights how the accumulation of objects is transient while "what endures are the social ties that are reaffirmed with each exchange and the prestige conferred upon both the recipient and the giver in enacting it" (Becker 1995: 24).

Nancy Pollock responds to what she sees as a stereotype of Pacific Islanders only eating energy-dense imported foods. She explores the meaning of food and food preparation and argues:

> I am challenging the philosophy that asserts that traditional food habits in Pacific Island cultures have undergone major changes with Westernization. Observing how food habits have changed has been the usual approach. Here I will stress the continuities by asking the alternative questions: In what ways have food habits persisted, and why? Do "traditional" food habits have a place in the Pacific Islands of the 1980s and 1990s? (1992: 21).

Pollock draws our attention to how feasting events are more than just large meals but are expressions of respect and love that sustain emotional and structural connections between groups. Pollock explains that health is not limited to the individual but focused on the well-being of the group (see Rosen, this volume). Pollock states succinctly: "In the Pacific, health was a shared sense of well-being, not the individual feeling as Westerners see it. It was built on the basis of sharing food as a symbol of caring and mutual support" (1992: 201). I build on Pollock's examination of food practices by exploring how many Samoans are responding to disease stereotypes and health demands through fasting. I argue that fasting needs to be understood not in contrast to food as a mode of relating, but as an extension of this idea.

Concerns with eating among Samoan evangelical Christians both challenge assumptions connecting care, eating, body size, and health while also reinforcing these ideas. Obesity and chronic diseases are embedded in a larger etiological narrative about the relationship between self-care and social care (cf. McMullin 2010). Losa, a woman active in a Hawaii-based evangelical ministry, explained the reasons for the steady growth of chronic illness amongst Samoans: "There is a lack of care, amongst the islanders.... Everything is being given to them, you want something, go to the store. You don't have to hunt for it, you don't have to work for it. You don't have to care for the family or the land when you go to the store to buy your pisupo, 'tinned corn beef.' Just yourself." As we can see from Becker (1995) and Pollock (1995), idioms of large body size often connote positive values attached to care, nurturance, and social networks.

However, in a context where large body size can also reveal lack of labor and reliance on cash and imported foods, this commentary can also be a potential criticism of viewing the body as a repository and highlights an immoral state of selfishness. From Losa's comments we see that food abundance and large body size may communicate deep social connections, but, it is just as likely to reveal alienation from families. The idiom of large body size can be flipped to connote the same symbolic scheme but in the negative—lack of care, illegitimate use of power, and immoral wealth—thus providing a mode of critical engagement (see Figure 5.1 and 5.2).

Fasting ameliorates this tension because fasting appropriates social efforts toward relationship building and places the emphasis onto a divine domain. Fast-

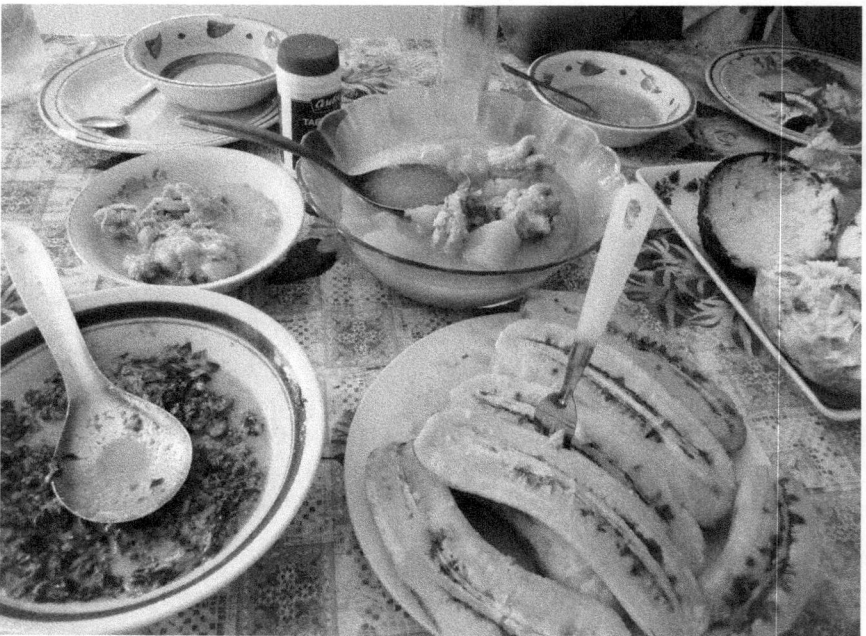

Figure 5.1. To'ona'i, "Sunday Lunch." Photograph by Jessica A. Hardin.

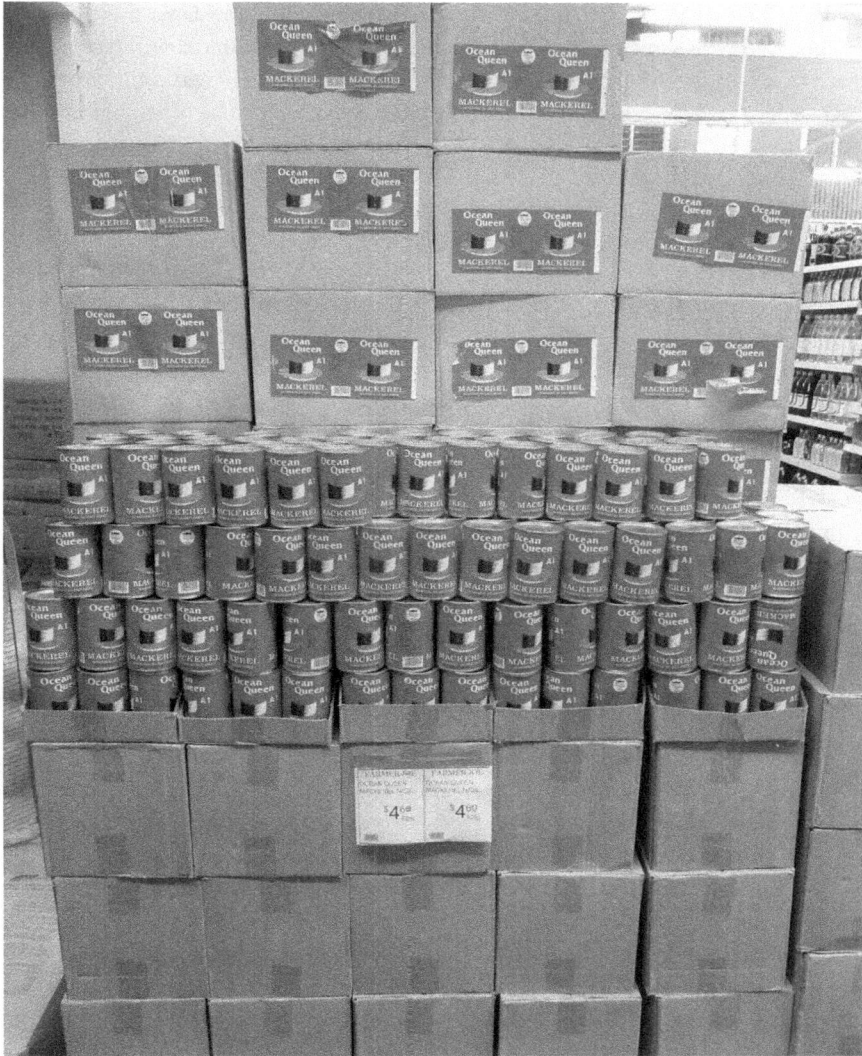

Figure 5.2. Tinned fish for sale at a supermarket in Apia. Tinned fish are fundamental objects of exchange in elaborate ceremonial exchange events called fa'alavelave. Photograph by Jessica A. Hardin.

ing in this context builds on concerns with eating as an appropriate way of being in the world but focuses instead on eating divine materials. Fasting discourses take idioms of consumption, tied to making social relationships, and re-focuses relationship building efforts with the divine, and subsequently strengthens congregation-based relationships at the expense of kin-based relationships.

It is not surprising that the meaning of consumption and large body size are in flux given the growing rates of chronic diseases heavily linked with large body size. In a context where there is an abundance of food, increasing competitive exchange, and less agricultural labor demands, disease can also be indicated by large body size and at times indicate selfishness, greed, and immoral interior states. Thus large body size indicates an ability to amass wealth, and consume that wealth, but the value of this is in question.

Multiple Translations of the Thrifty-Gene Hypothesis

Another approach to understanding obesity and chronic disease in Oceania is the thrifty-gene hypothesis, first developed by James Neel (1962). In Samoa and American Samoa, the thrifty-gene hypothesis is articulated in public health material as well as by my interlocutors in their temporal disease narratives. The thrifty-gene hypothesis has been widely applied to assist in understanding obesity and chronic disease in the Samoan islands (McGarvey 1995; Zimmet et al. 1997) and has been widely debated (see Brewis 2010 for a review). My point in bringing in ideas about the thrifty-gene to the fore is not to challenge or verify its existence but to examine how it is taken up by my interlocutors in their explanations of disease causation, as well in public health material. The following brief summary by Stephen McGarvey may illuminate the translations to follow:

> Neel speculated that the increase in the prevalence and incidence of diabetes mellitus in Western industrial populations, and those experiencing modernization, was associated with genetic factors which in the past had favored storage of calories in the form of adipose tissue in response to natural selection during food shortages. Individuals possessing tendencies towards "thriftiness" or metabolic efficiency might have been healthier, survived longer, and had more offspring. With lifestyle changes due to economic modernization there were increases in available food energy and decreases in energetic expenditure from lower physical activity. Thus, the advantage for a "thrifty" genotype in lean times became a disadvantage in times of plenty, leading to overweight, hyper-insulinaemia, and eventually development of glucose intolerance and diabetes mellitus (1995: 351).

This representation of the thrifty-gene is similar, if less technical, to etiological narratives that my interlocutors voiced about disease causation in Samoa.

In a report titled "Obesity in the Pacific: Too Big To Ignore," the World Health Organization (WHO) anticipates a local response that is skeptical of obesity by posing the rhetorical question "Aren't we just big people?" (2002: 8). The answer to this question reframes the thrifty-gene hypothesis by stating: "In the past, being overweight or large may have provided some protection against the periods of starvation and some common infectious diseases. Today being over-fat contributes to the most common illnesses of diabetes and heart disease" (2002: 8). This is one channel through which the thrifty-gene hypothesis is reframed in local ways. In this WHO report, obesity is framed as disadvantageous when compared to the past; disease is thus embedded in a temporal etiological narrative accounting for both genetic variability as well as cultural change. This is taken up by many Samoans as an explanation for the current state of disease, which in turn can circumvent blame discourses.

Among my interlocutors, the thrifty-gene hypothesis and its evolutionary explanation for obesity is often linked to larger politics of health research. When attending a research presentation on the results of a recent project documenting obesity in children in American Samoa, a Samoan man in the audience stepped up and explained his discomfort at listening to the findings of the research team. The man, whom I will call Manu, explained that he listened to a similar set of presentations on obesity at a conference in Guam; he noted he was the only Samoan at the conference. Manu explained that obesity can be understood as a "problem of cultural change" where change in lifestyle, from working in agriculture to working in offices, resulted in a situation where "Samoan bodies have not caught up yet."

Manu proposed the idea that Samoan bodies were maladapted to the current environment, which is a heightened concern when non-Samoans control research, statistics, and thus scientific representations of Samoans. He said: "People out there, they think Samoans are lazy, dependent on remittances, that we eat bad foods. It's a complicated issue. Samoa, though, looks bad out there in the academic world." Manu went on to explain that blaming cultural practices is not appropriate because this not only perpetuates stereotypes of Samoans, but also does not account for the different biological, evolutionary, and political economic realities within which many Samoans are embedded. Later I learned that Manu is a health research project manager, attained his BA from the National University of Samoa and has lived in Samoa, American Samoa, and California.

From his quote we see how Manu is concerned with the ethics of research, which is particularly important given how Manu understands the etiology of obesity for Samoan people. The comment highlights what I heard reiterated in many contexts: many people are concerned with stigmatizing health stereotypes of Samoans as fat and obese; this is compounded by the fact that many feel that the problem and solutions are out of their control or at least out of their reach, both in terms of biological and structural limitations. Manu was concerned that statistical and behavioral representations of Samoans outside of Samoa promote a vision of Samoan culture that is not only unflattering but untrue.

Others reiterated these concerns in a Christian idiom. One woman, whom I'll call Lea, an LDS church member, took a different stance. She said: "Palagi

[European/white people], they think we have always been like this, big people. But the problem is that Samoans they eat too much of the wrong food, not like in olden times where we had to work for our food and sometimes we didn't have food. That's why we have so much diabetes and obesity today. I think if you find God and live His way then you will make the right choices. They are ignorant without His help." Lea first embeds disease in a chronology that accounts for social and economic change and thus links consumption changes to the current state of health in Samoan today. Lea then explains chronic diseases as a faith issue where only Christians know the correct way to live. Reframing rates of chronic disease as a reflection of a lack spiritual knowledge locates the problems of disease squarely within the domain of the individual. These various iterations of the thrifty-gene hypothesis embed etiology into a temporal disease narrative, which simultaneously accounts for disease causation while also combats outsider explanations for disease by providing a Samoan response to individual responsibility.

Health and Well-Being in Christian Life

Investigating how health is experienced in religious contexts is of increasing anthropological interest (Klaits 2010; Zigon 2011). Simon Coleman and Peter Collins (2000) point out that studies of religious life should not be confined to church on Sunday; I add to this that the same is true of studying religious healing and health efforts. Examinations of healing efforts should not be confined to explicitly marked religious healing or biomedical encounters alone, but should include a vast array of everyday embodied efforts to maintain, sustain, or create health through faith-based practices. Everyday efforts toward cultivating health are especially visible in North American–oriented evangelical movements in which the so-called prosperity gospel links physical, spiritual, and financial success and health (cf. Griffith 2004). According to Stephen Hunt (2000) and James Bielo (2007), as signs of virtue, the related benefits of health and wealth represent a self that has achieved a personal relationship with Christ. Simon Coleman notes: "Physical and material well-being not only become an index of successful commitment to the Faith, but also help to constitute it" (2000: 151).

In other non–North American contexts, James Pfeiffer (2002) notes that evangelical churches in Mozambique do not separate illness from the political and economic context that result in disease. Thus by acknowledging the social life of disease, evangelical churches are able to heal afflictions of inequality. By not alienating the body in strictly biomedical terms these churches offer alternative strategies for healing. Pfeiffer's account points to how pressing everyday problems are appropriated by evangelical churches where individuals and communities are offered pragmatic and embodied solutions to pressing problems of economic, social, and political change.

Carolyn Schwarz's research among Galiwin'ku aboriginal people in Australia provides another case where evangelical Christian discourses about the self inflect health experiences and practices (2006). She writes that these churches offer a "repertoire of individualization that fosters self-reliance and self-actualization," which informs stances on health, lifestyle, and prevention of chronic diseases (2006: 71). Christian practices thus provide a basis for fashioning an alternative selfhood, which has implications for education and health efforts at the individual and community level. What we see in these cases is that health and well-being are measured beyond public health outcomes and are focused instead on cultivating a particular kind of Christian self that responds to contingencies and anxieties arising from various kinds of social change.

Fasting studies from Judaism, Islam, and medieval Christianity are helpful in exploring how food and eating practices come to be meaningful domains of religious activities (cf. Buitelaar 1993; Bynum 1987; Feely-Harnik 1981). Marjo Buitelaar (1993) realizes that the formulaic responses she elicited from Moroccan women during Ramadan on their motivations for fasting reveal very basic assumptions about religion and community. Buitelaar argues that Ramadan fasting unites Muslims, at least in a Moroccan imagination, through a shared practice across space and time. Buitelaar shows that fasting sustains a sense of an ideal Muslim nation because fasting organizes public and private time where the family and the religious community are also organized around efforts to purify both the spirit and the body. Fasting for Moroccan women is thus a community-building effort linking individuals through space and time.

Catherine Walker Bynum's work (1987) documents expressions of gendered piety within a schema of religious food symbols among pious medieval women. Bynum argues that medieval women's ascetic practices were a means of cultivating hyper-spiritual-bodily connections based on a symbolic system where food is constituted as flesh. She makes a corollary social argument that control of food was a useful symbolic endeavor that assisted women in manipulating their families and church authorities to expand their own agency. Rebecca Lester (2005) finds that among contemporary nuns in Mexico learning to manage the body is a key dimension of their habituation into religious life. While Lester does not examine fasting, she does find that the regulating of food and eating "are a specific arena in which desire and obligation are negotiated through bodily experience" (2005: 168).

Gillian Feely-Harnik (1981) explores fasting in a different historical context of early connections between Judaism, Christianity, and Islam to explore how dietary rules and eating practices were used to address ethical questions of identity and affiliation in a context of change. She argues: "[F]ood, articulated in feeding, eating, starving, and fasting, provided a powerfully concentrated 'language' for debating moral-legal issues and transforming social relations" (1981: xiii). Fasting is one practice among many food-related practices that was utilized to refashion symbolic indicators of identity and religiosity with practical and embodied effects in the world. Feeley-Harnik (1981) suggests that because of food's ability to pass through boundaries it might be a fruitful sign for thinking/embodying more abstract boundaries. In Samoa, fasting may be one such effort to take a practice with embodied effect in the world as a way of reifying specific, and novel, relationship-making efforts.

We see from these accounts that fasting, and eating practices, can be meaningful ways of making abstract concerns with community and social boundaries concrete. These social dynamics are reified through embodied experience, through the temporal ordering of the day, and by incorporating spiritual and religious concerns into profane dimensions of everyday life. In Samoa, fasting is not only made meaningful through a Samoan food ideology, where eating is central to everyday relationship-making efforts, but also as an everyday embodied practice aimed at transforming the self and self-care.

Fasting among Evangelical Samoans

Fasting takes many forms among the people I interviewed and conducted participant observation with in the islands and the diaspora. Primarily, both evangelical and mainline churches would choose a day of the week and every church member was supposed to fast. Others had family fast days or individual days of their choosing when they would fast. The amount of time and the food restrictions varied widely, from only fruits and vegetables for days at a time, or only water, to no food or drink between morning and dinner. Some of my interlocutors were keen to explain that fasting is an individual endeavor that one should not discuss or, worse, brag about. Others felt that fasting should be a collective effort where community members all fast for a particular reason, for example, for a sick family member. Among my interlocutors, fasting was directed toward a global concept of health where spiritual, physical, and financial dimensions are interdependent.[3]

Fasting as Eating

One of the most prominent themes to emerge from interview data was the idiom *ai le Upu,* "eat the Word," or *fafaga le Aga,* "feed on the Spirit." This idiom refers to a variety of spiritual practices including fasting, reading the Bible, and genres of prayer. Coleman (2000) finds the metaphor of eating the Word with his interlocutors in Sweden. He argues that the Word is vested with physical qualities, thus reading the Bible is akin to ingestion and eating. He notes, "In this view, the text is embodied in the person, who becomes a walking, talking representation of its power. Eating is an especially powerful image because it points to a notion of internalizing truth directly, bypassing the distorting effects of both social context and intellect" (2000: 128). Although the metaphor may be shared across evangelical churches, "eating the Word" in Samoa takes on literal qualities; it is phrase that builds on Samoan epistemology that to know something is to embody it or consume it. The idiom articulates this epistemology in a new context of efforts toward cultivating a Christian lifestyle.

Congregation members who use this phrase daily suggest that individuals should not just read the Bible, but eat it, ingest it, live it, and depend on it. One American Samoan woman explained: "Eating the Word is a substitute for eating food. You know, you make a relationship with God this way. You need to feed on the Spirit, eat the Word." Using the metaphor of eating the Word as opposed to eating actual physical food has the effect of constituting a particular kind of relationship with God (one of intimacy, interdependence, and commensality) while also challenging worldly relations as secondary to spiritual eating. Fasting as eating helps reproduce church relationships, while potentially challenging kin-based responsibilities and commitments.

One particularly articulate woman explained eating the Word through an analogy between desire and consumption. In the following excerpt, we see how these features are key to creating a sustainable relationship with God. Eating, for this interlocutor, is to produce action and desired outcomes over time.

> To eat the Word means to partake of it everyday, it means to act out the Word. Normally, when you're thinking of it you have to put something in and something comes out. But it's the eating of the Word, it's the consuming of it, it's making your everyday bread the Word....biblically it means, your eyes, your ears, everything is to partake of it. So you read it out loud so you can see it, and hear it and your mouth says it. So it's a whole consuming of that one thing…it means to almost gorge on it—right now we are gorging on the wrong kinds of foods. So often we miss the part that we need to crave it. We need to desire it. There needs to be a fragrance in the Word so that people will be drawn to it. Like any kind of meal, people are drawn to the fragrance of the meal, what it smells like. You know you're drawn to the kitchen because it smells so good. So we as Christians, or born again believers, those of us that love the Word, and love Jesus Christ as our Lord, need to get to the point where the fragrance of the Word is consuming you every day. You know it's like a craving, like a desire that won't go away, no matter how much you get of it. It's that desire, you've got to just eat so much of it that your busting opening and then you want to eat it again.

This interlocutor uses the metaphor of eating the Word and feeding spiritually to reconstitute a hierarchy of human social relations by placing this kind of eating as primary and worldly eating with kin as secondary and even potentially suspect.

Although this interlocutor is focused on explaining how spiritual eating should occur, midway through she reveals a critique that many Samoans are engaging in the wrongs kinds of eating and therefore socially relating in a morally undesirable manner. As an aside she notes, "[R]ight now we are gorging on the wrong kinds of foods"; she continues to explain that her fellow congregation members need to learn how to crave the right kind of eating, foods, and relationships. The urgency with which she speaks highlights the transformative role she hopes that consuming the Word of God will have on individuals. Using eating as a metaphor for connecting with God lends intimacy and materiality to this abstract spiritual condition and idea. Abstaining suggests that individuals should reconsider their eating practices in their everyday lives. Abstaining from food thus places foods, sharing, and eating within a space for questioning individual motivations, experiences, and consumption.

By placing worldly eating within questionable brackets new habits can be formed by questioning old ones. One pastor's wife in Samoa explained: "Through fasting we teach the church, like children, the ways of God. We need to affirm them, and keep teaching them to do the right thing. This has it a lot to do with changing habits, changing their thinking." This woman continued to explain that to change how one eats is to change how one thinks. From our conversation it became apparent that this effort to remake daily eating practice calls into question how one eats, what one eats, and with whom. For the above interlocutor, by focusing on prayer and fasting as the "twin tools of leading a Christian life," individuals are able to ameliorate the social and spiritual problems that arise from reciprocity. Through these tools many evangelical Christians are able to carve out distinctive modes of morality by reconceptualizing responsibility, respect, and social care in terms of an individual relationship with God, a focus on personal commitment, and a questioning of the ethical effects of giving and sharing practices.

The Experience of Hunger

A second theme to emerge is that the experience of hunger is evidence of immorality. David Howes's research on fasting is helpful here because he shows how "sensory experience is also an arena for structuring social roles and interactions" (2003: xi). Howes conducts a sensory analysis of the ceremonial exchange system known as kula in the Massim Valley, Papua New Guinea, with special attention to fasting during travel. Howes explores why men who are kula traveling abstain from eating in three points: (1) Because eating interferes with one's capacity for giving, fasting is preferable; (2) According to local ideology, eating slows the body and makes it heavy. Fasting thus makes the body more productive, light and buoyant, which are desirable qualities when one is kula traveling; (3) Eating also effects the body's image by making the body less beautiful, clean, and light. Body size is not the issue as much as the cleanliness of the exterior, which might be soiled by consumption. From this case we can see how fasting is a way to manipulate the body to heighten one's capacity for particular kinds of social relationships.

While Howes explores the sensory experiences of hunger, the moral dimension of hunger in Oceania has also been explored in Oceania (Schieffelin 1990; Throop 2010; Young 1972). Jason Throop (2010) explores hunger as one dimension of a moral sensibility in Yap where suffering is not mere suffering, but rather individuals suffer for their families and clan through labor. In Yap, the ability to cultivate mastery over one's somatic states is part of a larger process of cultivating and enacting endurance (Throop 2010: 97–98). Mastery over one's hunger reflects a larger "ethical mode of being" where "pain is understood to arise or result from an individual's effort to provide for, contribute to, and help his or her family, village, or community" (Throop 2010: 183). This contrasts to hunger among my interlocutors, where in the context of fasting, hunger is a negative sign. Hunger while fasting, contrary to Yapese cultivations of endurance, indicates something is wrong, revealing that one's motivations are not aligned with one's actions. The lack of hunger while fasting and the witnessing of effects, i.e., the safe return of a friend from military service, are evidence that one is motivated for the appropriate reasons. Lack of hunger, or comfort in a state of abstention from eating, reveals the ethical state of the self.

Not experiencing hunger while fasting is evidence of God's presence and correct moral motivation. Fasting is said to be easy, without feelings of hunger, when you are feeding on the Word of God. A young woman attending the American Samoa Community College explained: "You don't feel hungry because God steps in. You don't feel hungry if you are patient and pray because fasting is a way to commit to God. It won't be difficult if you feed on the Word of God." Another man in his thirties, who was active in church ministry in Hawaii, explained: "You don't feel hungry, you feel strong and clean because you are connecting to God's spirit." If one feels hungry while not eating, this is more likely the result of dieting or not having enough food, not the experience of fasting. Thus feeling hunger becomes somatic evidence that one is fasting for selfishly oriented desires (like losing weight), whereas fasting produces healthful spiritual and physical effects. The effects reveal that one's motivations are aligned with one's prayers, and this balance leads to spiritual and physical health.

Fasting versus Dieting

Fasting was often compared to dieting as a foil for understanding meaningless hunger. Comparing dieting to fasting is a common activity for youth church members in Hawaii, even outside interviews. One young woman, who was a leader in the youth ministry, explained: "It's not like when you diet, you feel weak and angry." Another woman, in this same church, noted: "If I fast for diet it's weak, it's just for food. You always go to sleep if you don't eat for diet. But if you fast for the Word and the inner person to feel, you don't want to sleep. You can go for the whole night, three days. Awake." Dieting can be seen as a selfish practice that is meaningless because it is not productive except to potentially better the individual. Fasting, on the other hand, is abstaining from eating to build a relationship with God and better the community. Fasting, while it can better the individual's moral and spiritual state, is largely discussed as having a social effect in the world—for sick family members or, more complexly, as a way to become spiritually and morally upright, which will lead to better collective health for the community. Hunger then is a cultivated productive moral state where personal efforts are directed toward spiritual-social life.

Fasting for health reasons, where spiritual, physical, and financial dimensions are interconnected, embeds disease concerns within a moral and religious set of strategies and solutions. When individuals fast, instead of diet, they circumvent public health and biomedical efforts to modify lifestyle by addressing health in a specifically spiritual way, thus avoiding discussions about food availability and the social pressures to eat (cf. Rosen, this volume). One particular case may illuminate the differences between dieting and fasting. When interviewing a doctor about the current state of chronic disease in Samoa, she volunteered a story about her friend who had lost a substantial amount of weight. Moana, the doctor, explained that her friend asked for God's help and He responded that the friend must do the biblical Daniel fast, a fast derived from the book of Daniel that describes a diet of fruits and vegetables only. Moana reported the story during a discussion about her own struggles with weight and "self-discipline." Despite her biomedical knowledge and her acceptance of Jesus Christ, Moana was frustrated because she believed that as a doctor and a Christian she should have enough knowledge and faith to change her lifestyle, and yet she still struggles.

Moana's story of her friend's triumph in changing her size provided a balanced narrative of biomedical knowledge and spiritual motivations that Moana found inspiring. The friend asked for God's help because she recognized she could not change her life alone. Moana reported that her friend, also a health care professional, said she needed to align her knowledge about health with her spiritual priorities. After completing the forty-day and forty-night fast the friend prayed again and the Holy Spirit told her to continue to eat this way but to also eat fish and avoid fatty meats. Moana continued: "She received this knowledge through the Holy Spirit. She is happy and bright now. The fast strengthened her faith through discipline."

This narrative provided Moana evidence of the Holy Spirit's intimate presence in daily life and as a support and provider of knowledge in times of physical and spiritual need. For Moana there was no "magic" in how and why her friend lost the weight and continued to maintain her weight loss: the Holy Spirit strengthened her friend's already present knowledge (that she should modify her diet) but it was the Holy Spirit that provided her friend the discipline to persist in changing her life. The narrative of the friend who has lost weight, regained her health, and is spiritually strengthened provides evidence of individuals who live according to contemporary biomedical knowledge (diet) but who have the discipline and the will to live by this knowledge with the help of the Holy Spirit.

Moana explained that dieting alone cannot be maintained long term because the effects could be one of the following: (1) dieting is too hard; (2) dieting cannot be maintained because one does not have the assistance of the Holy Spirit; or (3) there may be negative repercussions for dieting for worldly reasons. Whereas experiencing hunger indicates that something is not right in the self, fasting allows the experience of hunger to manifest positively by its absence. Fasting thus can be seen as a productive activity not geared toward the self directly but toward maintaining a relationship with the divine, thus imbuing the embodied experience of hunger with moral meaning.

Fasting and New Understandings

From Moana's narrative we see that fasting provides a special mode of changing one's life through the Holy Spirit and this is recognized by somatic shifts in the body as mamafa, "heavy," or *mama,* "clean," as free from worldly wants and as alert to the words of the Holy Spirit. The metaphor of eating the Word of God and feeding on the Spirit are taken to be avenues for understanding and sharing knowledge. Fasting is an embodied practice aimed toward interior transformation. One pastor explained: "You need to feed yourself spiritually in order to think spiritually." Fasting helps clear the mind of distractions, which is particularly helpful to students. One student from the National University of Samoa explained: "If I have an exam, and you know I want to get an A, I will fast to help with my concentration."

Whereas these are activities geared toward transforming the interior state of the self, fasting also prepares the self to do community work directed outward from the self. Another pastor from Samoa told me: "When I am preparing to give a speech I will fast. This prepares me for spreading the Word of God. Fasting anoints me, it allows the Word of God to reveal himself through me." His wife tacked on: "Fasting is a way to help you understand His plan. It allows you to concentrate an understand what's happening in your life." Fasting thus provides a special avenue for new types of learning and understanding.

Individuals come to a new kind of knowledge of the self and God's plan for the self by attenuating the connection to the world of the body through depravation of food; this can be seen as an extension of food based modes of social relating where abstaining from eating can be seen as one way to separate oneself from the social relations of everyday life. Food is situated as a deterrent to knowledge; food fills the body and thus inhibits a focused experience of an intimate relationship with God and the Holy Spirit. So while eating and the sharing of food allow individuals and families to sustain social networks and relationships, abstaining from eating heightens one's sensitivity and interior alertness to the Holy Spirit and God. These two different modes of feeding, on food and on the Word of God, are both modes of knowledge and understanding about relationships, with family or with the divine.

Conclusions and Implications

Anthropologists and public health practitioners know little about how indigenous body idioms and food ideology are challenged and negotiated in changing epidemiological contexts. Examining how food ideologies are reshaped in contemporary (and growing) evangelical Christian communities provides an opportunity to understand how pressing health issues are articulated and appropriated as moral and practical concerns; Samoa is a case in point. By examining fasting in Samoa today, I argue that fasting omits critical attention directed at the structural problems of food availability by placing health responsibility on the individual's spiritual life. Additionally, focusing on fasting also circumvents global discourses of Pacific Islander obesity and stereotypes of "big" Polynesians by articulating the epidemiological problem in specifically Samoan terms and responses. Fasting also reveals that health is not always measured in terms of disease outcomes but in cultivating particular kinds of relationships with others and with the divine.

Examining fasting practices also speaks to the complexity of personhood (Hollan 1992; Lamb 1997; McIntosh 2009) where models of personhood cannot be reduced to individual or sociocentric orientations. On the surface, Samoan fasting practices convert sociocentric modes of being in the world to individualized modes for creating and sustaining social relations. Fasting highlights individual efforts to access the Holy Spirit and new knowledge. Simultaneously though, fasting is made meaningful because it is an inherently social activity aimed at moral transformation of self and society. When fasting is evoked it is as a practice that will improve the moral state of individuals and community, and conversely ameliorate attendant diseases. Fasting socializes abstaining from eating, which without this moral meaning is considered an uncomfortable and selfish practice. Thus fasting takes an individualistic activity of abstaining from eating and reformulates it as a social activity concerned with cultivating Samoan persons.

Public health programming and interventions might learn something from this process. As Rochelle Rosen points out (this volume), is it very difficult for Samoans to abstain from eating in the household and during ritual exchange.

In this chapter, I have explored the various dimensions through which fasting is a meaningful mode of abstaining from eating while also socially engaging, with moral purpose, with the community. Public health programming and interventions should consider working closely with Samoan community members to frame disease prevention and intervention activities as socially driven, community oriented everyday practices that not only improve the health of individual persons but also aim toward improving the health of the community at large. Embedding prevention and intervention activities in socially oriented discourses, which are locally created, may help to make lifestyle changes not only more palatable but potentially more effective.

In returning to my original conundrum: why is it that scholars and public health practitioners do not know of or engage with the practice fasting among Samoan evangelical Christians, I surmise that this problem may reflect a limited definition and conception of health. Throughout this volume we see health as inextricably linked to measurement-based understandings. As I struggled to describe and analyze an evangelical Samoan concept of health, I ran up against the loadedness of the word *health* in Euro-American folk ideologies, which permeate public health messaging. Thus in writing about a Samoan concept of health, it is possible to view in relief a widely circulating strictly defined concept of health in anthropology, public health, and certainly biomedicine; this concept of health is marked by notions of personal responsibility and rationality, individually control, and a state to be worked toward and achieved.

My work challenges a singular concept of health. This paper provides an ethnographic account of one specific cultural construction of health while also drawing attention to a dearth of anthropological concepts for understanding health defined by alternative, non-metric-based, measures and meanings. Samoan evangelical Christian health-seeking behaviors, like fasting, are moral and spiritual ways of training the individual and social body into health and Christianity, as the two cannot be uncoupled or comprehended separately. By limiting analysis to those features tied to a metric-based understanding of health, including, but not limited to diet, exercise, and consumption, researchers, anthropologists, and public health practitioners often partition off a host of religious and spiritually based practices aimed toward maintaining and sustaining health and well-being. Not only are the intersections of health and religious beliefs and practices critical domains for use in health interventions, but they may actually provide new ways for thinking about the multiple meanings of health and alternative modes of measuring health.

Notes

1. From 2008 to 2010, I have conducted preliminary fieldwork in American Samoa, Samoa, Hawaii, and California. These field trips total to nine months of preliminary fieldwork, which provides the basis for this paper.

2. This research is based in an Assemblies of God (AOG) Congregation, which is considered Pentecostal, according to the mother institution website. However, my interlocutors in Samoa refer to the AOG as an evangelical institution. I will use the Samoan categorization even though this does not neatly match with global evangelical classifications or emerging scholarly distinctions (Anderson et al. 2010).
3. More research and sustained participant observation are necessary to understand variation in fasting practice.

References

Anderson, A., M. Bergunder, A. Droogers, and C. Van Der Laan. 2010. "Introduction." In *Global Pentecostalism: Theories and Methods*. Berkeley: University of California Press, 1–12.

Becker, A. E. 1995. *Body, Self and Society: The View from Fiji*. Philadelphia: University of Pennsylvania Press.

Besnier, N. 1995. *Literacy, Emotion and Authority: Reading and Writing on a Polynesian Atoll*. New York: Cambridge University Press.

Bielo, J. S. 2007. "'The Mind of Christ': Financial Success, Born-again Personhood, and the Anthropology of Christianity." *Ethnos* 72, no. 3: 315–338.

Brewis, A. 2010. *Obesity: Cultural and Biocultural Perspectives*. New Brunswick: Rutgers University Press.

Buitelaar, M. 1993. *Fasting and Feasting in Morocco: Women's Participation in Ramadan*. Oxford: Berg.

Bynum, C. W. 1987. *Holy Feast and Holy Fast: The Religious Significance of Food to Medieval Women*. Berkeley: University of California Press.

Codrington, R. H. 1915. "Melanesians." In *Encyclopedia of Religion and Ethics*, ed. J. Hastings. Edinburgh: T. and T. Clark, 529–538.

Coleman, S. 2000. *The Globalization of Charismatic Christianity: Spreading the Gospel of Prosperity*. Cambridge: Cambridge University Press.

Coleman, S., and P. Collins. 2000. "The 'Plain' and the 'Positive': Ritual, Experience, and Aesthetics in Quakerism and Charismatic Christianity." *Journal of Contemporary Religion* 15, no. 3: 317–329.

Durkheim, E. 2001. *The Elementary Forms of Religious Life*. Translated by Carol Cosman. New York: Oxford University Press.

Feely-Harnik, G. 1981. *The Lord's Table: The Meaning of Food in Early Judaism and Christianity*. Washington, DC: Smithsonian Books.

Firth, R. 1940. "The Analysis of Mana: An Empirical Approach." *Journal of Polynesian Society* 49 no. 196: 483–512.

Griffith, R. Marie. *Born Again Bodies: Flesh and Spirit in American Christianity*. Berkeley: University of California Press, 2004.

Hardin, J. "'God Is Your Health': Healing Metabolic Disorders in Samoa." In *Conflicts and Convergences: Critical Perspective on Christianity in Australia and the Pacific*, ed. C. Schwarz and F. Magowan: Brill, under review.

Hocart, A. M. 1922. "Mana Again." *Man* 22: 139–141.

Hollan, D. 1992. "Cross-cultural Differences in the Self." *Journal of Anthropological Research* 48, no. 4: 283–300.

Howes, D. 2003. "On the Pleasures of Fasting, Appearing, and Being Heard in the Massim World." In *Sensual Relations: Engaging the Senses in Culture and Social Theory,* Ann Arbor: University of Michigan Press.

Hunt, S. 2000. "'Winning Ways': Globalization and the Impact of the Health and Wealth Gospel." *Journal of Contemporary Religion* 15, no. 3: 331–347.

Klaits, F. 2010. *Death in a Church of Life: Moral Passion during Botswana's Time of AIDS.* Berkeley, Los Angeles, and London: University of California Press.

Lamb, S. 1997. "The Making and Unmaking of Persons: Notes on Aging and Gender in North India." *Ethos* 25: 279–302.

Lester, R. J. 2005. *Jesus in Our Wombs: Embodying Modernity in a Mexican Convent.* Berkeley: University of California Press.

McGarvey, S. T. 1995. "Thrifty Genotype Concepts and Health in Modernizing Samoans." *Asia Pacific Journal of Clinical Nutrition* 4: 351–353.

McIntosh, J. 2009. "Stance and Distance: Social Boundaries, Self-lamination, and Metalinguistic Anxiety in White Kenyan Narratives about the African Occult." In *Stance: Sociolinguistic Perspectives,* ed. A. M. Jaffe. Oxford: Oxford University Press, 72–91.

McMullin, J. 2010. *The Healthy Ancestor: Embodied Inequality and the Revitalization of Native Hawaiian Health.* Walnut Creek, CA: Left Coast Press.

Neel, J. V. 1962. "Diabetes Mellitus: A 'Thrifty' Genotypes Rendered Detrimental by 'Progress'?" *American Journal of Human Genetics* 14, no. 4: 353–362.

Pfeiffer, J. 2002. "African Independent Churches in Mozambique: Healing the Afflictions of Inequality." *Medical Anthropology Quarterly* 16: 176–199.

Pollock, N. 1992. *These Roots Remain: Food Habits in Islands of the Central and Eastern Pacific since Western Contact.* Laie: The Institute for Polynesian Studies.

———. 1995. "Cultural Elaborations of Obesity: Fattening Practices in Pacific Societies." *Asia Pacific Journal of Clinical Nutrition* 4: 357–360.

Sahlins, M. 1981. *Historical Metaphors and Mythical Realities: Structure in the Early History of the Sandwich Islands Kingdom.* Vol. No. 1, ASAO Special Publications. Ann Arbor: University of Michigan Press.

Schieffelin, B. B. 1990. *The Give and the Take of Everyday Life.* Cambridge: Cambridge University Press.

Schwarz, C. 2006. "Christianity, Identity, and Employment in an Aboriginal Settlement." *Ethnology* 45, no. 1: 71–86.

Shore, B. 1989. "Mana and Tapu." In *Developments in Polynesian Ethnology,* ed. A. Howard and R. Borofsky. Honolulu: University of Hawaii Press, 137–173.

Throop, C. J. 2010. *Suffering and Sentiment: Exploring the Vicissitudes of Experience and Pain in Yap.* Berkeley, Los Angeles, and London: University of California Press.

Tregear, E. 1904. *The Maori Race.* Warganvi: A. D. Willis.

WHO (World Health Organization). 2002. "Obesity in the Pacific: Too Big to Ignore." Paper presented at the Workshop on Obesity Prevention and Control Strategies in the Pacific, Apia.

Yates-Doerr, E. 2012. "The Weight of the Self: Care and Compassion in Guatemalan Dietary Choices." *Medical Anthropology Quarterly* 26, no. 1: 136–158.

Young, M. W., and W. E. H. Stanner. 1972. *Fighting with Food: Leadership, Values and Social Control in a Massim Society.* New York: Cambridge University Press.

Zigon, J. 2011. *HIV Is God's Blessing: Rehabilitating Morality in Neoliberal Russia.* Berkeley, Los Angeles, and London: University of California Press.

Zimmet, P. Z., D. J. McCarty, and M. P. de Courten. 1997. "The Global Epidemiology of Non-insulin Dependent Diabetes Mellitus and the Metabolic Syndrome." *Journal of Diabetes and Its Complications* 11: 60–68.

Acknowledgments

I need to thank many people for their help through the many stages of this project. This preliminary research has been supported by a Fulbright-Hays group project, a Mellon and Sachar Dissertation Grant, and the Women's and Gender Studies Graduate Student Grant from Brandeis University. An earlier draft of this chapter was presented at the American Anthropological Association meetings in Philadelphia, along with other chapters that form this volume. Before the AAA, a version of this chapter was presented at the National University of Samoa; comments from the Samoan Studies Department were extremely helpful. I would like to thank John Mayer, Samoan Studies faculty at the University of Hawaii-Manoa, Brian Alofaituli, Jackie Fa'asislia, Jessica Garlock, Silao Kasiano, Christina Kwauk, Leah Stucky, and Brent Vickers for their generous feedback on this project and translation assistance. I would also like to thank my doctoral committee Richard Parmentier, Sarah Lamb, and Elizabeth Ferry for their continued support. Special thanks to Megan McCullough and Hanna Garth for helpful comments on earlier drafts. *Muamua ona si'i le fa'afetai i le alofa o le Atua ua fa'aiu manuia ai lenei su'esu'ega. Fa'afetai fo'i i e na fesoasoani mai, aemaise lava ou aiga i Samoa fa'apea ali'i ma tamaitai faiaoga. A iai ni sese po o ni upu ua sasi, ia lafo i fogavaa.*

III

Cultures of Practice and Conflicting Interventions

CHAPTER **6**

Perspectives on Diabetes and Obesity from an Anthropologist in Behavioral Medicine

Lessons Learned from the "Diabetes Care in American Samoa" Project

Rochelle K. Rosen

✛ ✛ ✛

From 2006 to 2012 I was a co-investigator on a translational research project that adapted an existing diabetes self-management intervention based in the United States and implemented it in American Samoa. I am an anthropologist trained in behavioral medicine, and during the project I developed a strong appreciation for how anthropological perspectives on human health behavior can contribute to behavioral health research. This chapter articulates some of the tensions I perceive between my two disciplines. Anthropology and social science perspectives could, I argue, contribute more fully to behavioral medicine research generally. Furthermore, I will provide concrete suggestions as to how anthropology and social science can be crucial in shaping the effective development of models for health behavior change in collectivist or sociocentric cultural contexts.

"Diabetes Care in American Samoa"

"Diabetes Care in American Samoa" was an NIH-funded translational research grant testing the effectiveness of an intervention designed to help Samoan diabetes patients develop and maintain the self-management activities essential to living with this difficult chronic disease.[1] Results published elsewhere (DePue et al. 2013).

In this randomized controlled trial, participants received regular visits from a team of community health workers and a nurse case manager. The team counseled them about healthy diet and exercise behaviors and also helped them learn about diabetes, understand their medications, and make and keep related medical appointments (McGarvey 2009; DePue et al. 2010). Diabetes Care in American Samoa (DCAS) is an adaptation of Project Sugar 2, a successful diabetes intervention conducted with African-American patients in urban Baltimore, Maryland (Gary et al. 2004; Gary et al. 2005).

To translate that intervention for Samoans, the project first conducted formative qualitative work, including focus groups with diabetes patients to hear about their experiences living with, and getting care for, their illness. We also conducted individual interviews with clinic staff and providers about their experiences providing care to people with diabetes. As behavioral researchers are trained to do, we sought to identify the barriers and facilitators of diabetes care and identify effective local strategies for disease management with input from the local research staff of four community health workers and one nurse case manager; we created intervention materials and adapted protocols.

This formative research and analysis also prompted us to incorporate appropriate collectivistic cultural components to the materials and trainings we gave to the staff. For example, we emphasized the role of family and encouraged the staff to enlist family support during intervention visits by inviting all family members to participate in them. In addition we problem-solved with focus group participants about the dietary challenges they encountered at Samoan cultural occasions. We included quotes from the focus groups and interviews throughout the intervention materials; we sought to give those materials a local voice to make them appropriate and useful to participants (DePue et al. 2010).

The intervention focused on enabling staff members to support diabetes self-management in their patients. But since those formative focus groups and interviews were conducted and initially analyzed in 2007–2008, I have begun to question whether self-management, a common component of behavioral interventions, is the most effective way to approach Samoan health behavior. The anthropology of the Samoas, and other Pacific Island communities, suggests that the cultural construction of health extends beyond individual well-being to balance in one's social relationships (Capstick et al. 2009; Mishra et al. 2003; MacPherson and MacPherson 1990; Norris et al. 2009). Shared food consumption, along with informal and formal communal behaviors related to diverse domains—from religious congregations to village and extended family settings—are ways American Samoans create and maintain those relationships. Asking people to eat, move, and behave differently from others, even for health improvements, may put those relationships at risk.

Diabetes self-care requires intense individual-level behaviors and time management, which in turn may decrease available resources for culturally salient sociocentric or communal relationships that are the cornerstone of health for many Pacific peoples. While the steps of self-care are necessary for individual health, they may not be the most successful way to build an intervention in an environment where social health is as, or perhaps even more, important than physical health. Yet when I began to look for alternative models on which to build future interventions, I discovered a paucity of health behavior theories that allow researchers to look beyond individual or self-care for intervention design.

Background: Samoa and Diabetes

American Samoa is a U.S. territory, population 67,242 (CIA 2011), located in the South Pacific about halfway between Hawaii and New Zealand. The independent nation of Samoa is just to the west, and together they form an island chain populated by the same linguistic and ethnic group of native Pacific Islanders. American Samoa has been a U.S. territory since 1900. For much of this history the U.S. military maintained a significant presence on the island. Governors were U.S. Navy or U.S.-government appointed until 1977. American Samoans are U.S. nationals, and the territory's government derives a major portion of its annual budget from U.S. Department of Interior Grant-in-Aid and other federal grants. It is designated a "medically underserved" and "health professional shortage area" (HRSA 2010).

Before World War II, American Samoans worked primarily in subsistence farming and fishing. Diabetes, hypertension, and other noncommunicable diseases were rare. The increase in dietary intake and the reduction of physical activity that are hallmarks of the nutrition transition began after World War II and accelerated from 1970 to 2000 (Baker et al. 1986; McGarvey and Baker 1979; McGarvey et al. 1993; Galanis et al. 1999; Popkin and Gordon-Larsen 2004). As a result, noncommunicable disease risk factors and prevalence are rising in both adults and children (Keighley et al. 2006; Keighley et al. 2007; DiBello et al. 2009a; DiBello et al. 2009b; WHO 2007).

Type 2 diabetes has reached epidemic proportions: in 1990 its prevalence in twenty-five- to fifty-four-year-old men was 13 percent; by 2002 it had increased to 17 percent. Among women of the same age, the prevalence doubled from 8 percent in 1990 to 17 percent in 2002. Type 2 diabetes prevalence among all adults in 2002 was 22 percent in men and 18 percent in women (Keighley et al. 2007). More recent data are not available, but in 2007 the World Health Organization reported that 47 percent of the population had been told that they had diabetes in the twelve months before they were surveyed or had a fasting blood glucose $\geq$ 110 mg/dl—which the report identifies as one of the highest rates in the world (WHO 2007). For comparison, in 2011 the CDC identified 11 percent of the U.S. (mainland) adult population as having diabetes (CDC 2011) (The CDC's criteria for diagnosis in the United States is $\geq$ 126 mg/dl, pre-diabetes is considered 110–125 mg/dl.)

The levels of overweight and obesity have likewise risen and are extremely high in the territory. Between 1976 and 2002 body mass index (BMI) levels and the prevalence of obesity increased significantly among both men and women in American Samoa. In 1976–1978 McGarvey and colleagues found that 51 percent of women were obese. In 2002 71 percent of American Samoan women were obese and another 19 percent were overweight, leaving fewer than 10 percent of American Samoan women within the range of normal BMI. Among American Samoan men the prevalence of obesity rose from 28 percent in 1976–1978 to 61 percent in 2002 (Keighley et al. 2007; Keighley et al. 2006; McGarvey 1991).

In addition to the reductions in physical activity that come with a transition away from an agricultural economy, other factors are directly connected to these increases in obesity and its related diseases such as diabetes. Food choices have changed from a traditional plant and fish-based diet to one with a heavy reliance on highly processed imported foods, resulting in higher consumption of calories, protein, simple carbohydrates, cholesterol, sodium, and saturated fat (Galanis et al. 1999; DiBello et al. 2009b). Fast food consumption has also increased, and as of this writing the main American Samoan island of Tutuila has several fast food outlets, including two McDonald's. In 2011 the local franchises began advertizing a Samoan Burger: a Big Mac sandwich to which a fried egg is added (SamoaNews 2011). Although the fast-food franchises are a recent phenomenon, high-fat non-Samoan foods have been part of the island's diet since the early twentieth century, when tinned meats imported by U.S. servicemen became high-status items used in the reciprocal food exchanges that are essential to many cultural events (Galanis et al. 1999; DiBello et al. 2009b).

Exercise levels have dropped as the shift away from agricultural and subsistence labor eliminated a regular source of physical activity (Keighley et al. 2007; Keighley et al. 2006). Although epidemiological research is underway and may provide evidence for novel genetic influences, modernization, American culture, and other lifestyle changes in the last thirty to fifty years have all contributed to the epidemic levels of obesity and diabetes (McGarvey and Baker 1979; McGarvey 1991, 1994, 2001; Keighley et al. 2007).

Samoan Concepts of Health, Body Image and the Individual

Previous body image studies among Samoan adults have indicated an acceptance of large body size. Traditionally as well as in the recent past, a larger body size was seen as beautiful and correlated with social prestige (Brewis et al. 1998; Drozdow-St. Christian 2002; Shore 1998). More recent data, however, has suggested that this pattern is beginning to shift, perhaps influenced by the increase in obesity-related diseases. Brewis and colleagues have measured rates of obesity-related stigma in Samoa that are among the highest in the world (Brewis 2010 Brewis et al. 2011).

A variety of significant cultural barriers to healthy eating and health behavior change have been identified in the ethnographic and intervention literature of Pacific cultures. Many of these barriers were also raised by participants in our qualitative research. Food features prominently in cultural events in American Samoa, including *fa'alavelave*, required cultural gatherings for such life-cycle events as funerals, marriages, investitures of new chiefs, and the consecration of a new building. High calorie consumption also occurs at *to'ona'i*, weekly family- and village-based Sunday meals. Food at these cultural events was traditionally distributed according to status, with those of high status served first, making it particularly difficult to decline offered food (Braun et al. 2002). Fa'alavelave were identified as a source of stress by our participants, as well as in other research (Elstad et al. 2008), because they take time and require monetary contributions, sometimes making less money available for purchasing healthy food or for medical appointment and prescription co-payments. The requirement to contribute money to them is absolute, for if a household fails to make the required contribution, "this is taken as a sign of their withdrawal from the family or village circle. The threat is actually an eviction order" (Tcherkézoff 2008).

Fa'alavelave and to'ona'i are also challenging from the perspective of health behavior change for diabetes patients. Some of our participants indicated that these events relied heavily on meat, including pigs and canned or tinned meat, both of which have a very high fat content. Many of the providers we interviewed suggested strategies for healthy eating at these events, including eating traditional items like banana, taro, or vegetables with smaller portions of meat, yet acknowledged that this could be difficult.

Deeper cultural concepts contribute to the challenge of changing food-related health behavior. In adapting diabetes messages to the Pacific, Braun et al. observed that people had some difficulty eating in a manner different from others. There was also a belief that food is a gift that should not be refused and that feasting is an important part of the culture that cannot be altered (Braun et al. 2002). Shovic also identified related cultural attitudes about food, including its especially important role at social functions. Family activities and ceremonies center on eating, often to an excess; large quantities of food provided by the host family signified their prosperity, and guests are expected to eat lest they offend the hosts. Jessica Hardin's work highlights many related and relevant concerns about body size and the Samoan cultural ideology in which eating together and sharing food creates and sustains social relationships. In particular, the eating of heavy Samoan foods is phenomenologically connected to key concepts in *fa'asamoa* (the Samoan cultural way of life) including *fa'aaloalo* and *alofa* ("respect" and "love") (Hardin, this volume).

Writing in 1994, Shovic observed a heavy reliance on imported food products, including canned meat, fruit in heavy syrup, processed foods, and foods with a high sugar content (Shovic 1994). Recent research shows that this reliance on processed and imported foods continues in the region. Deborah Gewertz and Frederick Errington document the presence of inexpensive, poor-quality, and very high fat cuts of meat like lamb flaps and turkey tails, which are byproducts of industrial meat processing in New Zealand that are regularly imported to American Samoa and other Pacific cultures as a source of inexpensive, but high-fat, protein (Gewertz and Errington 2011).

The idea that American Samoans consume large amounts of food was expressed often enough in our qualitative data that it evolved into a code, which I titled simply "Samoans eat a lot of food." Over and over, clinicians and diabetes patient said some version of that phrase, so that it almost seemed to be part of their cultural identity; both an admitted problem, yet also a source of pride. The latter perhaps explains why a McDonald's advertisement touts the Mega Burger with its "extra meat patties at no cost" (SamoaNews 2010): it's a selling point to name a sandwich with added fat and protein as especially Samoan.

Other themes intermix with this notion of food consumption. One was that although previous generations may have also eaten heartily, they did not have diabetes—because they ate differently, moved more, or didn't eat *palagi* (European/white people) food. Throughout our discussions of food behavior and choices, many of the diabetes patients also showed a clear understanding that some foods are unhealthy and that they knew that overconsumption is directly related to diabetes. For example:

> The life of a Samoan, like I said, it's all about food; yeah people just eat so much food. There were no disease like this [in] those days, but now, we have this disease called diabetes. Since the doctors have researched, and from what I understand it is thought that food is another cause of this disease. But from our ancestor's time, I don't know about the other fathers that are here tonight, but the truth is there was no disease like ... diabetes [in] those days. Life went on, but nowadays there are changes. Diabetes has become common, as well as high blood pressure. This is why food is so bad. ...

The mix of identity, frustration, and pride about the consumption of large amounts of food in our qualitative data echoes what Drozdow-St. Christian wrote in his ethnography of health in (Western) Samoa:

> Samoans are remarkable eaters. They can consume monumental amounts of food every day. The food is heavy in starches, such as taro and rice, and also has a high fat content because so many dishes are prepared using beef tallow. At the same time, as a person matures into their 40s they are expected to do less and

less physical labour. The normative status which attaches to maturity means that middle-aged Samoans supervise manual labour, rather than participate directly in it. A combination of an increasingly sedentary lifestyle and a high fat, high carbohydrate diet, results in mid-life obesity in almost all Samoans (Drozdow-St. Christian 2002).

This ethnographer described the Samoan body type as a large and imposing physical presence: "a combination of mass, strength and stillness" (Drozdow-St. Christian 2002) in which adult weight gain accompanies the increase in dignity and status that occurs as Samoans age (Drozdow-St. Christian 2002; Shore 1998). Like food consumption, attitudes about physical activity are also shaped by cultural values. Elders, who hold power in this status-based gerontocracy, traditionally did not have high activity levels: "The Samoan view of age accords the diminished physical powers of the elderly a kind of cultural respectability in terms of an ideology of power that valorized passivity and inactivity" (Shore 1998). In this analysis, power comes, in part, from inactivity and from having the status to have other people move on your behalf. This concept, too, was articulated in our qualitative data:

> See we have a custom here, if you are married and have kids you stay home. You don't walk. Period. And you may walk to church but they laugh at you they [say] 'oh, that [is] for the kids' [because] the kids are the ones that go play. If you are married and you are an adult you are not supposed to do those things. It is believed that you should stay at home. They look at you in a very funny way, especially the older ones. They say 'what is this old man doing?' But now they are realizing there is a lot of benefits and lot of older folks are walking. Before you [would] never see an older man or woman walk.

In these comments we see traditional concepts about food and exercise changing, perhaps brought about by the very high rates of obesity and noncommunicable diseases like diabetes.

Examining Communalism and Collectivism

As challenging as all of these barriers to health behavior changes are, there is another element that I overlooked in the initial analysis of our data: little consideration has been paid to how the communal nature of this Polynesian culture has driven health behavior management. Anthropologists eschew the application of such global terms as *collectivistic* and *individualistic* because they are overbroad and indistinct. I, as an anthropologist myself, find it problematic—and even against the spirit of relativism—to apply broad generalizations to any particular culture or group of people. Yet these global concepts are often used in behavioral medicine, and I recognize that to participate in global public health debate and effective intervention design, we need to find language, as well as models and theories, that work in both arenas.

Within the Samoan belief system, health is communal. In this understanding, social well-being is essential to physical well being (Pollack 1992). Health is developed by several factors: being spiritually healthy, morally healthy, and in balanced social and interpersonal relationships (Capstick et al. 2009; Mishra et al. 2003; MacPherson and MacPherson 1990; Norris et al. 2009; Sobralske 2006; Hardin, this volume). When the cultural construction of health includes social relationships, individuals are not physically healthy if social relationships and requirements are not met first, and one of the ways those relationships are maintained is by eating together in a culturally relevant way.

In collectivistic cultures such as Samoa, individual goals are subordinate to those of the collective (Triandis et al. 1988), whereas in individualistic societies people define themselves according to how they are different from others, seeing the self as a set of unique internal attributes. In collectivistic cultures the self is defined according to how people are similar to, and fit in with, the larger group. The collectivistic self emphasizes status, social role, and relationships; belonging and fitting in; occupying one's proper place; engaging in appropriate action; and being indirect in communication (Shore 1982; Poasa et al. 2000). Anthropologists make a similar distinction between sociocentric and egocentric cultures (Geertz 1974) in which the Samoan self is clearly sociocentric (Mageo 1998). That self has been described as being relational, a part of an interconnected family and community, and specifically a self that is not an isolated or independent individual (Capstick et al. 2009; Hardin, this volume; Norris et al. 2009; Pollack 1992).

In behavioral and public health, we know little about how or why collectivism facilitates positive or negative health behaviors, yet some research suggests that being a member of collectivistic societies amidst modernization does in fact confer both health and well-being advantages via social support (Hanna 1998; Janes 1990a, 1990b). This raises the question of how we might harness the positive aspects of such social structures while managing negative influences on health behavior choices.

Theory and the Self in Behavioral Medicine

Diabetes is a particularly salient illness for this challenge precisely because living with it is so complex. Patients need to take medication, lose weight, change their eating habits, increase their physical activity, and monitor blood glucose levels to prevent complications such as neuropathy, retinopathy, nephropathy, cardiovascular disease, and amputations. These lifestyle changes are particularly challenging when family and cultural norms differ from the structured regimes that good diabetes control requires. In its early stages diabetes has few symptoms, so the complexity and burden of the recommended behavioral changes may actually seem worse than the disease or its complications (Wing et al. 2001). Our intervention was specifically designed to teach participants the complex self-management skills needed, and we know that understanding blood glucose changes, medication taking, and healthy food choices were challenging for many of our participants.

Diabetes Self-Management Education (DSME) seeks to support patients in acquiring the knowledge and skills to change unhealthy behaviors and to live with diabetes. DSME was introduced in the 1940s (Ford 1949; Osborne and Fisher 2008) and has become a dominant treatment paradigm. While diabetes has increased in disproportionately high rates in ethnic minority communities, DSME programs have been criticized for using a "one size fits all" approach developed for use with white populations (Osborne and Fisher 2008). The very behaviors that people with diabetes most need to change are those that are abundant in cultural meaning: eating, sharing food, moving, and attitudes about the body. Diabetes care programs need to address these cultural values, and some interventions do so (Sarkisian et al. 2003). Yet many still follow the principles of DSME, in which the self is centric and which is therefore an individualistic paradigm.

Increasingly, researchers are calling for behavioral interventions that begin with an understanding of population-specific attitudes and barriers to self-management behaviors and that are informed by health behavior change theory (Glazer et al. 2006; Osborne and Fisher 2008; Sarkisian et al. 2003). Behavior change theories and models identify methods for supporting healthy behaviors and amending unhealthy ones. Behavioral scientists have emphasized the importance of using health behavior change theories to design interventions because those that do are more effective (Painter et al. 2008; Rothman 2004). Yet these theories focus on how individual cognitions and perceptions affect health behavior change. Interventions for collectivist cultures require theories that incorporate social and contextual factors. Tamasese and colleagues have observed: "The Samoan self ... is a relational self. ... [I]t cannot be assumed that developmental theories, therapeutic interventions and mental health service practices that have evolved in cultures with individual concepts of self, will necessarily be relevant for people from collective based cultures" (Tamasese et al. 2005). We attempted to address these concerns by including family members in diabetes teaching provided by our staff to program participants. We also chose a model for the intervention that allowed us to include community perspectives in adaptation, implementation and evaluation.

In a recent systematic review of the use of theory in health behavior research, Painter and colleagues found that from 2000 to 2005, three-quarters of the articles using theory employed either individual- or interpersonal-level theories. Only one-quarter used community-based or multi-level theories such as the Socio-Ecological and Precede-Proceed models. The authors note that "the relative absence of applied community-level theory in the literature is surprising" (Painter et al. 2008). Our own study uses the Precede-Proceed model (DePue et al. 2010), and in a review article Kevin Cassel used the social-ecological model as a framework to understand obesogenic factors among Samoan populations (Cassel 2010).

Anthropology distinguishes between *emic* and *etic* approaches to culture, wherein the former seeks to understand categories of thought and behavior from within the cultural participants' point of view and the latter from a scientific or external perspective, allowing understanding of social and cultural structures that an insider might not see (Barrett 1984). These terms and perspectives are, however, not common in behavioral medicine. When, in behavioral medicine, interventions target barriers and facilitators to good health behavior or to health behavior change, those behaviors are being approached from what an anthropologist would term an etic perspective. Thus in Samoa, traditional attitudes about body size, inactivity in older adults, and frequent food-rich cultural events could be understood, as I initially saw them, as barriers to health and among the causes of obesity and its related diseases. But from an emic perspective these very same behaviors provide fulfilling opportunities to create and maintain social relationships in a culturally appropriate way—which in turn promotes well-being and health. Clearly we need both perspectives, and truly translational research cannot proceed without them. Anthropologists are particularly well placed to provide insights needed to balance cultural and evidence-based perspectives.

Anthropological Contributions to Culturally Salient Diabetes Care

In 2006 Mariana Leal Ferreira and Gretchen Chesley Lang edited a volume dedicated to community responses to the high prevalence rates of diabetes in many indigenous peoples (Ferreira and Lang 2006). In that volume, Dennis Wiedman considers the specific contributions of medical anthropologists to diabetes research, noting they have been researching, publishing and giving conference presentations on diabetes since the 1970s, and that native communities in Canada, the United States, and the Pacific have received particular attention (Weidman 2006). Anthropologists have argued that diabetes and other noncommunicable illnesses are diseases of civilization because of their strong association with modernization and the transition to processed food (c.f. Brewis 2010; Ferreira and Lang 2006; McGarvey and Baker 1979; McGarvey 1991, 2001; Weidman 2006).

Wiedman notes that because the breadth of the anthropological perspective incorporates everything from genetics to system-wide structures, it is well suited to understanding how much the environment and culture contribute to human development. He suggests four specific areas to which anthropological contributions are particularly appropriate: (1) providing groups and leaders with relevant knowledge of environmental and cultural dynamics, (2) influencing healthy food choices within communities, (3) enhancing activity levels with exercise facilities and transportation system design, and (4) influencing health and food policies (Weidman 2006). In this chapter I have argued that there is another place where an anthropological perspective specifically, and a social science perspective more broadly, is particularly needed: the design and implementation of translational behavioral research and the development of theories in behavioral medicine that incorporate culture in a way that respects sociocentric dynamics around health.

Ways Forward: Anthropology and Cultural Models of Diabetes Care

Many anthropologists have identified specific cultural models of diabetes. Rebecca Hagey and Linda Garro each worked in Canada with the Anishinaabe/Ojibway, Chippewa and Cree first nations (Garro 1995; Hagey 1984, 1989). They identified different cultural models of illness and native explanations essential for understanding diabetes, including that it is a form of sickness unknown prior to European contact, an observation that resonates with the comments of participants in our project. Their work incorporated appropriate cultural metaphors and used relevant means of communication, including dancing, drumming and ceremonies, in diabetes intervention. Many other anthropologists have worked within specific communities and the health care setting to ensure the delivery of culturally appropriate medical care (Ferzacca 2000; Hunt et al. 1998; Hunt and Arar 2001). They have documented the use of allopathic and traditional medicine (Hunt et al. 2000) and the effects of stress and acculturation (Dressler et al. 1996; Scheder 2006[1988]), they have identified local understandings of care provision within the context of a demand-sharing economy (Dussart 2009), and they have influenced policy development and intervention design (Ritenbaugh et al. 2003).

These anthropologically informed projects, along with our diabetes intervention in American Samoa, illustrate how to effectively incorporate local or native perspectives and knowledge. But they have not yet fully influenced the theories of health behavior change and behavioral medicine, which continue to focus heavily on individual self-care and individual behavior change rather than on culture, community, and environment. To be fair, there are such theories as the Social Ecological Model and the Precede-Proceed approach that focus on the individual in the culture and environment. But as I discovered in the Diabetes Care in American Samoa project, we need to go beyond these models to fully connect to collectivistic cultures (see Rosen et al, forthcoming).

Recently there has been an encouraging increase in efforts to include culturally relevant perspectives into behavioral theory and interventions. In 2009 the journal *Health Education and Behavior* published an entire special issue on behavioral theory and culture. Two perspectives may be particularly relevant for future research that incorporates culturally informed theory development and intervention design, especially among Polynesian populations: community-based participatory research (also called community engaged scholarship), and research that incorporates social network theory. Our own work has recently begun to inquire into the perspectives of participants, providers and staff about self-management support used in the diabetes care in American Samoa intervention. These perspectives will increase the relevance of translational behavioral research.

Where health is communal, interventions predicated on individual self-care may fail to help. To view culturally informed behaviors as a barrier or facilitator of self-care misses the very point of those behaviors and the motivations that lead people to continue them. Until we can access those behaviors from the emic perspective of the people who engage in them, we cannot hope to alter them or find culturally appropriate solutions to them. Anthropologists and other social scientists should address the absence of relevant, community-level, even community-specific, theories so we create behavioral interventions that are not just translated to new environments, but effectively created for them.

Notes

1. This project was funded by NIDDK grant number 5 R18 DK075371-03. Stephen T. McGarvey, Ph.D., MPH, was the principle investigator. Co-investigators include Judith D. DePue, EdD, MPH, Rochelle K. Rosen, Ph.D., John Tuitele, MBBS, MS, and Michael G. Goldstein, MD.

References

Baker, P.T., J. M. Hanna, and T. S. Baker. 1986. *The Changing Samoans: Behavior and Health in Transition.* New York: Oxford University Press

Barrett, R. A. 1984. *Culture and Conduct: An Excursion in Anthropology.* Belmont, CA: Wadsworth Publishing Company.

Braun, K. L., R. L. Kuhaulua, H. M. Ichiho, and N. T. Aitaoto. 2002. "Listening to the Community: A First Step in Adapting Diabetes Today to the Pacific." *Pacific Health Dialogue* 9: 321–328.

Brewis, A. 2010. *Obesity: Cultural and Biocultural Perspectives.* New Brunswick: Rutgers University Press.

Brewis, A. A., S. T. McGarvey, J. Jones, and B. A. Swinburn. 1998. "Perceptions of Body Size in Pacific Islanders." *International Journal of Obesity* 22, no. 2: 185–189.

Brewis, A. A., A. Wutich, A. Falletta-Cowden, and I. Rodrigues-Soto. 2011. "Body Norms and Fat Stigma in Global Perspective." *Current Anthropology* 52, no. 2: 269–276.

Capstick, S., P. Norris, F. Sopoaga, and W. Tobata. 2009. "Relationships between Health and Culture in Polynesia—A Review." *Social Science and Medicine* 68: 1341–1348.

Cassel, K. D. 2010. "Using the Social-ecological Model as a Research and Intervention Framework to Understand and Mitigate Obesogenic Factors in Samoan Populations." *Ethnicity and Health* 15, no. 4: 397–416.

CDC. 2011. "National Diabetes Fact Sheet: National Estimates and General Information on Diabetes and Prediabetes in the United States." U.S. Department of Health and Human Services, available at http://www.cdc.gov/diabetes/pubs/pdf/ndfs_2011.pdf.

CIA. 2011. "CIA World Factbook: American Samoa." Available at https://www.cia.gov/library/publications/the-world-factbook/geos/aq.html, accessed July 19, 2011.

DePue, J., R. K. Rosen, M. Batts-Turner, N. Bereolos, M. House, R. F. Held, O. Nu'usolia, J. Tuitele, M. G. Goldstein, and S. T. McGarvey. 2010. "Cultural Translation of Interventions: Diabetes Care in American Samoa." *American Journal of Public Health* 11: 2085–2093.

DePue, J., S. Dunsiger, A. D. Seiden, J. Blume, R. K. Rosen, M. G. Goldsein, O. Nu'usolia, J. Tuitele, and S. T. McGarvey. 2013. "Nurse-Community Health Worker Team Improves Diabetes Care in American Samoa: Results of a Randomized Controlled Trial." *Diabetes Care* 36: 1947–1953.

DiBello, J. R., A. Baylin, S. Viali, J. Tuitele, L. Bausserman, and S. T. McGarvey. 2009a. "Adiponectin and Type 2 Diabetes in Samoan Adults." *American Journal of Human Biology* 21: 389–391.

DiBello, J. R., S. T. McGarvey, P. Kraft, R. Goldberg, H. Campos, C. Quested, T. S. Lauloli, and A. Baylin. 2009b. "Dietary Patterns are Associated with Metabolic Syndrome in Adult Samoans." *Journal of Nutritional Epidemiology* 139: 1922–1943.

Dressler, W. W., J. R. Bindon, and M. J. Gilliland. 1996. "Sociocultural and Behavioral Influences on Health Status among the Mississippi Choctow." *Medical Anthropology* 17, no. 2: 165–180.

Drozdow-St. Christian, D. 2002. *Elusive Fragments: Making Power, Propriety, and Health in Samoa.* Durham, NC: Carolina Academic Press.

Dussart, F. 2009. "Diet, Diabetes and Relatedness in a Central Australian Aboriginal Settlement: Some Qualitative Recommendations to Facilitate the Creation of Culturally Sensitive Health Promotion Initiatives." *Health Promotion Journal of Australia* 20, no. 5: 202–206.

Elstad, E., C. Tusiofo, R. K. Rosen, and S. T. McGarvey. 2008. "Living with Ma'i Suka: Individual, Familial, Cultural, and Environmental Stress among Patients with Type 2 Diabetes Mellitus and Their Caregivers in American Samoa." *Preventing Chronic Disease* 5, no. 3.

Ferreira, M. L., and G. C. Lang, eds. 2006. *Indigenous Peoples and Diabetes.* Carolina Academic Press Medical Anthropology Series, ed. P. J. Stewart and A. Strathern. Durham: Carolina Academic Press.

Ferzacca, S. 2000. "'Actually, I Don't Feel that Bad': Managing Diabetes and the Clinical Encounter." *Medical Anthropology Quarterly* 14, no. 1: 28–50.

Ford, M. J. 1949. "Diabetic Patient Education." *Public Health Nursing* 41: 527–530.

Galanis, D. J., S. T. McGarvey, C. Quested, B. Sio, and S. Afele-Fa'amuli. 1999. "Dietary Intake among Modernizing Samoans: Implications for Risk of Cardiovascular Disease." *Journal of the American Dietetics Association* 99, 184–190.

Garro, L. C. 1995. "Individual or Societal Responsibility? Explanations of Diabetes in an An-ishinaabe Ojibway Community." *Social Science and Medicine* 40, no. 1: 37–46.

Gary, T. L., M. Batts-Turner, L. R. Bone, H. C. Yeh, N. Y. Wang, F. Hill-Briggs, D. M. Levine, N. R. Powe, M. N. Hill, C. Saudek, M. McGuire, and F. L. Brancati. 2004. "A Random-ized Clinical Trial of the Effects of Nurse Case Manager and Community Health Worker Team Interventions in Urban African Americans with Type 2 Diabetes." *Controlled Clini-cal Trials* 25: 53–66.

Gary, T .L., F. Hill-Briggs, M. Batts-Turner, and F. L. Brancati. 2005. "Translational Research Principles of an Effectiveness Trial for Diabetes Care in an Urban African American Popu-lation." *Diabetes Educator* 31: 880–889.

Geertz, C. 1974. *The Interpretation of Cultures.* New York: Basic Books.

Gewertz, D., and F. Errington. 2011. *Cheap Meat: Flap Food Nations in the Pacific Islands.* Berkeley: University of California Press.

Glazer, R. H., J. Bajcat, N. R. Kennie, and K. Wilson. 2006. "A Systematic Review of Inter-ventions to Improve Diabetes Care in Socially Disadvantaged Populations." *Diabetes Care* 29: 1675–1688.

Hagey, R. 1984. "The Phenomenon, the Explanations and the Responses: Metaphors Sur-rounding Diabetes in Urban Canadian Indians." *Social Science and Medicine* 18, no. 3: 265–272.

———. 1989. "The Native Diabetes Program: Rhetorical Process and Praxis." *Medical Anthro-pology* 12, no. 1: 7–33.

Hanna, J. M. 1998. "Migration and Acculturation among Samoans: Some Sources of Stress and Support." *Social Science and Medicine* 46, no. 10: 1325–1336.

HRSA. 2010. "Shortage Areas." Health Research Services Administration.

Hunt, L., and N. H. Arar. 2001. "An Analytical Framework for Contrasting Patient and Provider Views of the Process of Chronic Diabetes Management." *Medical Anthropology Quarterly* 15, no. 3: 347–367.

Hunt, L., N. H. Arar, and L. L. Akana. 2000. "Herbs, Prayer, and Insulin: Use of Medical and Alternative Treatments by a Group of Mexican American Diabetes Patients." *Journal of Family Practice* 49, no. 3: 216–223.

Hunt, L., N. H. Arar, and A. C. Larma. 1998. "Contrasting Patient and Practitioner Perspec-tives in Type 2 Diabetes Management." *Western Journal of Nursing Research* 20, no. 6: 657–682.

Janes, C. R. 1990a. *Migration, Social Change and Health.* Stanford: Stanford University Press.

———. 1990b. "Migration, Changing Gender Roles and Stress: The Samoan Case." *Medical Anthropology* 12: 217–248.

Keighley, E. D., S. T. McGarvey, C. Quested, C. McCuddin, S. Viali, and U. A. Maga. 2007. "Nutrition and Health in Modernizing Samoans: Temporal Trends and Adaptive Perspec-tives." In *Health Change in the Asia-Pacific Region: Biocultural and Epidemiological Ap-proaches,* eds. R. Ohtsuka and S. J. Ulijaszek. Cambridge: Cambridge University Press, 147–191.

Keighley, E. D., S. T. McGarvey, P. Turituri, and S. Viali. 2006. "Farming and Adiposity in Samoan Adults." *American Journal of Human Biology* 18: 12–121.

MacPherson, C., and L. MacPherson. 1990. *Samoan Medical Belief and Practice.* Auckland: Auckland University Press.

Mageo, J. M. 1998. *Theorizing Self in Samoa: Emotions, Genders and Sexualities.* Ann Arbor: University of Michigan Press.

McGarvey, S. T. 1991. "Obesity in Samoans and a Perspective on its Etiology in Polynesians." *American Journal of Clinical Nutrition* 53: 1586S–1594S.

———. 1994. "The Thrifty Gene Concept and Adiposity Studies in Biological Anthropology." *Journal of the Polynesian Society* 103: 29–42.

———. 2001. "Cardiovascular Disease (CVD) Risk Factors in Samoa and American Samoa, 1990–95." *Pacific Health Dialogue* 8, no. 1: 157–162.

———. 2009 "Interdisciplinary Translation Research in Anthropology, Nutrition and Public Health." *Annual Review of Anthropology* 38: 233–249.

McGarvey, S. T., and P. T. Baker. 1979. "The Effects of Modernization and Migration on Samoan Blood Pressure." *Human Biology* 51: 461–479.

McGarvey, S. T., P. D. Levinson, L. Bausserman, D. J. Galanis, and C. A. Hornick. 1993. "Population Change in Adult Obesity and Blood Lipids in American Samoa from 1976–78 to 1990." *American Journal of Human Biology* 5: 17–30.

Mishra, S. I., J. Hess, and P. H. Luce. 2003. "Predictors of Indigenous Healer Use among Samoans." *Alternative Therapies* 9, no. 6: 64–69.

Norris, P., F. Fa'alau, C. Va'ai, M. Churchward, and B. Arrol. 2009. "Navigating between Illness Paradigms: Treatment Seeking by Samoan People in Samoa and New Zealand." *Qualitative Health Research* 19, no. 10: 1466–1475.

Osborne, C. Y., and J. Fisher. 2008. "Diabetes Education: Integrating Theory, Cultural Considerations, and Individually Tailored Content." *Clinical Diabetes* 26, no. 4: 148–150.

Painter, J. E., C. P. C. Borba, M. Hynes, D. May, and K. Glanz. 2008. "The Use of Theory in Health Behavior Research from 2000–2005: A Systematic Review." *Annals of Behavior Medicine* 35, no. 3: 358–362.

Poasa, K. H., B. Mallinckrodt, and L. Suzuki. 2000. "Causal Attributions for Problematic Family Interactions: A Qualitative, Cultural Comparison of Western Samoa, American Samoa, and the United States." *Counseling Psychologist* 28, no. 1: 32–60.

Pollack, N. 1992. *These Roots Remain: Food Habits in Islands of the Central and Eastern Pacific since Western Contact.* Laie: The Institute for Polynesian Studies.

Popkin, B. M., and P. Gordon-Larsen. 2004. "The Nutrition Transition: Worldwide Obesity Dynamics and Their Determinants." *International Journal of Obesity* 28, Suppl 3: S2–9.

Ritenbaugh, C., T. I. Teufel-Shone, M. G. Aickin, J. R. Joe, S. Poirier, C. Dillingham, D. Johnson, S. Henning, S. M. Cole, and D. Cockerham. 2003. "A Lifestyle Intervention Improves Plasma Insulin Levels among Native American High School Youth." *Preventative Medicine* 36, no. 3: 309–319.

Rothman, A. J. 2004. "'Is There Nothing More Practical than a Good Theory?' Why Innovations and Advances in Health Behavior Change Will Arise if Interventions Are Used to Test and Refine Theory." *International Journal of Behavioral Nutrition and Physical Activity* 1, no. 11: 11.

SamoaNews. 2010. *Samoa News,* 15 November, 9.

———. 2011. *Samoa News,* 23 March, 8.

Sarkisian, C. A., A. F. Brown, K. C. Norris, R. L. Wintz, and C. M. Mangione. 2003. "A Systematic Review of Diabetes Self-care Interventions for Older, African-American or Latino Adults." *Diabetes Educator* 29, no. 3: 467–479.

Scheder, Jo. 2006 [1988]. "A Sickly-sweet Harvest: Farmworker Diabetes and Social Inequality." In *Indigenous Peoples and Diabetes: Community Empowerment and Wellness*, M. L. Ferreira and G. C. Lang. Durham, NC: Carolina Academic Press.

Shore, B. 1982. *Sala'ilua: A Samoan Mystery.* New York: Columbia University Press, 1982.

———. 1998. "The Coming of Aging in Samoa." In *Welcome to Middle Age,* ed. R. Shweder. Chicago: University of Chicago Press, 101–137.

Shovic, A. C. 1994. "Development of a Samoan Nutrition Exchange List Using Culturally Accepted Foods." *Journal of the American Dietetics Association* 94, no. 5: 541–543.

Sobralske, M. 2006. "Olakino Maika'i: Health Care in Pacific Island Culture." *Journal of the American Academy of Nurse Practitioners* 18: 81–82.

Tamasese, K., C. Peteru, C. Waldegrave, and A. Bush. 2005. "Ole Taeao Afua, the New Morning: A Qualitative Investigation into Samoan Perspectives on Mental Health and Culturally Appropriate Services." *Australian and New Zealand Journal of Psychiatry* 39: 300–309.

Tcherkézoff, S. 2008. *'First Contacts' in Polynesia: The Samoan Case (1722-1848) Western Misunderstandings about Sexuality and Divinity.* Canberra: Australian National University Press.

Triandis, H. C., H. Bontempo, M. J. Villareal, M. Asai, and N. Lucca. 1988. "Individualism and Collectivism: Cross-cultural Perspectives on Self-ingroup Relationships." *Journal of Personality and Social Psychology* 54, no. 2: 323–338.

Weidman, D. 2006. "Striving for Healthy Lifestyles: Contributions of Anthropologists to the Challenge of Diabetes in Indigenous Communities." In *Indigenous Peoples and Diabetes: Community Empowerment and Wellness,* ed. M. L. Ferreira and G. C. Lang. Durham, NC: Carolina Academic Press, 511–534.

WHO (World Health Organization). 2007. *American Samoa NCD Risk Factors STEPS Report.* World Health Organization and American Samoa Government.

Wing, R. R., M. G. Goldstein, K. J. Acton, L. L. Birch, J. M. Jakicic, J. F. Sallis, D. Smith-West, R. W. Jeffery, and R. S. Surwit. 2001. "Behavioral Science Research in Diabetes: Lifestyle Changes Related to Obesity, Eating Behavior, and Physical Activity." *Diabetes Care* 24, no. 1: 117–123.

Acknowledgments

I extend a hearty thanks to my co-investigators on the Diabetes Care in Samoa Project, especially to PI Stephen McGarvey and to Judy DePue, as well as to Michael G. Goldstein, Kelley Smith, John Tuitele, and Nicole Bereolos. I am grateful to our staff and CHWs in American Samoa as well as the participants in the project, who so graciously shared their experiences and rich cultural knowledge. Special thanks to Megan McCullough and Jessica Hardin for their leadership in organizing the session on obesity at the American Anthropological Association, and for their thoughtful editorship of this volume.

CHAPTER 7

Body Image and Weight Concerns among Emirati Women in the United Arab Emirates

Sarah Trainer

✛ ✛ ✛

Much has been written in the last half century, both in scholarly and popular literature, about obesity—as a public health concern, as an individual health concern, and as an example of development gone awry. Obesity has also been understood as a source of body image dissatisfaction, as a sign of social status or disadvantage, and as an indicator of a body under stress. Despite its popularity as a topic (or perhaps because of it), many issues relating to obesity remain uninterrogated and underexplored. This volume seeks to explore these underexplored questions, to problematize commonly held assumptions regarding weight and health, and to introduce new perspectives on the purported problem that obesity presents in the world today by providing case studies and narratives rooted in local specificities. As Becker (this volume) points out, obesity and overweight are dramatically increasing worldwide, with undeniable implications for the health of an increasingly diverse array of communities and groups, at the same time that popular and medical preoccupation with fatness and fat people has intensified. In the midst of all of this noise, many assumptions go unchallenged (or less challenged), beginning with "the presupposition that health can be located in the metrics of body size" (Yates-Doerr, this volume). Additional myopic perspectives that stress the role of individual lifestyle and agency in weight gain remain unquestioned while neglecting larger structural forces at work. Casual but widespread stigmatization of large body size continues to inform assumptions—both popular and medical—of an essentialized "fat body," one that takes in too many calories and expends too few in exercise. In this chapter, therefore, I examine some of these assumptions by delving into the very particular experiences of a specific population, but also by situating this case study within larger patterns and structural influences.

This chapter explores issues relating to fatness and thinness in the United Arab Emirates (UAE), in the Arab Gulf (Al Khaleej). Using biological data, as well as data gathered on the attitudes, ideas, and concerns Emirati women expressed about health and body image, I locate this information within the larger context in which these young Emirati women are embedded. This chapter localizes and contextualizes the nutrition transition occurring in the UAE as the state experiences an accelerated but patchy modernity, as well as notes how significant gender and age are in this nutrition transition. As a medical and biocultural anthropologist, I bring the perspectives and methods of both these disciplines to bear on the often unproblematized discussions and activities taking place in the UAE with respect to the obesity epidemic on the one hand and the concerns with weight, beauty, and the body expressed by local women on the other. These concerns are particularly important in light of the fact that emic perspectives on and from Emirati women represent an underexplored area in the anthropological and public health literature (see Bristol-Rhys 2010, 2009, 2007 for an important exception).

Theoretical Background

I begin with the concept of the nutrition transition (and the closely linked but not interchangeable health transition), drawing on the literature focusing on changing patterns of disease in the world today, a shift that is also linked to increases in overweight and obesity within and across populations, both of which are in turn associated with systemic changes in food consumption patterns. There is a prolific epidemiological and public health–oriented body of literature on these topics (including Brownell and Yach 2006; Cassels 2006; Hawkes 2006; Popkin 2011, 2009, 1999; WHO 2009, 2008; WHO-EMRO 2011, 2007, 2003), but anthropologists, including Carol Worthman (Worthman and Kohrt 2005) and Andrea Wiley (2007a, 2007b), have also weighed in, as have increasing numbers of human biologists (e.g. Brewis 2012; Wells 2012). I mention this literature at the outset because I think it is important, in a volume that aims to critique the current state of obesity research, to highlight the fact that however much we may critique moralistic overtones in the literature (McNaughton, this volume), we are nonetheless experiencing a profound shift in average weights and epidemiologies in societies across the world today.

In the region the World Health Organization designates as the Eastern Mediterranean (WHO-EMRO), 52 percent of deaths were due to chronic diseases in the last estimate made by that organization.[1] Furthermore, overweight rates for men (thirty-plus years) in the WHO-EMRO Region are 42 percent and for women (thirty-plus years) have risen to 54 percent (WHO 2011a, 2011b). Of course, the countries that make up the WHO-EMRO range from Egypt to Afghanistan to Saudi Arabia and thus are extremely diverse economically, politically, socially, religiously, linguistically, etc.; this makes generalizations problematic. Statistical representations of the WHO-EMRO region necessarily flatten economic, political, cultural, social, and economic differences and render many complexities invisible, or at least, less visible. These statistics are effective in capturing the rapid, massive changes affecting the area and are thus useful despite their limitations, but the gaps and simplifications are vital. They can also be tenacious: statistics from the UAE itself still retain many unexplored gloss-overs. I wish, therefore, to insert critical perspectives concerning the repercussions at a political and societal level of the burgeoning public health and medical sectors in the UAE, to pull apart the epidemiological and population statistics that have been amassed on the UAE, to place them in context and to introduce an ethnographically rich set of data that problematizes many of the assumptions made by the public health literature with respect to nutrition/health transitions, obesity, and lifestyle, etc.

UAE Background

Within the WHO-EMRO region, Bahrain, Kuwait, Oman, Qatar, Saudi Arabia, and the UAE are all designated as high-income countries and are all located along the Arab Gulf. Interestingly, "high-income country" is a term that is often used interchangeably with "developed country" by the World Bank (2011), just as low- and middle-income countries are often classified as developing, but the Arab Gulf states are both developing and high income. Much of the Gulf has experienced a period of accelerated development and urbanization in recent decades, stimulated by enormous oil and gas revenues, and this development and urbanization underpins the equally dramatic changes in health that they have experienced. These trends are all the more striking because the Arab Gulf had very little infrastructure (health care or otherwise) until quite recently. Historically, in Trucial Oman (as the UAE was known prior to independence in 1971), medicine was an informal, largely home-based affair (Al-Fahim 1995; Al-Gurg 1998; Heard-Bey 2004 [1982]). Biomedical products and services were mostly lacking, although there were exceptions. In the 1940s, a British-run Dubai Government Dispensary opened and was replaced in 1951 with the British-run Al Maktum Hospital; visitors to the Dispensary and Hospital during the 1950–1951 period most often presented with malaria, although whooping cough and mumps were also a problem among the local children (Persian Gulf Administrative Reports 1951–1950). The Persian Gulf Administrative Reports for 1950 mention that there were no infectious disease epidemics that year, which was a significant improvement over past decades, when outbreaks of smallpox and cholera necessitated appeals to the British Political Agent by the ruler of Abu Dhabi. Fast-forward to the present—only sixty years later—and the epidemiological profile for the UAE is profoundly different. The UAE—and indeed, all of the Arab Gulf—has experienced a very marked increase in chronic disease-related illness and death, with rates of death from infectious diseases and the like falling equally rapidly (WHO 2002; WHO-EMRO 2011).

The UAE has thus experienced an immense amount of change in an unprecedentedly short period of time, with oil-revenue-fueled development and urbanization transforming the physical and socioeconomic landscapes, as well as the epidemiological ones (Bristol-Rhys 2010, 2009, 2007; Davidson 2009, 2008; Al-Fahim 1995; Fenelon 1973; Ghose 2008; Al-Gurg 1998; Kakande 2010; Lawson and Al-Naboodah 2008; Mourtada-Sabbah et al. 2008; Musaiger 2003, 1994; Musaiger and Miladi 1995; Al-Qasimi 2009a, 2009b; Rahman 2008; Al-Sharekh 2007, 2008; Shihab 2000; Thesiger 1959). The population of the UAE has experienced profound changes: official statistics recently placed the total population of the Emirates at over 8 million (a 65 percent increase over the past four years), of which less than 20 percent are local Emiratis and the rest are foreign-born temporary residents (UAE Interact 2011).

The changes wrought by rapid modernization and development make many locals in the UAE exceedingly anxious, even as they have benefited materially from them. This anxiety manifests in several interesting forms that directly impact my research. The first strand of this anxiety takes the form of concern over the obesity epidemic that, according to official medical and public health literature, is devastating the Emirati population (Carter et al. 2004; DHA 2011; Eapen et al. 2006; HAAD 2009; Al-Haddad et al. 2005; Harrison 2010; Hasab 2007; Malik and Bakir 2007; Malik et al. 2005; Tomeh 2002; WHO 2002; WHO-EMRO 2011, 2010, 2007, 2003). Popular media sources echo the public health literature's concern with obesity, with articles on the subject appearing in the major English-language newspapers on at least a weekly basis throughout my fieldwork period (e.g., Career mums 2009; Issues in the news 2003; Musharrakh 2000 Muslim 2007a, 2007b; Rathke 2007; RCA launches 2006; Underwood 2009). Such concern also manifested regularly in my conversations with locals, who would reference articles from both English-language and Arabic-language newspapers, as well as TV news programs and their own observations, when discussing local increases in obesity.

The second strand of this anxiety focuses on a supposed loss and/or corruption of local culture and traditions. This loss is linked in popular publications to intense exposure to foreigners and globalizing influences (Al-Asoomi 2008; Attwood et al. 2008; Ghose 2008; Gulf News Report 2008; Ismail 2011; Issa 2010; Kakande 2010; Al-Kitbi 2008; Mikiewicz 2010; Morris 2009; Al Saayegh 2008). I also heard similar sentiments from individuals, both from the study participants and from older female and male Emiratis, during my research. Changes in eating patterns and food use are sometimes cited in these discussions of disappearing local culture.

The third strand of this anxiety focuses on young Emirati women's supposed unhealthy overfocus on their appearances and documents their overspending, overconsumption, increasing battles with eating disorders and plastic surgery, etc. This last concern has appeared recently in popular media sources (Gerson 2010; Al-Hinai 2011; Menon 2010; Moussly 2010; Al-Qasimi 2010; Shaheen 2010; Thomas 2009). Many Emiratis with whom I spoke were aware of some of these body issues as they related to young Emirati women, and yet most of these issues remain unexamined and poorly understood. All three of these strands of anxiety intersect at multiple points and indeed, it is these intersections that provide some of the most illuminating insights into the often unexplored discussions taking place in the UAE concerning obesity, overweight, fatness, thinness, chronic disease, body image, and disordered eating on the one hand and issues of modernity and development on the other.

Methods, Field Sites, and Participants

It was in this larger context, therefore, that my research took place. As I already mentioned, I situated my research within the local Emirati community and in particular, I focused on young Emirati women, aged eighteen to thirty years, who live in the UAE and attend an institution of higher education. Employing the perspectives of medical and biocultural anthropology, as well as a mixed-methods approach, in the study of the obesity epidemic taking place in the UAE—and the reactionary concerns with thinness and fatness voiced by local women—proved invaluable. The many contradictory and complicated behaviors and attitudes that my study examined are products of a web of social and biological processes and need to be examined as such.

Fieldwork lasted from August 2009 to July 2010 and from December 2010 to January 2011. Within the UAE, my two primary institutional affiliations were Zayed University in the city/emirate of Dubai (ZU-Dubai) and UAE University (UAEU) in the small town of Al Ain (in Abu Dhabi Emirate). Both are public universities and this means they cater almost exclusively to Emiratis, for whom education is free. This allows a far greater range of Emiratis to access higher education and this, plus the UAE government's promotion of higher education amongst its citizens over the last three decades, has greatly increased the percentage of Emiratis who continue with education past secondary school. Interestingly, this is particularly marked among Emirati women: 70 percent of the female population go on to higher education, whereas the numbers for Emirati men are a fraction of this (Embassy of the UAE 2010, UAE Ministry of State 2008).

For this project, I recruited eighty students from ZU-Dubai and twenty-three students from UAEU. Over the course of two semesters (August 2009 to June 2010), as well as a portion of a third semester (December 2010 to January 2011),

I obtained measurements (body fat percentages, height, weight, and body mass indices), data from 24-Hour Food and Activity Recalls (Biro et al. 2002; Sallis and Saelens 2000), and structured and semi-structured interview data (Nichter 2000) from all of the participants at ZU-Dubai: at least one set of measurements, recalls, and interviews per woman. Fifty-eight of the eighty women (self-select-ing) at ZU-Dubai also participated in a second set of measurements and recalls and interviews and of these, thirteen women (again, self-selecting) returned for one to three additional interviews. At UAEU, the timeframe was shorter: one semester (January to June 2010), plus a portion of the following semester (De-cember 2010 to January 2011). I collected one set of measurements, recalls, and interviews from all of the UAEU participants and subsequently conducted two additional interviews each with three women from the original sample of twenty-one (again, self-selecting).

The participant data was supplemented with interview data from a range of nonparticipants (local and expatriate) working in the education and health care sectors of Dubai, Al Ain, and Abu Dhabi. All of the interview information was, in turn, situated within the data I gathered via participant observation in the UAE during the thirteen months of my fieldwork.

Results and Discussion: Weight Among Young Emirati Women

As I have discussed elsewhere (Trainer 2012, 2010), in a national context of in-creasing rates of overweight and obesity among many cohorts of Emiratis (Carter et al. 2004; DHA 2011; HAAD 2001; Malik et al. 2005; Musaiger 2003, 1994; Musaiger and Miladi 1995; WHO 2002), the young Emirati women in my study showed a preponderance of underweight and (low) normal weight. This finding was based both on the body fat percentages and on the BMIs I collected, and it highlights the importance of obtaining such measurements, despite the signifi-cant limitations inherent in these biological measures (and that Yates-Doerr, this volume, describes so well). It also adds a vital nuance to the literature on the obesity epidemic supposedly occurring in the UAE, for it is a step toward add-ing the complexity that I remarked at the outset is missing from larger statistical samples of the region and country. If these women are living in an obesogenic environment, riddled with fast food outlets, surrounded by rapidly urbanizing neighborhoods with little opportunities for physical activity, etc., then why are so few of them obese, especially when data shows that other age cohorts of Emiratis do carry excess weight (Carter et al. 2004; DHA 2011; HAAD 2001; Malik et al. 2005; Musaiger 2003, 1994; Musaiger and Miladi 1995; WHO 2002)? Does this mean that these young women are healthier and more concerned with health?

The ethnographic information provides further insights into such questions. (see figures 7.1 and 7.2). The women in this study were all aware of the health risks as-

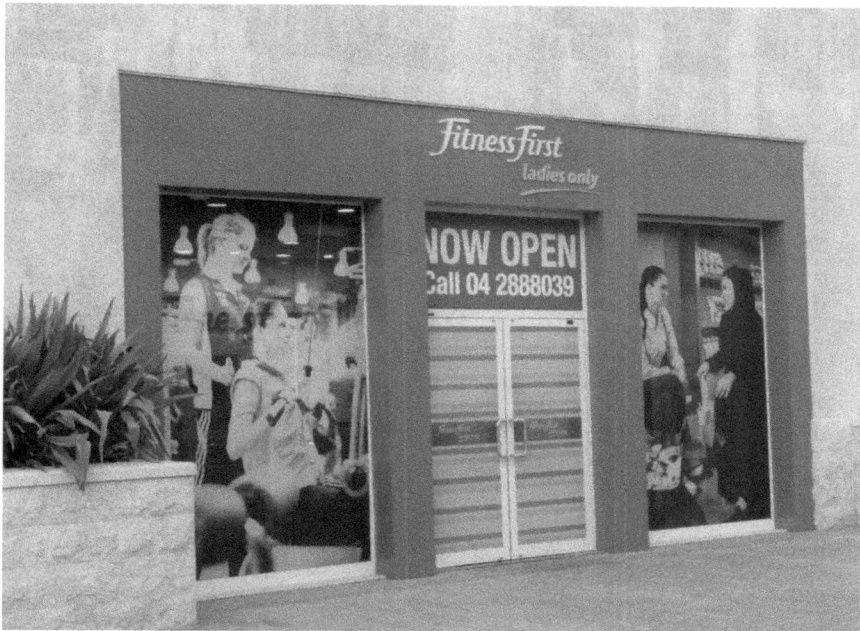

Figure 7.1. A ladies-only gym in Dubai. Photograph by Sarah Trainer.

sociated with overweight and obesity and knew that overweight and obesity had become far more common in the UAE in recent decades. Increasing rates of overweight and obesity were commonly framed as a problem for the country at large and the Emirati community/communities specifically by participants, echoing what they heard in the media, at school, from parents, and from health personnel. However, participants were universally firm in their feedback that what drove young Emirati women to lose weight was not fear of ill-health but fear of being fat and thus unattractive. All of the university students I spoke with during my research (including, but not limited to, participants) agreed that young Emirati women now equate attractiveness with being "thin but curvy," citing Hollywood stars like Beyonce, Kim Kardashian, and Angelina Jolie as having beautiful bodies worth trying to copy. This adherence to the "cult of thinness" (Talukdar 2012, quoting Hesse-Biber) is all the more remarkable, given that forty years previously, the beauty ideal for local women had been quite different, as one participant pointed out, saying, "The traditional idea of what looks good was a girl who 'filled out her skin' because it showed her family had enough to feed her well."

Participants all cited their constant exposure to international media as the root cause behind the shift in local beauty ideals. The magazines that women read, the TV shows and movies they watched, and the Internet sources they used all reinforced the same messages about beauty and glamour, showing a parade of beau-

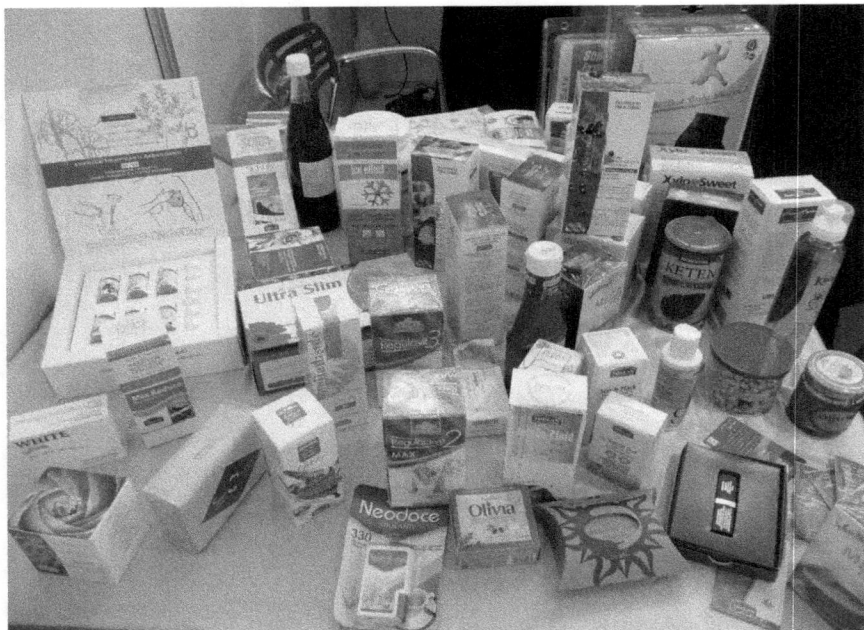

Figure 7.2. Weight-loss aids for sale at a campus "Health Fair." Photograph by Sarah Trainer.

tiful, thin women in beautiful, expensive dresses. I follow Talukdar (2012) in arguing that local traditions did still retain power in many areas of women's lives, including appearance; Nichter (2000), for example documented how American high school students consistently described "the perfect girl" as blond, tall, and thin, whereas my participants were more likely to discuss the "traditional" ideal of black hair and big eyes. Dress was another body-oriented source of negotiation, because Emirati women were usually expected (by the community and their families) to wear the black abaya and shayla coverings in public but the forms that these garments took—as well as the clothes that the women wore under the garments—were very much products of interactions between local ideas about tradition, the global Islamic fashion industry, Western couture, and Western brands (Abaza 2007; Deeb 2006; Moors 2009, 2007; Moors and Tarlo 2007; Out of the public eye 2012; Al-Qasimi 2010). With respect to body weight and achieving the ideal (slender) body, however, expectations were both rigid and heavily influenced by Western norms.

Women expressed considerable stress about their weight, especially those who fell into higher BMI categories. For instance, a participant—extremely pretty but class 3 obese—said in her very first interview with me, "I will tell you the honest truth, Ms. Sara—I am thinking about my weight every second of every day, even when I'm studying or doing other things. . . . It is like a stone in my heart." Such stress was framed both in terms of current negative feedback from female peers and family members, but also in terms of worry over future romantic and marital prospects, in a society where marriage is still considered an important step for most young women. This same participant told me that her cousin backed out of a marriage agreement with her because he thought she was "too fat," as did another man: "I was particularly shocked my cousin would do that to me but he works out and has four-packs [abs] and he doesn't think much of me." She said that she worries that she is never going to get married because of her weight.

At the same time, of course, public health messages within the UAE continue to focus on the obesity epidemic and the importance of weight loss: several health and beauty fairs held on the ZU and UAEU campuses during my fieldwork also focused on weight loss (including through weight-loss products like diet pills, aloe vera drinks, and cellulite creams) and beauty regimes (skincare and hair products, make-up, etc.). I became increasingly impatient with such venues over the course of my fieldwork. What worried me even more, however, were the reports I received from participants concerning their interactions with private nutritionists and spas/clinics. At the time of my fieldwork, private clinics were not well regulated within the UAE but frustratingly, from my perspective, participants tended to prefer patronizing private clinics to public, government hospitals and clinics. I was not unsympathetic to the desire to avoid the long lines and minimal attention characteristic of many of the public hospitals; I was also aware that private clinics have upper-class associations and public ones have the opposite for many residents in the UAE. However, many of the private clinics were dispensing advice that I found highly problematic. For example, one participant—who moved from normal weight to underweight during my study and who I became increasingly concerned about over the course of the year—reported that her mother was also worried enough to send her (my participant, that is) to a private nutritionist in the spring of 2010. According to my participant, however, the nutritionist told her, "I can help you lose two to three more kilos" and then spent the rest of the session trying to sell her diet products.

In the midst of all of this very vocal stress about weight and body, concern over health and nutrition often subsided into the background or was lost entirely. The pressure many women felt to achieve an idealized thin-but-not-skinny body for aesthetic reasons, without an accompanying concern with health and nutrition, results in worrying patterns among the students: pervasively inactive lifestyles; poor diets; and reportedly high rates of anemia, micronutrient deficiencies, and even muscle and bone loss. In an interview with a nurse on one university campus, for instance, she stated that in a blood drive conducted on campus in 2007–2008, 250 of the 300 women who volunteered to give blood were rejected due to anemia. Nurses at both ZU and UAEU also mentioned having students frequently brought in for fainting, as a result of skipping meals, becoming dehydrated, and underlying cases of abnormal blood sugar and blood iron levels. In interviews with the athletic directors at ZU and UAEU, the directors reported seeing muscle degeneration and bone loss in students as young as seventeen and eighteen, due to inactivity and poor diets. The data from my 24-Hour Food and Activity Recalls certainly would seem to support this, showing overwhelming rates of sedentary daily patterns coupled with nutritionally poor diets among the participants. Frustratingly, however, there appears to be very little research on the issue of micronutrient deficiencies in the Arab Gulf, perhaps because of the overwhelming focus on obesity in that region. Those few articles I was able to locate do tend to reinforce my ethnographic findings, with a study at the University of Sharjah indicating that anemia was a problem among the female university students (Sultan 2007); a study in Abu Dhabi of pregnant women showing good folic acid intake during pregnancy but poor intake prior (Al-Hossani et al. 2010); and a large-scale assessment of the Eastern Mediterranean region as a whole pointing out that "anaemia, particularly attributed to iron deficiency, among infants, preschool children and women of childbearing age has remained a widespread public health problem, irrespective of the family economic status and income level in most countries of the Region" (Bagchi 2004: 754). None of these possible threats to health, nor the verbally expressed stress of many young women, would be obvious in data that relied exclusively on BMI and body fat percentage data.

Public Health, Surveillance, and Governmentality in the UAE

Worthman and Kohrt (2005) point out that the dangers of chronic disease were "unmasked" once rates of illness and death from infectious diseases decreased and that epidemiology, public health, and biomedicine are ill-equipped to deal with this alteration. They also argue (along with Farmer 2003 and Krieger 2000) that diseases are structured by a wide range of socioeconomic factors, saying that "socialized" diseases reflect practices and social situations that affect exposure to health insults, as well as political or structural factors that affect exposure and vulnerability. According to Worthman and Kohrt (2005), obesity is a health risk that is profoundly socialized, one that comes with the changes in diet and activity patterns that characterize a nutrition/health transition. They echo the WHO (2009, 2008) in arguing that the traditional orientation of biomedical health services cannot adequately address the complex problems posed by chronic diseases. Wells (2012) develops several of these points further, arguing that susceptibility and exposure to what he terms "the obesogenic niche" are shaped by socioeconomic forces associated with modern forms of capitalist economies and that an overfocus on the biological mechanisms underlying susceptibility and exposure often leads scientists and medical personnel to ignore the structural forces at work.

Most of the countries in the Khaleej have the resources to embark on major renovations and extensions of their medical and public health services and indeed, many have already begun very ambitious projects involving the construction of medical facilities and the extension and codification of health care services, as well as actively pursuing data gathering and research into the populations they serve. These processes and projects have been far from cohesive and unidirectional, but are nonetheless accomplishing interesting goals. Public health campaigns and interventions designed to increase awareness concerning the health problems associated with overweight/obesity and chronic disease, and to change individual behaviors, have also become common (Carter et al. 2004; DHA 2011; HAAD 2010; Al-Haddad et al. 2005; Harrison 2010; Hasab 2007; Musaiger 2003, 1994; Muslim 2007a, 2007b; RCA launches 2006). The UAE is a case in point.

As I mentioned earlier, the first hospital in Dubai was built in 1951; very little health care infrastructure was created in the emirate in the subsequent years before Federation—and even fewer services were available in Abu Dhabi and the northern emirates. The situation began to change after Federation in 1971, but it has only been in the last thirty years that health care services and regulations have really expanded. Even with this expansion, the nature of the Federation has meant that the provision of these services and regulations is often far from cohesive, particularly in the northern emirates of Fujairah, Umm al Quaim, and Ras al Khaimah. Davidson (2009, 2008) points out that although the seven emirates have been federated for forty years, it is only in the past decade that there has been a concerted effort to work together, and these efforts are again, often problematic. Dubai and Abu Dhabi have impressive facilities, modeled after the latest products of Western biomedicine, and impressive safety and quality regulations, produced by various health authorities and again modeled on Western standards. Even in Dubai and Abu Dhabi, however, actual access to these facilities by patients, the care patients receive in them, and the regulation and enforcement of standards is far from uniform.

Currently, there are several institutional bodies that oversee health care and medicine in the UAE, principally the UAE Ministry of Health, the Abu Dhabi Health Authority (HAAD), the Dubai Health Authority (DHA) and, most recently, the Sharjah Health Authority. The projects that institutions like HAAD and the DHA are implementing with respect to health include amassing databases on their populations, implementing public health campaigns to raise awareness about health risks among their populations, creating interventions to change behaviors with respect to lifestyle risks, attempting to steer people into certain patterns of self-discipline, and employing medical and health experts. Such "knowledges, techniques, and procedures" are the hallmarks of modern governance and rely on dispersed forms of power and surveillance (Chatterjee 2004; Foucault 2008, 1983a, 1983b; Miller and Rose 2008; Mitchell 2002).

They reinforce the notion of the UAE as a modern state, a creation that the leaders of Abu Dhabi and Dubai in particular, have been at great pains to foster in the Western public imaginary (Davidson 2009, 2008; Al-Sharekh 2008, 2007). Anthropologists such as Lupton (2000, 1995), following in the tradition of Foucault, might point out that the clinics (and universities) in the UAE are sites of biopower and that health education in the UAE is attempting to produce modern subjects through specific types of moral training involving *good* nutrition and self-regulation. Scheper-Hughes and Lock's observation that "health is increasingly viewed ... as an achieved rather than ascribed status, and each individual is expected to 'work hard' at being strong, fit, and healthy" (Scheper-Hughes and Lock 1987: 25) is also relevant. So too is Featherstone's (1982) observation that dietary management is integral to the production of Foucault's docile bodies.

On the other hand, the UAE does not, in fact, govern from a distance in many respects—personal, family, and tribal networks remain very important, especially for the local populations. Thus, the "knowledges and technologies" that index modernity in public discussions of development in the UAE coexist with older networks (Bristol-Rhys 2010; Davidson 2009, 2008; Al-Sharekh 2008, 2007). Many of my interviewees talked about the level of surveillance that most Emiratis experience every day: from their families, from their friends, from the Emirati community, and from the state. Much of this surveillance and discipline has to do with "proper" behavior for Emirati women: wearing the black abaya and shayla, especially in public environments; living at home, either with the natal family or the husband's family; refraining from interacting with men outside the family; praying five times a day, fasting during Ramadan, and following other basic Islamic tenets; etc. The reasons for following these strictures are sometimes attributed to Islam, sometimes to Emirati culture and traditions, and sometimes to a conflation of the two. Some participants endorsed these whole-heartedly, others to a certain degree, and still others chafed under the regulations. Many students at both ZU and UAEU were very strategic in terms of how/what they chose to adhere to. This included having relationships online with men while physically staying at home with their families, and seeming to obey societal strictures about gender-mixing; dressing one way on campus and another way in front of their parents; arranging to visit a female friend or cousin and then going somewhere else with someone else; and smoking or drinking in certain very private contexts, despite cultural and religious prohibitions.

It is within a very interesting larger national context, therefore, that the public health initiatives already mentioned are taking shape. These are adding another layer of oversight to an already watched population and are doing so in an area—food, consumption, weight, health risks—that was relatively unmonitored until recently. Aside from following basic Islamic food restrictions (abstaining from alcohol and pork, fasting during Ramadan, etc.), there were fewer moralistic overtones associated with "overconsumption," "overeating," "overweight," and the like twenty and even ten years ago in the UAE. This has since changed, most profoundly in the younger generations but even leaking upward into the older ones as well. Within-country public health campaigns and exposure to international (principally Western, but also Bollywood, etc.) cultural mores and standards have changed Emirati attitudes toward weight and consumption; they are also increasingly affecting behaviors, as my fieldwork demonstrates. The introduction to this volume references Collier and Ong's (2005) term, global assemblages, saying, "The concept of 'global assemblages' aids us in tracing obesities as local cultural understandings of bodies change and morph in a constant tide of exchange with the global flows" (see Hardin and McCullough, this volume). Such global exchanges are having an overwhelming effect on young women in the UAE today, as my research demonstrates, interacting in a variety of unpredictable ways with local traditions and mores.

Emirati Culture versus the Problem of Location

The situation that the women in this sample are living in is thus rife with complications, inconsistencies, and constant changes. This, as mentioned earlier, creates a great deal of anxiety; it also produces a great deal of musing on the subject of global versus local culture. One striking aspect of living in the UAE is how often the subject of Emirati culture and Emirati tradition is raised. Thus, rapid development and change in the UAE (and in the region more generally) seems to be accompanied by active attempts to preserve local culture and traditions, or at least certain interpretations of these. As one researcher puts it, "As the world shrinks… as a result of such as iPods, Internet downloads and satellite television, all of which contribute to a universal popular culture, many natives of the GCC cling to a manufactured, glorious past to reduce anxieties" (Al-Sharakh 2008: 181). What makes this debate and anxiety all the more interesting is the confusion over what Emirati culture and/or Emirati traditions are. Before the 1970s, there were no Emirates, and although cultural similarities and familial links pulled the groups living in the region together, they were for the most part a heterogeneous assortment of fishermen, traders, pearl divers, herders, and merchants originating from all over the Gulf and beyond. Current attempts, usually spearheaded by the federal government, to stress a unified and consistent Emirati culture end up relying on simplistic images—usually involving the noble Bedouin of the desert with his horse, camel, hunting falcon, and coffee pot—and gloss over the divisions, both past and present, that underlie "Emirati-ness."

Anxiety over global versus local influences, along with uncertainty over what exactly constitutes local, and nostalgic attempts to reconstruct local traditions manifest in all kinds of different realms. National dress—the white kandora that Emirati men wear and the black abaya and shayla worn by Emirati women—the most visible sign of Emirati-ness and belonging, is much more strictly adhered to now than it was thirty or forty years ago. A similar process of codification of supposedly "traditional Emirati foods" (Appadurai 1988; Heine 2000) also appears to be taking place. Articles (e.g., Al-Qasimi 2009a), cookbooks (e.g., Brock-Al Ansari 1994), and organizations like the Sheikh Mohammed Center for Cultural Understanding highlight foods such as harees (ground wheat and goat or mutton are beaten and then cooked together to a porridge-like consistency) and machbous (not unlike osso buco) as national dishes but, according to participant reports on their grandparents' lifestyles, these time-intensive dishes were never typical everyday fare.

Confusing and contradictory accounts of the past also appeared in interviews when the subject concerned the recent development-linked changes in health in the UAE. Emirati culture was often deployed as an explanation for the health issues this chapter focuses on, but these explanations were messy and contradictory—and rife with unexplored assumptions (see Hardin, this volume, for a similar discussion of assumptions about Somoan culture). For example, participants and other interviewees, foreign and Emirati, would often cite local culture as a culprit in the observed increases in obesity rates and in lifestyles perceived to be unhealthy: traditional foods are too heavy and oily, traditional obligations of hospitality toward visitors commonly center on food consumption, traditional eating patterns involve huge family meals, traditional attitudes concerning women's activities limit their movements in the public sphere and also condemn their playing certain sports, traditional attitudes toward women's bodies endorse a heavier body size, traditional attitudes dictate the wearing of the black abaya and shayla by local women, further restricting their movements… variations in these themes were expressed repeatedly, but the notion of what constitutes tradition was usually left unexplored.

Confusingly, perceived loss of Emirati culture and traditions as a result of development and modernization was also cited, both by participants and other Emirati and foreign interviewees, as causing the surge in obesity and associated diseases like type 2 diabetes among locals in the UAE. This later perspective sees the shift toward eating more fast foods and convenience foods at the expense of family meals and the increasing material wealth (which has brought servants, cars, other labor-saving devices, and office jobs) of many Emiratis as responsible for the current health issues, making many locals "lazy" and "spoiled." At the same time, however, cultural loss is also often blamed for the reported increases in disordered eating, plastic surgery and diet aid use, and perceived overconsumption of clothes and other fashion-related material goods among young Emiratis, with the young people frequently being cast as more interested in global popular culture than in local traditions and thus losing their roots and becoming, once again, lazy and spoiled.

By contrast, there is one issue that both locals and local public health programs in the UAE often overlook in their rhetoric, and that is the basic problem posed by the location of the United Arab Emirates in the Arab Gulf. Most countries in the Middle East spent the previous century grappling with the problem of food production and nowhere are the problems more pronounced than in the Arab Gulf. The Middle East as a whole is mostly desert, but it was not until fairly late in the twentieth century that its natural resources began to prove insufficient to feed the populations living there, as a result of rapid overall increases in population, large-scale urbanization and development projects, and changing dietary demands among the inhabitants (i.e., demand for meat skyrocketed) (Allan 2000, WHO-EMRO 2003). In the last decades of the twentieth century, all of these trends were particularly pronounced in the Arab Gulf—a region that (with the exception of Iran, which is not Arab anyway) had far fewer natural resources to begin with.

The UAE currently imports more than 80 percent of its food (AOAD 2010; Austrade 2011). Hypermarkets like Lulu's, markets like Spinney's, and the (heavily restructured) so-called "traditional" souqs—as well as two recent shops in Dubai that market themselves as organic—all sell an incredible range of food, aimed at the diverse array of palates (British, Indian, American, Arab) of the population in the emirates. The vast majority of the food is imported, with the exception of a very small percentage of the produce, seafood, meat, and dairy that is locally sourced. Carrots come from Australia, beans from Kenya, okra from India, peppers from Belgium, eggplants from China, mutton from Pakistan, etc.

My personal experience was that very little of the imported foodstuffs, especially the produce, retained much flavor; most participants made similar comments, and a common complaint among the young women was that they knew they should eat "boiled vegetables," but they didn't usually care for the taste. Of course, heavily processed foods survive the trip to the UAE without losing their (heavily constructed) taste and therefore make for more pleasurable eating. A very few Emiratis—who have had a great deal of exposure to the movements in the United States and Europe that stress local, organic, slow-food, etc., and can cite people like Jamie Oliver and Michael Pollen—told me in personal conversations and interviews that they are attempting to bring a similar movement to the UAE but they have an uphill battle. While the foods available are very diverse and the eating venues—transnational fast food outlets (e.g., Dunkin' Donuts, Baskin Robbins, Pizza Hut, Nandos), expensive multi-star restaurants with big-name chefs, food courts in the malls, cheap cafeterias (usually serving South Asian food), family homes, petrol stations selling packaged foods, and family homes—equally so, the emphasis seldom is on fresh ingredients or healthy eating options. The participants in my study most commonly ate at home (eating foods usually prepared by the family maid), on campus, or picked food up from petrol stations or fast food restaurants while in transit between home and university. Despite the bewildering apparent diversity of cuisines available in the UAE, especially in Dubai, participants showed very little diversity in their food tastes.

Therefore, despite constantly hearing Emirati women make self-critical statements like, "Arabs love sweets, khalaas," or "Most Emiratis aren't interested in eating healthy, even though they know they should," I would argue that the reason a local, slow-food movement is going to be difficult for the UAE does not stem from some unhealthy tendency inherent to Emiratis but to the seemingly insurmountable problem of location: the UAE's population in its desert location must rely primarily on heavily traveled food. This obstacle also makes the public health messages about individual responsibility and healthy lifestyles (e.g. DHA 2010, HAAD 2010, Musaiger and Miladi 1995) problematic.

Conclusion

Overall, public health and medical surveillance—with the focus on the dramatic increases in weight and associated chronic diseases in the UAE—is not resulting in better health for the young women I met, although it certainly seems to be contributing to their heightened feeling that fat = bad. Most of my participants also knew enough about nutrition and health to talk about the fact that they knew they "should" be getting exercise and "should" be eating more vegetables and less fat. Nuanced understandings of nutrition, however, were less common. Furthermore, the increased public health and medical surveillance was accompanied by increased self-surveillance (and also, in many instances, of surveillance by peers) but the focus and concern of most of the women's surveillance was on being thin, where the outcome often justified the means used.

Two other factors further exacerbate the situation. On the one hand, the profound rupture between this age cohort and its parents' generation (Bristol-Rhys 2010, 2009) in terms of life experiences, attitudes, education, etc. (as a result of the exponentially rapid socioeconomic and physical changes the UAE has undergone) has meant that the older generation is often not viewed as a helpful source of advice. On the other, there are a host of competing voices in the UAE offering advice and health with respect to health and beauty, and this can be very confusing. The plethora of weight/beauty/health "clinics" and salons offering help and advice, for example, as well as the mind-numbing number of related products available in these clinic and salons, in pharmacies and other, considerably less formal and regulated settings, means that women can access whatever messages and services and products they deem helpful, with very little guidance in many instances as to what this help entails and how risky some of them are.

Notes

1. These designations, as well as all of the health-related statistics quoted in this narrative, predate the upheavals that took/are taking place throughout the Middle East and North Africa since 2011.

References

Abaza, M. 2007. "Shifting Landscapes of Fashion in Contemporary Egypt." *Fashion Theory* 11, no. 2/3: 281–298.

Allan, T. 2000. "Food Production in the Middle East." In *A Taste of Thyme: Culinary Cultures of the Middle East,* ed. S. Zubaida and R. Tapper. London and New York: Tauris and Co.

Appadurai, A. 1988. "How to Make a National Cuisine: Cookbooks in Contemporary India." *Comparative Studies in Society and History* 30, no. 1: 3–24.

Arab Organization for Agricultural Development (AOAD). 2010. "UAE Has Over 2,800 sq km in Sudan Farms." Posted 13 October, available at http://www.aoad.org/index_en.htm.

Al-Asoomi, M. 2008. "Identity in the Balance." *Gulf News,* 28 May.

Attwood, K., H. Dajani, and H. Naylor. 2008. "What Does It Mean to be an Emirati?" *The National,* 17 April.

Austrade: Australian Government. 2011. "Food to the UAE." Available at http://www.austrade.gov.au/Food-to-the-United-Arab-Emirates/default.aspx, accessed May 1, 2011.

Bagchi, K. 2004. "Iron Deficiency Anaemia—An Old Enemy." *Eastern Mediterranean Health Journal* 10, no. 6: 754–760.

Biro, G. K. F., L. Hulshof, J. A. Ovesen, and C. Amorim. 2002. "Selection of Methodology to Assess Food Intake." *European Journal of Clinical Nutrition* 56, no. Supplement 2: S25–32.

Brewis, A. 2012. "Obesity and Human Biology: Toward a Global Perspective." *American Journal of Human Biology* 24: 258–260.

Bristol-Rhys, J. 2007. "Weddings, Marriage and Money in the United Arab Emirates." *Anthropology of the Middle East* 2, no. 1: 20–36.

———. 2009. "Emirati Historical Narratives." *History and Anthropology* 20, no. 2: 107–121.

———. 2010. *Emirati Women: Generations of Change.* New York: Columbia University Press.

Brock-Al Ansari, C. A. 1994. *The Complete United Arab Emirates Cookbook, Including Local Customs and Traditions.* Abu Dhabi: Emirates Airlines Publication.

Brownell, K. D., and D. Yach. 2006. "Lessons from a Small Country about the Global Obesity Crisis." *Globalization and Health* 2, no. 11.

Career Mums—Fat Kids? 2009. 7 Days in Dubai, 6 October. Available at http://www.7daysindubai.com/Career-mums-fat-kids/story-15441562-detail/story.html

Carter, A. O., H. F. Saadi, R. L. Reed, and E. V. Dunn. 2004. "Assessment of Obesity, Lifestyle, and Reproductive Health Needs of Female Citizens of Al Ain, United Arab Emirates." *Journal of Health, Population, and Nutrition* 22, no. 1: 75–83.

Cassels, S. 2006. "Overweight in the Pacific: Links between Foreign Dependence, Global Food Trade, and Obesity in the Federated States of Micronesia." *Globalization and Health* 2, no. 10.

Chatterjee, P. 2004. *The Politics of the Governed: Reflections on Popular Politics in Most of the World.* New York: Columbia University Press.

Collier, S. J., and A. Ong. 2005. "Global Assemblages, Anthropological Problems." In *Global Assemblages: Technology, Politics, and Ethics as Anthropological Problems,* ed. S. J. Collier and A. Ong. Malden: Blackwell Publishing, 3–21.

Davidson, C. M. 2008. *Dubai: The Vulnerability of Success.* New York: Columbia University Press.

———. 2009. *Abu Dhabi: Oil and Beyond.* New York: Columbia University Press.

Deeb, L. 2006. *An Enchanted Modern: Gender and Public Piety in Shi'i Lebanon.* Princeton: Princeton University Press.

Dubai Health Authority (DHA). 2011. Homepage. Available at http://www.dha.gov.ae/EN/Pages/default.aspx, accessed May 1, 2011.

Eapen, V., A. A. Mabrouk, S. Sabri, and S. Bin-Othman. 2006. "A Controlled Study of Psychosocial Factors in Young People with Diabetes in the United Arab Emirates." *Annals of the New York Academy of Science* 1084: 325–328.

Embassy of the United Arab Emirates in Washington, D.C. 2010. "Women in the UAE." Available at www.uae-embassy.org/uae/women-in-the-uae?id=65, accessed January 1, 2012.

Al-Fahim, M. 1995. *From Rags to Riches: A Story of Abu Dhabi.* London: The London Centre of Arab Studies.

Farmer, P. 2003. *Pathologies of Power: Health, Human Rights, and the New War on the Poor.* Berkeley, Los Angeles, and London: University of California Press.

Featherstone, M. 1982. "The Body in Consumer Culture." *Theory, Culture and Society* 1: 18–33.

Fenelon, K. 1973. *The United Arab Emirates: An Economic and Social Survey.* London: Longman.

Foucault, M. 1983a. "Power, Sovereignty and Discipline." In *States and Societies,* eds. D. Held and J. Anderson. New York: New York University Press.

———. 1983b. "Afterword: The Subject and Power." In *Michel Foucault: Beyond Structuralism and Hermeneutics,* 2nd edition, ed. L. Dreyfus and P. Radinow. Chicago: University of Chicago Press, 208–226.

———. 2008. *The Birth of Biopolitics: Lectures at the College de France 1978–1979.* Edited by Michel Senellart, translated by Graham Burchell, New York: Palgrave Macmillan.

Gerson, J. 2010. "Women Pushed to Spend, Spend, Spend." *The National,* 16 April.

Ghose, G. 2008. "The Growth Problem: 'Economic Prosperity and National Identity Go Hand in Hand.'" *Gulf News,* 28 May.

Gulf News Report. 2008. "Rapid Growth Threatens to Erode Identity." *Gulf News,* 28 May.

Al-Gurg, E. S. 1998. *The Wells of Memory: An Autobiography.* London: John Murray Publishers Ltd.

Al-Haddad, F. H., B. B. Little, A. G. Abdul Ghafoor. 2005. "Childhood Obesity in United Arab Emirates Schoolchildren: A National Study." *Annals of Human Biology* 32, no. 1: 72–79.

Harrison, O. 2010. "Discussion of the Abu Dhabi Health Authority." Paper presented at the Global Health Conference, UAE University, Al Ain, UAE, January 6–12.

Hasab, Ali A.H. 2007. *Health in Dubai: Situational Analysis and Future Prospects.* Dubai: DOHMS.

Hawkes, C. 2006. "Uneven Dietary Development: Linking the Policies and Processes of Globalization with the Nutrition Transition, Obesity, and Diet-related Chronic Diseases." *Globalization and Health* 2, no. 4.

Health Authority of Abu Dhabi (HAAD). 2009. "Health Statistics." Available at www.haad .ae/statistics, accessed September 25, 2010.

Heard-Bey, F. 2004 [1982]. *From Trucial States to United Arab Emirates: A Society in Transition.* Dubai: Motivate Publishing.

Heine, P. 2000. "The Revival of Traditional Cooking in Modern Arabic Cookbooks." In *A Taste of Thyme: Culinary Cultures of the Middle East,* ed. S. Zubaida and R. Tapper. London: Tauris and Co. Ltd.

Al-Hinai, M. 2011. "Plastic Surgery for Good Looks and Upward Mobility." *The National,* 23 April.

Al-Hossani, H., H. Abouzeid, M. M. Salah, H. M. Farag, and E. Fawzy. 2010. "Knowledge and Practices of Pregnant Women about Folic Acid in Pregnancy in Abu Dhabi, United Arab Emirates." *Eastern Mediterranean Health Journal* 16, no. 4.

Issues in the News. 2003. *Washington Report on Middle East Affairs* 22, no. 2.

Ismail, M. 2011. "More Emirati Women Marrying Foreigners." *The National,* 10 April.

Issa, W. 2010. "Grand Mufti of Dubai Calls for Curb on Mixed Marriages." *The National,* 24 August.

Kakande, Y. 2010. "Arabic is Key to Identity: Sharjah Ruler." *The National,* 16 April.

Al-Kitbi, E. 2008. "Prevent Being Side-lined." *Gulf News,* 29 May.

Krieger, N. 2000. "Epidemiology and Social Sciences: Towards a Critical Reengagement in the 21st Century." *Epidemiologic Reviews* 11: 155–163.

Lawson, F. H., and H. H. Al-Naboodah. 2008. "Heritage and Cultural Nationalism in the United Arab Emirates." In *Popular Culture and Political Identity in the Arab Gulf States,* ed. A. Al-Sharekh and R. Springborg. London: SAQI Books and the London Middle East Institute SOAS.

Lupton, D. 1995. *The Imperative of Health: Public Health and the Regulated Body.* London: Sage Publications.

———. 2000. "The Social Constrution of Medicine and the Body." In *Handbook of Social Studies in Health and Medicine,* ed. G.L. Albrecht, R. Fitzpatrick, and S. Scrimshaw. London: Sage Publications.

Malik, M., and A. Bakir. 2007. "Prevalence of Overweight and Obesity among Children in the United Arab Emirates." *Obesity Review* 8, no. 1: 15–20.

Malik, M., A. Bakir, B. A. Saab, and H. King. 2005. "Glucose Intolerance and Associated Factors in the Multi-ethnic Population of the United Arab Emirates: Results of a National Survey." *Diabetes Research and Clinical Practice* 69, no. 2: 188–195.

Menon, P. 2010. "Police Raid Illeagal Plastic Surgery Clinic." *The National,* 9 February.

Mikiewicz, G. 2010. "Marriage Can Wait for Many Emirati Women." *The National,* 19 June.

Miller, P., and N. Rose. 2008. *Governing the Present: Administering Economic, Social and Personal Life.* Cambridge: Polity Press.

Mitchell, T. 2002. *Rule of Experts: Egypt, Techno-Politics, Modernity.* Berkeley: University of California Press.

Moors, A. 2007. "Fashionable Muslims: Notions of Self, Religion, and Society in San'a." *Fashion Theory* 11, no. 2/3: 319–347.

———. 2009. "'Islamic Fashion' in Europe: Religious Conviction, Aesthetic Style, and Creative Consumption." *Encounters,* Dubai: Zayed University.

Moors, A., and T. Emma. 2007. "Introduction." *Fashion Theory* 11, no. 2/3: 133–143.

Morris, L. 2009. "Preserving the Essence." *The National,* 26 September.

Mourtada-Sabbah, N., M. Al-Mutawa, J. W. Fox, and T. Walters. 2008. "Media as Social in the United Arab Emirates." In *Popular Culture and Political Identity in the Arab Gulf States*, ed. A. Al-Sharekh and R. Springborg. London: SAQI Books and the London Middle East Institute SOAS.

Moussly, R. 2010. "Falling Prey to Eating Disorders: A Study Suggests Women Students in the UAE are Heavily Influenced by the Media and the Pressure to Look Good." *Gulf News*, 23 May.

Musaiger, A. O. 1994. "Diet-related Chronic Diseases in the Arab Gulf Countries: The Need for Action." *Ecology of Food and Nutrition* 32: 91–94.

———. 2003. "Recommendations of the First Conference on Obesity and Physical Activity in the Arab Countries, Held in Bahrain, 24–26 September, 2002." *Nutritional Health* 17, no. 2: 117–121.

Musaiger, A. O., and S. S. Miladi, eds. 1995. *Food Consumption Patterns and Dietary Habits in the Arab Countries of the Gulf.* Cairo, Egypt and UAE University: FAO Regional Office for the Near East.

Musharrakh, Z. 2000. "Lifestyle Takes its Toll of Women more than Men." *Gulf News*, 5 November.

Muslim, N. 2007a. "I am Seeing Children as Young as 10 with Adult-onset Diabetes." *Gulf News*, 7 March.

———. 2007b. "UAE Sitting on Diabetes 'Timebomb.'" *Gulf News*, 7 March.

Nichter, Mimi. 2000. *Fat Talk: What Girls and their Parents Say about Dieting.* Boston: Harvard University Press.

Out of Public Eye, Arab Women Power Haute Couture. 2012. Elite Daily: For the Aspiring, Successful and Established, posted 15 April, available at http://elitedaily.com/elite/2011/out-of-public-eye-arab-women-power-haute-couture/

Persian Gulf Administrative Reports. 1950–1951. Cambridge: British Archives.

Popkin, B. 1999. "Urbanization, Lifestyle Changes and the Nutrition Transition." *World Development* 27: 1905–1916.

———. 2009. "What Can Public Health Nutritionists Do to Curb the Epidemic of Nutrition-related Noncommunicable Disease?" *Nutrition Reviews* 67 (Supplement): S79–S82.

———. 2011. "Agricultural Policies, Food and Public Health." *EMBO Reports* 12: 11–18.

Al-Qasimi, Noor. 2010. "Immodest Modesty: Accommodating Dissent and the Abaya-as-Fashion in the Arab Gulf States." *Journal of Middle East Women's Studies* 6, no. 1: 46–74

Al-Qasimi, Nouf. 2009a. "Country cooking." *The National*, 23 September.

———. 2009b. "Out to Lunch about Well-nourished Kids." *The National*, 14 October.

———. 2010. "How Emotions Affect our Relationship with Food." *The National*, 16 April.

Rahman, N. 2008. "Place and space in the memory of United Arab Emirates elders." In *Popular Culture and Political Identity in the Arab Gulf States*, ed. A. Al-Sharekh and R. Springborg. London: SAQI Books and the London Middle East Institute SOAS.

Rathke, K. 2007. "Review: Childhood Obesity in the Emirates." Almisbar: *UAEU Library Newsletter*, 10, Al Ain: UAE University.

RCA Launches 25 Kiosks to Offer Diabetes Test. 2006. *Gulf News*, 6 November.

Al Saayegh, F. 2008. "How Can We Maintain a National Identity?" *Gulf News*, 27 May.

Sallis, J.F. and B.E. Saelens. 2000. "Assessment of Physical Activity by Self-report: Status, Limitations, and Future Directions." *Research Quarterly for Exercise and Sport* 17: 1–14.

Scheper-Hughes, N. and M. Lock. 1987. "The Mindful Body: A Prolegomenon to Future Work in Medical Anthropology." *Medical Anthropology Quarterly* 1: 6–41.

Shaheen, K. 2010. "Emirati Girls Starve Themselves 'To Look Pretty in a Dress.'" *The National,* 19 April.

Al-Sharekh, A., ed. 2007. *The Gulf Family: Kinship Policies and Modernity.* London: SAQI Books and the London Middle East Institute SOAS.

———. 2008. "Conclusion." In *Popular Culture and Political Identity in the Arab Gulf States,* ed. A. Al-Sharekh and R. Springborg. London: SAQI Books and the London Middle East Institute SOAS.

Shihab, M. 2000. "Economic Development in the UAE." In *United Arab Emirates: A New Perspective,* ed. I. Al Abed and P. Hellyer. UAE: Trident Press Ltd.

Sultan, A. H. 2007. "Anemia among Female College Students Attending the University of Sharjah, UAE: Prevalence and Classification." *Journal of the Egyptian Public Health Association* 82, no. 3–4: 261–271.

Talukdar, J. 2012. "Thin but not Skinny: Women Negotiating the 'Never too Thin' Body Ideal in Urban India." *Women's Studies International Forum* 35, no. 2, 109–118.

Thesiger, W. 1959. *Arabian Sands.* London: Penguin Books.

Thomas, J. 2009. "Too Fat, Too Thin, Two Sides of the Same Coin." *The National,* 1 October.

Tomeh, L. A. 2002. "Regional Overview of Obesity." Paper at the WHO Eastern Mediterranean Regional Office, Cairo, Egypt.

Trainer, S. 2010. "Body Image, Health, and Modernity: Women's Perspectives and Experiences in the United Arab Emirates." *Asia-Pacific Journal of Public Health* 22: 60S–67S.

———. 2012. "Negotiating Weight and Body Image in the UAE: Strategies among Young Emirati Women." *American Journal of Human Biology* 24: 314–324.

UAE Interact. 2011. "UAE Up by 65 Percent in Four Years." Available at http://www.uaeinteract.com/news/default.asp?ID=134, posted on 4 March.

Underwood, M. 2009. "Children Eating their Way to Obesity." *The National,* 6 September.

United Arab Emirates Ministry of State for Federal National Council Affairs. 2008. "Women in the UAE: A Portrait of Progress." UAE.

Wells, J. C. K. 2012. "Obesity as Malnutrition: The Role of Capitalism in the Obesity Global Epidemic." *American Journal of Human Biology* 24: 261–276.

Wiley, A. 2007a. "Transforming Milk in a Global Economy." *American Anthropologist* 109, no. 4: 666–677.

———. 2007b. "The Globalization of Cow's Milk: Biocultural Perspectives." *Ecology of Food and Nutrition* 46, no. 3–4: 281–312.

World Bank. 2011. "Countries and Economies." Available at http://data.worldbank.org/country, accessed May 1.

World Health Organization (WHO). 2002. "The Impact of Chronic Disease in the United Arab Emirates." Available at http://www.who.int/chp/chronic_disease_report/en/

———. 2008. "World Health Report: Primary Healthcare—Now More than Ever." Geneva: World Health Organization Publication.

———. 2009. *Global Health Risks: Mortality and Burden of Disease Attributable to Selected Major Risks.* Geneva: World Health Organization Publication.

———. 2011a. "Chronic Diseases and Health Promotion." Available at http://www.who.int/chp/en/index.html, accessed May 1.

―――. 2011b. "Preventing Chronic Diseases: A Vital Investment." Available at http://www
.who.int/chp/chronic_disease_report/en/, accessed May 1.

World Health Organization, Eastern Mediterranean Region (WHO-EMRO). 2003. "WHO
Global Strategy on Diet, Physical Activity and Health." In Eastern Mediterranean Regional Consultation Meeting Report. Cairo, Egypt: World Health Organization.

―――. 2007. "Obesity, an Epidemic." Nutrition Division of Health Protection and Promotion, WHO-EMRO. Available at http://www.emro.who.int/nutrition/, accessed July 3.

―――. 2010. "Eastern Mediterranean Regional Health System Observatory—Health System
Databases." Available at http://gis.emro.who.int/HealthSystemObservatory/Database/
Forms/Database.aspx, accessed January 1.

―――. 2011. "Noncommunicable Diseases." Available at http://www.emro.who.int/ncd/,
accessed May 1.

Worthman, C. M., and B. Kohrt. 2005. "Receding Horizons of Health: Biocultural Approaches to Public Health Paradoxes." *Social Science and Medicine* 61: 861–878.

Yach, D., D. Stucklet, and K. Brownell. 2006. "Epidemiologic and Economic Consequences
of the Global Epidemics of Obesity and Diabetes." *Nature Medicine* 12: 62–66.

CHAPTER **8**

"Not Neutral Ground"

Exploring School as a Site for Childhood Obesity Intervention and Prevention Programs

Tracey Galloway and Tina Moffat

⁜ ⁜ ⁜

School-based programs are widely acknowledged as fundamental tools for monitoring and improving child health (Florencio 2001; Hay 1999; Institute of Medicine 2010). Ensuring good health requires a lifespan approach to intervention, and school-based programs are key components of an overall public health strategy for school-age children. Evidence suggests good health is a prerequisite for learning readiness in young children (Bundy et al. 2006), and the organizational structure of school—classes, teachers, and curriculum—offers opportunity for social and behavioral marketing, in essence the delivery of health-based curriculum to a largely captive audience. Internationally, school-based programs reach students from across the socioeconomic spectrum. Schools also offer a controlled environment conducive to intervention in the areas of dietary intake and physical activity, whether through school foodservice or curricular requirements for health knowledge and physical education.

For these reasons, and in response to calls for multi-level, multi-sector obesity prevention approaches (Bundy et al. 2006), the majority of current obesity surveillance and prevention programs targeting children incorporate a school component. Many of these employ behavioral models, with changes in dietary intake among their key outcome variables (see table 8.1). For example, there are numerous evaluations of local- and state-level initiatives to provide breakfast (Hooper and Evers, 2003; Wesnes et al. 2003), increase fruit and vegetable consumption (Bell and Swinburn 2004; French and Wechsler 2004; Gortmaker et al. 1999; Lowe et al. 2004; Reynolds et al. 2000; Sadeno et al. 2000), and decrease sweetened beverage consumption (Cullen and Thompson 2005; James et al. 2004; James and Kerr 2005) among schoolchildren. Recently such programs have expanded their mandate to include increasing physical activity, decreasing sedentary behaviors, and improving academic performance among school-aged children (de Silva-Sanigorski et al. 2010; Greening et al. 2011; Lubans et al. 2010; Maynard et al. 2009).

Global analysis of school-based obesity interventions indicates that many of these programs originated in the United States. Programs, such as Coordinated Approach to Child Health (CATCH) and Planet Health (Hoelscher et al. 2010; Madsen et al. 2009), have a behaviorist orientation, explicitly linking poor health outcomes with unhealthy food and physical activity choices on the part of children and their parents. Contento et al. (2010) explore "choice," "personal agency," and "autonomous motivation" as the prime determinants of healthy growth and nutrition outcomes in children (cf. Rosen, this volume). Even those programs that include an environmental component (Chomitz et al. 2010; Hoelscher et al. 2010, for examples) tend to define "environment" as merely the sphere within which children and parents exercise autonomous decision making.

The behaviorist approach that underlies the majority of North American interventions is reflected in other school-based interventions in, for example, Norway, Brazil, Turkey, and India (Table 8.1). In fact, a number of U.S. programs have been adapted for use in international settings such as the UK (Kipping et al. 2010). A notable exception is the Kiel Obesity Prevention Study (Platcha-Danielzik et al. 2011), which is designed to explore the wider determinants of program efficacy among German schoolchildren. Results from this eight-year follow-up indicate that although the overall impact of school-based health promotion is modest, favorable effects are significantly more pronounced among high socioeconomic status (SES) students. This suggests that among the determinants of childhood obesity are factors which are beyond an individual's control.

The pattern of modest results is generally consistent among studies of school-based interventions. Since the early 1990s, the U.S. CATCH and Planet Health programs have resulted in decreases in obesity prevalence in the range of 1–5 per-

Table 8.1. Recent School-Based Interventions Targeting Childhood Obesity

Intervention	Location	Age range	Outcome measures	Source
Kiel Obesity Prevention Study	Germany	6 and 14 years	BMI	Platcha-Danielzik et al. 2011
HEALTHY Study	USA	10–14 years	dietary behavior, dietary intake	Siega-Riz et al. 2011
TEAM Mississippi Project	USA	6–10 years	nutritional knowledge, BMI, WC, % body fat, fitness level, dietary intake, physical activity	Greening et al. 2011
Obesity Prevention Program	Brazil	11–17 years	dietary behavior	da Silva Vargas et al. 2011

Intervention	Location	Age range	Outcome measures	Source
Choice, Control and Change	USA	11–13 years	dietary behavior, dietary intake, physical activity, sedentary behavior	Contento et al. 2010
HEalth In Adolescents (HEIA)Study	Norway	11–13 years	dietary behavior, dietary intake, physical activity, sedentary behavior	Lien et al. 2010
Nutrition and Enjoyable Activity for Teen Girls (NEET) Study	Australia	13 years	BMI, muscular fitness, dietary behavior, dietary intake, physical activity, sedentary behavior	Lubans et al. 2010
Obesity Reduction Program	Turkey	9 years	BMI	Toruner and Savaser 2010
Get Fit with the Grizzlies	USA	8–11 years	nutritional knowledge, dietary behavior, dietary intake, physical activity, sedentary behavior	Irwin et al. 2010
Kids—"Go for your life" (K-GFYL)	Australia	5–12 years	nutritional knowledge, dietary behavior, dietary intake, lunchbox surveys, physical activity, sedentary behavior	de Silva-Sanigorski et al. 2010
Active for Life Year 5	UK	9–10 years	dietary intake	Kipping et al. 2010
Fitwits School Program	USA	10–11 years	nutrition knowledge, dietary behavior	McGaffey et al. 2010
Healthier Options for Public Schoolchildren (HOPS)	USA	6–13 years	BMI, academic performance	Hollar et al. 2010
Healthy Living Cambridge Kids (HLCK)	USA	5–14 years	BMI, fitness level	Chomitz et al. 2010
Coordinated Approach To Child Health (CATCH) Trial	USA	9–11 years	BMI, dietary behavior, dietary intake, physical activity, academic performance	Hoelscher et al. 2010
Nutrition and lifestyle Intervention	India	15–17 years	BMI, WC, WHR, dietary behavior, dietary intake, blood glucose	Singhal et al. 2010
DiEt and Active Living (DEAL) Study	UK	10–12 years	nutritional knowledge, dietary behaviour	Maynard et al. 2009

BMI: Body Mass Index   WC: Waist Circumference   WHR: Waist Hip Ratio cent (Hoelscher et al. 2010; Madsen et al. 2009). Gortmaker et al. (1999) observe a reduction in obesity prevalence for girls but not boys, which was attributable to decreased time spent watching television. Coleman et al. (2005) do not report a reduction in child obesity prevalence, although they do observe the intervention program at least slowed the rate of obesity increase among participating children. While these modest gains are a step in the right direction, the limited overall success of school programs has led researchers to explore issues constraining their effectiveness, including teacher type and lesson location (McKenzie et al. 2001), overall school climate (Parcel et al. 2003), social support (Johnson et al. 2000), and lack of community involvement (Hoelscher et al. 2010).

To date, despite the limited success of school-based obesity interventions, the implementation of programs in schools continues apace. The purpose of this chapter is to explore issues arising from use of school as a site for obesity intervention and prevention. The school environment, broadly conceived, is a conceptual space in which a number of conflicting models of childhood and personhood prevail. School is an institution historically designed to train children's bodies and minds. It is a place where an entrenched hierarchical model of authority explicitly and implicitly constrains children's autonomy. Moreover, at school children are exposed to institutionalized, normalized, and gendered notions of the body and personhood. Punishment and discipline are commonplace, though as Michel Foucault (1975) outlines, this is not the punishment and discipline of an earlier era that relied on a physical demonstration of punishment to maintain discipline—in the case of schools, corporal punishment—but rather the control of individual bodies as "docile bodies," through a "policy of coercions that act upon the body, a calculated manipulation of its elements, gestures, its behavior" (1975: 138). We argue that, taken together, these aspects of the school environment make intervention in the area of obesity a rather more delicate consideration than heretofore understood.

At the same time, obesity is an issue built around societal models of identity and the body. Lay understandings of obesity causation, which are widespread among health and education professionals, include the belief that obesity is a genetic or heritable condition and the sense that obesity arises from a lack of self-control on the part of the obese child or adult (Bryant et al. 2010; Urquhart and Mihalynuk 2011; van Strien and Bazelier 2007). Add to this the relative inaccuracy of epidemiological tools such as BMI to assess adiposity in children (Williams et al. 2007; Yates-Doerr, this volume), a lack of consensus on the degree of health risk posed by childhood obesity (Freedman et al. 1999; Herman et al. 2009; Hesketh et al. 2004; Williams 2001), and the problematic framing of childhood obesity as an epidemic (Moffat 2010), and it is clear that the adoption of school-based obesity programs requires a cautious approach (see part I, this volume).

Methods

The present study undertakes an examination of the factors in the school environment which necessitate a rethinking of current practices surrounding school-based obesity prevention and intervention. As an illustration of the issues under consideration, we report findings from the Bluewater Nutrition Project, a school-based study of children's growth and nutrition conducted in rural Ontario, Canada. Our sample was drawn from the populations of seven elementary schools in the Bluewater District School Board, located in the Georgian Bay region of Southern Ontario. The schools serve a diverse range of community sizes: the smallest school communities are entirely rural, with all children bused from surrounding townships; the largest school is located in a small city, population twenty-one thousand. Ethics approval for the research was provided by the McMaster Research Ethics Board, McMaster University, as well as the Bluewater District School Board and the Grey Bruce Health Unit.

Letters of information were distributed to 1,042 students in grades 2–8 (ages eight to thirteen years); the guardians of 535 children returned written consent for children's participation in the study (51.3 percent participation rate). Between January and March 2004, children with parental consent participated in anthropometric measures of height and weight. Children were measured by the researcher in a private room located on school premises. A research assistant was present to record data. Verbal assent was obtained from children prior to measurement. Twenty-nine children were absent from school or involved in school activities that prevented their participation. Two children declined to be measured and were excluded from the sample. Measurements were completed for 504 children (253 boys and 251 girls).

Between March and May 2003, children with parental consent participated in dietary recalls. The number of participants was limited by school activities and the length of time required for each dietary recall interview (fifteen to twenty minutes). Efforts were concentrated on children in grades 4–8, resulting in a dietary recall sample of 364 children.

From each classroom's pool of study participants with parental consent, four children were randomly selected to participate in the focus group discussions. A total of 144 children (72 boys and 72 girls) took part in thirty-seven focus groups. Verbal assent was elicited from children prior to each focus group. Focus groups were led by the investigator (Galloway) and conducted in private on school premises during school hours. Each discussion took approximately twenty minutes. Individual and small group interviews were also done with teachers and members of school parent groups. Interviews and focus groups were transcribed verbatim and the transcripts were examined for concepts, categories, descriptions and patterns of conceptual ordering used in participants' responses.

Food Rules: Controlling Children's Bodies and Behavior

The seven study schools displayed a wide variety of food-related rules and practices. The results of focus group discussions revealed that children perceived many rules and restrictions on food-related activities in the school. For the sake of brevity, we will provide only a few examples.

There were numerous rules about the order, timing, and location of food consumption that dominated young children's accounts: "Lunch at 12:15 to 12:25…if you're not finished you have to take it outside with you" (ten-year-old girl). Children reported eating "in our room" (eight-year-old boy); "at our desk" (nine-year-old girl); "with no getting up" (eight-year-old boy). Analysis by age reveals that younger children reported far more food prescriptions, restrictions, and ordinal rules, as well as more rules governing their physical movement and the level of noise in the environment.

Children reported having their lunches inspected by the teacher and, on occasion, having foods removed from their lunches and returned at the end of the day. For example, one child reported that "if you have a sandwich and the teacher sees you eating a snack then sometimes they'll check your lunch" (eleven-year-old boy). In interviews, teachers explained this activity as a form of preventive behavior management. Teachers associated classroom disruptions with consumption of pop and sugary snacks. Young children were required to eat their sandwiches first and leave unhealthy or sugary snacks to the end of their meal. The majority of students under the age of twelve were required to eat at their desks in their classrooms, either reading or engaging in quiet social interaction. In some instances, the freedom to move within the classroom was viewed as a privilege that was withdrawn by teachers as punishment for loud or inappropriate behavior.

Children reported both positive and negative qualities of food and drink: "Snack gives us energy to play, like basketball or soccer" (ten-year-old boy), but "juice makes me hyper" (eleven-year-old girl). Analysis of these food rules by gender reveals a number of interesting differences. Girls were much more likely than boys to describe rules and restrictions around what they should or shouldn't eat: "Water is better for you" (twelve-year-old girl); "If we buy too much [junk food] we could get sick" (eight-year-old girl). Indeed paradoxically, while girls described prescriptive and restrictive food rules with greater frequency, teachers reported more concerns with the content of boys' lunches and food-related behavioral issues in boys. Girls made far more statements about the nutritive value of food and the relationship between diet and health. And girls were far less likely than boys to report rules governing their physical location or bodily movement.

Conversely, the majority of food rules reported by boys governed the physical movement and location of their bodies. Boys reported restrictions on their mobility within the classroom and even at their own desks, where they were not permitted to stand up or to "fiddle" or "play" with objects such as their lunch items or water bottles. For the majority, any deviation from the default, such as visiting a friend's desk or going to the washroom, required special permission from a teacher or lunch monitor.

For children of either gender, the issues of cleanliness and noise control pervaded discussions of lunch and snack time rules. Many food restrictions involved controlling the potential for spills and messes in the classroom. Almost all children reported restrictions on the contents of their drink bottles, but children's perceptions of the reasons behind teachers' preference for water were almost universally associated with desktop and classroom cleanliness, rather than health: "If you spill [juice] on your book it will stain your book" (ten-year-old girl); "We have to drink water not juice…because if you spill juice it's sticky and it stains" (twelve-year-old girl).

Both boys and girls reported restrictions on the volume of noise permitted in their classrooms. The majority of children less than twelve years of age reported being required to eat either in silence (reading or being read to) or engaging in limited, whispered conversation: "No talking loud…you can whisper to your neighbor" (eight-year-old boy); "You have to whisper" (eight-year-old girl). As observers in the school, we can confirm that teachers frequently and emphatically enforced rules controlling the volume of children's voices.

Noise and cleanliness figure largely in students' descriptions of behavior, which garner food rewards: "If you clean up the floor or help [the teacher] she sometimes gives a treat" (nine-year-old boy). Food rewards are also given for general comportment and adherence to social conventions: "If you ask her [teacher] politely for a pencil she'll give you a candy" (nine-year-old girl). Students are rewarded for "putting up your hand" (twelve-year-old girl) and "not shouting out your answer" (twelve-year-old girl).

The social norms around meals are highly ritualized and differ widely among families and communities, but sociality is an almost universal element in meals (Douglas 1984; Meigs 1997). Schools and other institutions impose restrictive conditions on dining that are not present in the home. Meals and snacks are timed, and supervised, and take place in physical settings quite unlike those experienced elsewhere. In contrast, children view snack and lunch times as highly social occasions. Children, not surprisingly, seek to replicate aspects of the dining experience that are possible within the bounds of the institutional environment. Activities such as conversation, discussion, food sharing, and experimentation represent attempts by children to normalize the institutional meal experience. Requirements to read or be read to during lunch were viewed negatively by students as efforts by teachers to keep classrooms quiet, rather than provide a pleasant atmosphere. Although some children expressed complaints about the level of noise during lunch, the majority found noise rules intrusive and expressed a desire for social interaction and conversation.

The array of rules and restrictions addressing children's location, movement, and noise levels suggest that teachers and staff require children's comportment during snack and lunch times to closely mirror that of the larger school day. The majority of children sit in desks, in rows, in their classrooms during school meals. Their movements and the volume of their voices are closely regulated, thus limiting the degree of social interaction possible during meals. Simpson (1997) has described the myriad ways in which children's bodies are subjugated in the context of the school environment, to such an extent that formal instruction is given to teachers on such practices as "status-reducing exercises" designed to "strip the pupil of his assumed power" (Simpson 1997: 13). In contrast to the classroom environment, the lunchroom offers a period of noninstructional time that children view as a much more flexible, social occasion. Normative school rules governing their bodies impinge on their stated desires to move and vocalize freely.

The rules governing children's bodies limit their ability to engage in the social interactions that are the norm for adults and children outside the institution. Paradoxically, teachers at the study schools did not themselves experience the institutional restrictions imposed on the children. After supervising students' lunches, teachers left their classrooms and ate lunch in communal staff rooms, engaging in the highly social behaviors of conversation, discussion, food sharing, and experimentation.

Analyses of institutional regulation of children's bodies have not addressed the role of meals in social control and social reproduction. Willis (1977) and Haydon (1997) examine the role of schools in shaping a productive and disciplined workforce. Christensen and James (2001b: 214) describe school as one of a number of "socializing structures that will both foster children's autonomy, as well as their ability to conform." Although school is undoubtedly a site where the individual and civic identities of children are contested, research of this nature has largely focused on the instructional environment (Bryant 1989). To date there has been less emphasis on the role of the noninstructional school environment in the production and reproduction of normative values.

According to the UK's 1904 Elementary Code, "health education, social development and sound discipline would implant in the children habits of industry, self-control" (Haydon 1997: 104–105). These goals were explicitly linked to the goals of increasing economic competitiveness and viability in developing world markets. Elementary education was universalized, or offered to children of both sexes, with the express goal of broadening the pool of available productive labor. In the present study, the work habits rewarded are those that foster speed, "getting right down to work" (eleven-year-old girl), and diligence, "working hard" (twelve-year-old girl), qualities echoed in workplace demands for productivity (Willis 1977). Food rewards are given to students who "work independently" (eight-year-old boy), a practice that may discourage children from asking the teacher for help. Competition is encouraged, and winning individuals and groups are rewarded. Through these processes, food (primarily sweets that comprise the majority of food rewards) becomes associated with qualities that are highly valued both within and beyond the school: productivity, independence, competition, achievement, and success.

Food Rewards and Discipline

As Foucault (1975: 180) elaborates in *Discipline and Punish,* "In discipline, punishment is only one element of a double system: gratification-punishment." Control of student bodies is sometimes more effectively managed through rewards, and food is often used in this way in schools at both the group and individual levels. Teachers of all subjects encourage peer-discipline by offering food rewards such as pizza parties for overall classroom comportment. Many link individual behavior or achievement with group outcomes, by tools such as star charts or point systems. These tools are visibly displayed within the classroom, and the students exercise peer discipline on students whose columns fail to contribute to the aggregate. In some cases, food rewards are offered for circumstances beyond the student's control, such as the signing of planners or tests by parents. Similarly, the removal of items from a child's lunch may subject the child to discipline or reproof for circumstances beyond his or her control. Such actions on the part of teachers represent attempts to extend teachers' authority beyond the classroom and into the household or community.

On the individual level, small food reward items, such as hard candies, soft chewable candies, and licorice, were given to students by homeroom teachers, substitute teachers, and, occasionally, office staff. Food rewards given for academic work tended to reinforce work habits and foster competition among students: "If you do a really good story you can go to the office and she'll [secretary] give you a [candy] and you can read it to her" (eight-year-old boy). Students reported getting food rewards "if we answer the most questions or win a game" (eleven-year-old girl). Food rewards were also given to children for nonacademic tasks that foster communication between home and school, such as having parents sign tests and homework planners, and for participation in a range of civic duties within the school context, such as fundraising and helping in the cafeteria: "If you get your planner signed [by parents] for the whole month then you also get a treat" (ten-year-old girl); "Cafeteria helpers get to eat the leftovers" (twelve-year-old girl); "Office helpers and bus monitors get a pizza party at the end of the year" (thirteen-year-old girl).

Food serves as incentive to normative behavior and as disincentive to non-normative behavior. Substitute teachers in particular offered numerous food rewards. There is evidence that the subordinate professional status of substitute teachers is communicated to children and their parents (Weems 2003). It is likely substitute teachers resort to food incentives to achieve status and control in classrooms. Individual food rewards were also commonly dispensed by French teachers. In these English-language rural schools, French-language instructors face numerous challenges to child and parental engagement, not the least of which is significant geographic distance from a Francophone population center. French is simply a tough sell, and French teachers appear to be frequent users of food as incentive.

The use of food rewards by teachers has been documented by Kubik, Lytle, Hannan, Story and Perry (2002). In a survey of 490 elementary school teachers in Minneapolis-St. Paul, 73 percent of teachers reported using candy as incentive or reward for student behavior. Other commonly used food items were doughnuts, cookies, pizza, and sweetened beverages. Female teachers tended to use food rewards more frequently than did male teachers. By subject area, teachers of health-related curriculum, such as physical education and health, were the least likely to use food rewards or incentive. The use of rewards was negatively associated with years of teaching experience, suggesting that younger, less experienced teachers more commonly resort to food-related incentives or controls on children's behavior than their older, more experienced colleagues.

Nutrition Messages in Schools

It is immediately apparent that very few of the rules, restrictions, and rewards around food and beverage consumption in schools are related to nutrition or health. In the Canadian context, school curriculum requirements fall under the jurisdiction of the provincial Ministries of Education. The Ontario curriculum contains guidelines for nutrition instruction in the areas of healthy eating and daily physical activity (Ontario Ministry of Education and Training 2005). In addition, children's nutrition has been the subject of recent education policy initiatives aimed at reducing rates of childhood obesity (Ontario Ministry of Education and Training 2010). There is little doubt that, at an academic level, positive nutrition messages are being conveyed to children. But it is surprising that these messages are largely absent from children's perceptions of the rules and restrictions governing their lunch and snack times. For example, very few children referred to either positive or negative health consequences of consuming certain foods and beverages. Teachers' preference for water over juice was occasionally mentioned in association with either the hydrating effect of water or the negative effects of high-sugar beverage consumption. But the preference for water was overwhelmingly associated in children's minds with issues around environmental sanitation. In some classrooms, the "privilege" of having a water bottle at one's desk was denied or revoked. In many, the use of the water fountain was strictly regulated. The water bottle issue is clearly a case where teachers are missing an opportunity to reinforce nutrition curriculum with a broader contextual message about the positive health benefits of proper hydration.

In reference again to Simpson's study of schools and the control of students through rules that involve notions of spatiality and embodiment, this finding is not surprising. Indeed Simpson quite explicitly states: "[D]ue to their inability to resort to *corporal* punishment to control children, school staff are therefore forced to utilize a real or supposed concern with the welfare of pupils' actual *bodies* to enforce discipline, where the use of a body as a social signifier incorporates a perception that what the body does offers up a source of that body's identity" (Simpson 1997: 16–17). Students' knowledge about the negative health effects of junk food was at odds with the institutionalized presence of junk food in the schools: "At the cafeteria you have two lines and one is the hot food and the other is like the pop and chips" (eleven-year-old girl). Not only were students acutely aware of the negative health consequences of poor nutrition, but they associated those negative effects with the availability of junk food in the school: "Say the cafeteria was selling pixie sticks. Um, everybody would be buying like five or six…and they'd be eating them really quick and people would be getting diabetes" (ten-year-old girl).

Kubik et al. (2002) also observed that elementary school teachers, in general, do not role model healthy eating at school. In the Minneapolis-St. Paul study, teachers reported unhealthy cafeteria purchases and frequent vending machine use. In the present study, school administrators reported that soft drinks had recently been removed as a beverage option in school vending machines. Observation in this study proved that this was indeed the case in school lobbies, where the machines were accessible to children. However, soft drinks remained for sale in staff room vending machines. We observed that soft drinks were frequently purchased by staff and consumed in the classroom in front of children. In addition, we observed two occasions where teachers permitted students to purchase soft drinks from the staff room vending machines.

A number of authors have observed school nutrition environments that undermine nutrition and health education. Bauer et al. (2004), Neumark-Sztainer et al. (1999), and Story et al. (2002) report numerous barriers to healthy eating in U.S. schools, including high-fat cafeteria foods, limited availability of vegetables and fruits, and the presence of snack carts and vending machines selling non-nutritious snacks and beverages. According to students, parents, and teachers, soft drinks, candy, and fast foods are widely available in U.S. middle schools (Kubik et al. 2005a, 2005b). Similarly, Irish and Australian students cite the availability of junk food and junk food advertising in schools as contributors to poor diet (McKinley et al. 2005; O'Dea 2003).

With increasing global public awareness of childhood obesity, researchers and policy-makers are questioning the utility of existing school food programs (Bocquet et al. 2003) and the ethico-legal implications of foodservice that may have deleterious effects on schoolchildren's health (Bartlett 2004; Fox et al. 2005). As Crooks (2003: 191) observes: "[S]chool is a primary source of information about good nutrition, one that can affect snack consumption outside of school and has the potential to undermine both short- and long-term nutrition goals." Strategies to reduce obesity need to address not only the explicit nutrition messages contained in curriculum but the implicit messages about food and the body that are conveyed in the wider school environment.

A Gendered Environment

Counihan (1992) has described how food consumption patterns among U.S. college students unconsciously replicate hierarchies of gender and ethnicity observed in the broader American society: "By adhering to an ideology that values thinness and self-control and that permits well-off people to decide what poor people should eat and men to determine what women should eat, students uphold the stratification of US society, which elevates men, whites and the rich over women, people of color and the poor" (Counihan 1992: 55). The dietary patterns of U.S. college students are in turn formed by the cultural norms imposed by families, institutions, and the media. It is probable that gendered notions about food and the body are communicated to children and youth throughout their schooling through repeated exposure to the normative beliefs of school staff, administrators and volunteers.

In our study, there was little emotional reaction by children to the rules governing their bodily and vocal expression, suggesting these rules are longstanding and representative of institutionalized controls on children's, and especially boys', bodies. There was a significant gender disparity in the type and frequency with which these rules were applied. Boys reported significantly more restrictions on their physical movement than did girls. Boys reported more instances of discipline during school meals and were the target of teachers' concerns regarding the content of their lunches.

Haydon (1997) traces the historical roots of universal education in the UK and finds gendered notions of pedagogy that are reflected in current education practices. School has historically provided a form of "domestication" that is directed at taming boys' bodies. As late as 1975 in Britain, curriculum reinforced stereotypical values of "gender-appropriate" roles and responsibilities, preparing boys for full-time labor and girls for menial or domestic work (Haydon 1997; Corteen and Scraton 1997). Much has been written about the persistence of gender bias in British, North American, and Australian schools (Bannister 1993; Briggs and Nichols 2001; Connell 1989; Frank 1991; Goldstein 1987; Hasbrook and Harris 1999; Sargent and Harris 1998). In a particularly poignant ethnographic example, Jordan and Cowan (1995: 739) describe the institutional suppression of kindergarten boys' definitions of masculinity: through socialization to the school environment, boys' "warrior narratives" are replaced with a public-sphere masculinity of rationality and responsibility. Current teacher education texts include content that perpetuates gender stereotypes (Zittleman and Sadker 2002). Although children's exposure to gender bias is not limited to the school setting (Messner 2000; Murnen et al. 2003), school is a site where gendered treatment of boys and girls becomes institutionalized and normalized.

In our study, mealtime rules about bodily movement and comportment are a powerful illustration of the institutionalization of gender stereotypes. While the rules around physical movement and noise are purportedly the same for both boys and girls, boys appear to have much more difficulty adhering to them. Accordingly, the rules are reiterated and reinforced more frequently for boys. Boys are disciplined for violating the rules more frequently, and teachers are more likely to anticipate behavioral problems in boys. Girls, meanwhile, are largely exempt from this form of discipline, thus reinforcing their "self-control" and nonphysical play.

Despite recent increases in the number of male teachers, the overwhelming majority of elementary school teachers are female (Kovařík 1994). Messner (2000: 779) describes school as "an environment where mostly women leaders enforce rules that are hostile to masculine fantasy play and physicality." The effect is to create an environment in which both boys' and girls' physical behavior is "domesticated" or controlled. These expectations are communicated by the verbal and nonverbal language of teachers and, eventually, the children themselves, forming a gendered climate at school.

More frequent reports of food prescriptions and proscriptions among girls are likely associated with this gendered climate, in which academic performance is linked to gender identity. In such a climate, girls themselves are socialized to expect higher academic performance than they do from boys. Their responses associating food with health may be an attempt to please, to provide the "right answer" to the researcher. This process may constitute a form of researcher bias based on the gender of participants that is extremely difficult to control. Alternately, it may be the case that curricular health messages are less well received by boys due to the repetitive association between food and their behavior at school.

Discussion

To date there is limited evidence for biological effects associated with the social-cultural processes observed in our study. We suggest that this is due to limitations in the theory and methods underlying our research. To understand the breadth of influences shaping children's bodies, it may be necessary to step back from our present theoretical positions in health sciences or anthropology and widen the scope of our analysis to include multiple disciplinary perspectives. Although we as researchers understand that children's bodies are biologically and socially constituted, we continue to measure children's growth, development, and health in ways that elude complex understandings of the interaction of these variables (see Becker and Yates-Doerr, this volume).

Krieger (2005) observes that much of epidemiologic research is characterized by de-contextualized and disembodied bodies. In contrast, an embodied approach explores "how and why historically contingent, spatial, temporal and multilevel processes become embodied and generate population patterns of health, disease and well-being, including social inequalities in health" (Krieger 2005: 350–351). In the present study, we found demonstrable differences in growth (Galloway 2006) and nutrition (Galloway 2007) between boys and girls. The gendered climate observable in the schools may be one component of a larger set of interactions between biology and culture that is shaping schoolchildren's bodies (see McGarvey and Trainer, this volume).

While this study did not explicitly investigate an obesity intervention program, there are several corollary issues that are pertinent in the consideration of obesity prevention and intervention in schools:

Children's Autonomy

Children, as the constituents of school-based obesity programs, are rarely themselves consulted in the design, implementation or evaluation of school-based programming. A case in point is the U.S. CATCH program, the largest school-based intervention trial ever funded by the National Institutes of Health (Luepker et al. 1996). Begun in the early 1990s, the program has been implemented in ninety-six schools in California, Louisiana, Minnesota, and Texas. In 2003, in an effort to evaluate the tractability of negative health behaviors and the "school climate" of nutrition in study schools, researchers conducted interviews with 199 key informants (Lytle et al. 2003; Parcel et al. 2003); none of them were children.

The absence of child representation in the literature on school-based obesity interventions is representative of larger themes in research. Numerous authors observe that child informants are underutilized in child-centered research (Christensen and James 2001a; Corsaro 1997; Mayall 2000), despite their demonstrable reliability as interview and focus group participants after the age of seven years (Fine and Sandstrom 1988; Lytle et al. 1993; Mauthner 1997). In the school context, Jenks (2000: 64) contends that the absence of children's voices from education research unconsciously communicates the view that schools are populated by "passive, malleable and fundamentally non-intentional learners." This view permeates assumptions about the role of children in school-based research and wider research about children and childhood (James 1998; Qvortrup 2000; Schwartzman 2001).

Research has begun to incorporate children's voices in the area of adolescent health, where the impact of individual and group identity-making is widely acknowledged to have an effect on food purchasing and consumption. The results of this research have produced insights into the role of the school environment in shaping teens' and pre-teens' dietary habits. The food choices of 141 teens in a U.S. study were influenced primarily by taste, appearance, cost, and convenience (Neumark-Sztainer et al. 1999). In focus groups with twenty-six New England pre-teens, kids viewed the presence of high-fat convenience foods and sweetened beverages as a barrier to healthy eating in their schools: "How can we stay healthy when you're throwing all this in front of us?" (Bauer et al. 2004: 34).

Focus groups with younger children demonstrate the profound impact of the school environment in shaping children's eating habits. Children as young as seven years of age report a lack of school support for proper nutrition, proposing strategies for healthier eating such as "not taking money to school" due to the poor menu choices available (O'Dea 2003). In addition, children report gender differences in school food rules and practices. These include frequent admonishments to boys by teachers to finish their food or eat quickly, whereas similar instructions are less frequent or omitted for girls. Hart et al. (2002) suggest that through actions such as these, teachers socialize children early into the idea that boys should be fed to satiety while girls should exercise food restraint.

Among adults, ethnographic techniques such as interview and focus groups are becoming increasingly common in community-based research, as authors seek to understand the contexts underlying area-level variation in health outcomes (see Paluck et al. 2006; Towle, Godolphin and Alexander 2006, for examples). Aronson et al. (2007) and Worthman (1999) suggest that broad, anthropological and ecological approaches to research are required to fully explore the myriad levels at which health is determined, including among others genetics, biology, behavior, family, society, culture, economy, and environment.

Privacy

Children's privacy rights have often been overlooked since we view them as non-adult and thus not subject to the same rights and considerations. Alderson (1994) observes that the abrogation of children's privacy rights arises from a Western conceptualization that views the child as "incomplete." For example, both Jean Piaget and Sigmund Freud described childhood processually, invoking the notion that children are developing traits of cognition, personality, and identity (Sugarman 1987). This incomplete or non-adult conceptualization of childhood implies that children have a limited sense of their own identities and justifies actions that would violate adult boundaries of self.

Further, there is tension between the privacy and protection rights of children, which results in limited privacy, especially for young children. The notion of children's vulnerability is deeply embedded in Western society. Adults may violate children's privacy if the act of doing so is deemed in any way protective. This is especially the case in schools, where parental protection rights are assumed by principals and teachers (Bird 1994). For example, we observed one occasion in which a teacher held up a child's lunch contents to the class as an example of poor nutritional choices. It was an appalling invasion of the child's right to privacy, especially in light of the fact that the child may not have had any control over the contents of the lunch (see Rubin and Joseph, this volume). Although we have come a long way from the institutional practices and harsh remedial discipline of the 1940s and 1950s, children continue to be subjected to assessment, evaluation, verbal correction, and disciplinary measures in the public setting of the classroom. Much harm is still done to children in schools "for their own good" (see McCullough, this volume).

It is critical that we as researchers take steps to ensure that our research does not violate children's privacy. And we feel it should be stated that it is extremely easy to violate children's privacy in the school setting. The authority of the adult researcher, especially the adult female researcher, in the school setting is immediately recognized and rarely questioned by both children and parents. In the interests of achieving a large sample size, it is tempting for researchers to proceed quickly with the processes of explanation, assent, and measurement, giving children little or no opportunity to register their dissent. The physical spaces available for research use are rarely conducive to visual and auditory privacy. And the urgency with which obesity is portrayed in the media as an acute health problem means that school authorities are eager to partake in interventions targeting this health concern.

The measurement of children's weight has significant implications for children's privacy and self-esteem. Both children and parents cannot fail to be aware of social discourse on body size. The mainstream media certainly favors thinness over fatness (Neumark-Sztainer 1999). In the United States, health care providers' concerns over rising childhood obesity rates, such as the U.S. Surgeon General's "Call to Action to Prevent and Decrease Overweight and Obesity" (U.S. Department of Health and Human Services 2004), have prompted initiatives targeting childhood obesity. The response in Canada has been similar, with organizations such as the Heart and Stroke Foundation of Canada (2006) calling for increased governmental support for BMI screening programs.

In 2003, the Arkansas state legislature passed a law requiring schools to monitor students' weights and heights and send home periodic "BMI report cards" to parents (Ikeda et al. 2006). In Canada the British Columbia (BC) Medical Association (Legislative Assembly of BC Select Standing Committee on Health 2006) has recently proposed the creation of a child health registry that would track children's height, weight, and waist-to-hip ratio between kindergarten and grade 12. However numerous researchers have described the harmful effects of ill-advised screening programs on children's self-esteem and body image (Budd and Volpe

2006; Ikeda et al. 2006; Neumark-Sztainer 1999). Should jurisdictions proceed with school-based obesity screening, we recommend the measurement protocol include measures to safeguard the privacy and autonomy rights of children.

Peer Relations

After the family, school is perhaps the most significant social institution in children's lives. Research with children in the context of school plunges the researcher into the midst of numerous social relationships that are of great significance to children.

There is a large literature on the sociology of schoolchildren. Studies have illustrated the importance of children's social interactions (Alanen 2001; Bardy 1994; Belle 1989; Berndt 1989; Bryant 1994; Näsman 1994; Warde 2001; Youniss 1994) as well as the complexity and nuance of communication among children (Donaldson 1986; Opie and Opie 1992). Numerous researchers claim that peer relations are the most significant component of a child's socialization to school (Hirsch and Dubois 1989; Mayall 1994; Oswald et al. 1994).

In terms of overall quality of life, the social networks of children appear to have a significant impact on well-being. Children's peer relations at school have been correlated with self-esteem (Blyth and Traeger 1988) and the ability to cope with psychological stress (Sandler et al. 1989), as well as academic performance (Flook et al. 2005). Despite the widespread recognition in the sociological literature of the importance of children's social networks at school, the majority of the literature on school-based research fails to mention peer relations. An exception is a recent report of the influence of adolescent girls' social networks on dietary and physical activity behavior (Voorhees et al. 2005).

Obesity is an extremely sensitive topic for children, as evidenced by numerous reports of the stigmatization of overweight children (Brixval et al. 2011; Lumeng et al. 2010; McCormack et al. 2011; Robinson 2006). There is a real danger that introduction of obesity-related surveillance or screening into the school environment may formalize existing social patterns of stigmatization within the school or classroom, thereby worsening the suffering experienced by some children (see Rubin and Joseph, this volume). It is essential that all school staff receive training in the language and practices necessary to deal with this issue with sensitivity and respect and that this training be formulated and delivered in such a way that develops reflexivity among staff regarding the cultural norms of school.

Conclusions and Implications

Existing school-based interventions targeting childhood obesity tend to utilize the institutional model of education in the service of public health. Although this is certainly the intent of such programs, we argue that this approach constrains children's autonomy and privacy rights and replicates patterns of authority and gender construction and identity that may not be conducive to program goals of improving child health and reducing obesity.

The success of existing interventions tends to be framed in terms of improvement in children's dietary knowledge or behavior, reduction in sedentary activities, and increase in physical activity. The emphasis on behavioral approaches to obesity prevention is the result of a narrow conception of obesity as a public health problem (see McNaughton, this volume). Lay understandings of obesity causation, which are widespread among health and education professionals, include the belief that obesity is a genetic or heritable condition and the sense that obesity arises from a lack of self-control on the part of the obese child or adult (Birch and Davison 2001; Raynor et al. 2011). Despite a decade of calls for sweeping environmental changes, such as taxing or limiting fast food sales in public spaces (Institute of Medicine 2010), limiting advertising of junk food during children's television programming (Goris et al. 2010), and more attention to urban design to improve walkability and access to fresh, healthy food (Frank et al. 2004), individual and behavioral interventions continue to dominate public health rhetoric on child obesity (table 8.1) (see Rubin and Joseph, this volume, for a discussion of the individualized approach to obesity). An exception to this approach, however, can be found in an obesity prevention project in the UK called the Foresight Obesity Project, as outlined by Popkin (2011: 87). Included in this project among other initiatives is a national ban on media advertising to children of unhealthy foods and a school-based initiative for compulsory cooking classes for children aged six to eight years.

The expansion of outcome measures into the realm of academic performance (Hoelscher et al. 2010; Hollar et al. 2010) is a cause for concern. Matějček (1985, in Kovařík 1994) estimates that approximately 25 percent of children suffer chronic stress with regard to school performance and achievement. Research that explicitly links body size with academic performance may pose additional stress and suffering on children already stigmatized.

We suggest that the institution of school, permeated as it is with a culture of discipline through controlling bodies, is one that permits abrogation of children's autonomy and privacy rights and therefore is not the ideal location for childhood obesity intervention. Further, obesity itself is an issue requiring sensitivity in precisely the areas in which the cultural norms of school are entrenched: identity, autonomy, embodiment, and privacy for examples. In the present study, we observe that the institution of school enforces rigorous authority, a lack of autonomy, control of children's bodies and the cultivation of stereotypes that replicate societal patterns of gender identity. The context of school, therefore, is sensitive territory in which to embark on obesity surveillance and intervention.

The choice of the school setting is one that carries with it major implications for the overall health and well-being of children. It is not neutral ground.

References

Alanen, L. 2001. "Childhood as a Generational Condition: Children's Daily Lives in a Central Finland Town." In *Conceptualizing Child-Adult Relations,* ed. L. Alanen and B. Mayall. New York: Routledge/Falmer, 129–143.

Alderson, P. 1994. "Researching Children's Right to Integrity." In *Children's childhoods: Observed and Experienced,* ed. B. Mayall. London: Falmer Press, 45–62.

Aronson, R. E., A. B. Wallis, P. J. O'Campo, T. L. Whitehead, and P. Schafer. 2007. "Ethnographically Informed Community Evaluation: A Framework and Approach for Evaluating Community-based Initiatives." *Maternal and Child Health* 11, no. 2: 97–109.

Bannister, H. 1993. "Truths About Assessment and the Learning of Girls: From Gender Difference to the Production of Gendered Attainment." In *Gender Matters in Educational Administration and Policy,* ed. J. Blackmore and J. Kenway. London: Falmer Press, 101–115.

Bardy, M. 1994. "The manuscript of the 100-years project: towards a revision." In *Childhood Matters: Social Theory, Practice and Politics,* ed. J. Qvortrup, M. Bardy, G. Sgritta, and H. Wintersberger. Aldershot: Avebury, 299–318.

Bartlett, C. F. 2004. "You Are What You Serve: Are School Districts Liable for Serving Unhealthy Food and Beverages to Students?" *Seton Hall Law Review* 34, no. 3: 1053–1091.

Bauer, K. W., Y. W. Yang, and S. B. Austin. 2004. "How Can We Stay Healthy When You're Throwing All of This in Front of Us? Findings from Focus Groups and Interviews in Middle Schools on Environmental Influences on Nutrition and Physical Activity." *Health Education and Behavior* 31, no. 1: 34–46.

Bell, A. C., and B. A. Swinburn. 2004. "What Are the Key Food Groups to Target for Preventing Obesity and Improving Nutrition in Schools?" *European Journal of Clinical Nutrition* 58: 258–263.

Belle, D. 1989. "Gender Differences in Children's Social Networks and Supports." In *Children's Social Networks and Social Supports,* ed. D. Belle. New York: J. Wiley, 73–188.

Berndt, T. J. 1989. "Obtaining Support from Friends During Childhood and Adolescence." In *Children's Social Networks and Social Supports,* ed. D. Belle. New York: J. Wiley, 308–329.

Birch, L. L., and K. K. Davison. 2001. "Family Environmental Factors Influencing the Developing Behavioral Controls of Food Intake and Childhood Overweight." *Pediatric Clinics of North America* 48, no. 4: 893–907.

Bird, L. 1994. "Creating the Capable Body: Discourses about Ability and Effort in Primary and Secondary School Studies." In *Children's Childhoods: Observed and Experienced,* ed. B. Mayall. London: Falmer Press, 97–114.

Blyth, D. A., and C. Traeger. 1988. "Adolescent Self-esteem and Perceived Relationships with Parents and Peers." In *Social Networks and Social Support in Childhood and Adolescence,* eds. F. Nestmann and K. Hurrelmann. New York: de Gruyter, 171–194.

Bocquet, A., J. L. Bresson, A. Briend, J. P. Chouraqui, D. Darmaun, C. Dupont, M. L. Frelut, J. Ghisolfi, J. P. Girardet, O. Goulet, G. Putet, D. Rieu, J. Rigo, D. Turck, and M. Vidailhet. 2003. "The Morning Snack at School is Inadequate and Unnecessary." *Archives of Pediatrics* 10: 945–947.

Briggs, F., and S. Nichols. 2001. "Pleasing Yourself and Working for the Teacher: Children's Perceptions of School." *Early Childhood Development and Care* 170: 13–30.

Brixval, C. S., S. L. Rayce, M. Rasmussen, B. E. Holstein, and P. Due. 2011. "Overweight, Body Image and Bullying: An Epidemiological Study of 11- to 15-Year Olds." *European Journal of Public Health* 22, no. 1: 126–130.

Bryant, B. K. 1989. "The Need for Support in Relation to the Need for Autonomy." In *Children's Social Networks and Social Supports,* ed. D. Belle. New York: J. Wiley, 332–351.

———. 1994. "How Does Social Support Function in Childhood?" In *Social Networks and Social Support in Childhood and Adolescence,* ed. F. Nestmann and K. Hurrelmann. New York: de Gruyter, 23–36.

Bryant, E. J., K. Kiezebrink, N. A. King, and J. E. Blundell. 2010. "Interaction between Disinhibition and Restraint: Implications for Body Weight and Eating Disturbance." *Eating and Weight Disorders* 15, no. 1–2: e43–51.

Budd, G. M., and S. L. Volpe. 2006. "School-Based Obesity Prevention: Research, Challenges, and Recommendations." *Journal of School Health* 76, no. 10: 485–495.

Bundy, D. A. P., S. Shaeffer, M. Jukes, K. Beegle, A. Gillespie, L. Drake, S. F. Lee, A. M. Hoffman, J. Jones, A. Mitchell, D. Barcelona, B. Camara, C. Golmar, L. Savioli, M. Sembene, T. Takeuchi, and C. Wright. 2006. "School-based Health and Nutrition Programs." In *Disease Control Priorities in Developing Countries, 2nd ed.,* ed. D. T. Jamison, J. G. Breman, A. R. Measham, G. Alleyne, M. Claeson, and D. B. Evans. Washington, DC: World Bank, 1091–1108.

Chomitz, V. R., R. J. McGowan, J. M. Wendel, S. A. Williams, H. J. Cabral, S. E. King, D. B. Olcott, M. Cappello, S. Breen, and K. A. Hacker. 2010. "Healthy Living Cambridge Kids: A Community-based Participatory Effort to Promote Healthy Weight and Fitness." *Obesity* 18, Suppl. 1: S45–53.

Christensen, P., and A. James. 2001a. "Foreword." In *Research with Children: Perspectives and Practices,* ed. P. Christensen and A. James. New York: Falmer, xi–xii.

———. 2001b. "What are Schools For? The Temporal Experience of Children's Learning in Northern England." In *Conceptualizing Child-Adult Relations,* ed. L. Alanen and B. Mayall. New York: Routledge/Falmer, 70–85.

Coleman, K. J., C. L. Tiller, J. Sanchez, E. M. Heath, O. Sy, G. Milliken, and D. A. Dzewaltowski. 2005. "Prevention of the Epidemic Increase in Child risk of Overweight in Low-income Schools: The El Paso Coordinated Approach to Child Health." *Archives of Pediatric and Adolescent Medicine* 159: 217–224.

Connell, R. W. 1989. "Cool Guys, Swots and Wimps: The Interplay of Masculinity and Education." *Oxford Review of Education* 15: 291–303.

Contento, I. R., P. A. Koch, H. Lee, and A. Calabrese-Barton. 2010. "Adolescents Demonstrate Improvement in Obesity Risk Behaviors after Completion of Choice, Control and Change, a Curriculum Addressing Personal Agency and Autonomous Motivation." *Journal of the American Dietetic Association* 110, no. 12: 1830–1839.

Corsaro, W. 1997. *The Sociology of Childhood.* Thousand Oaks, CA: Pine Forge Press.

Corteen, K., and P. Scraton. 1997. "Prolonging 'Childhood': Manufacturing 'Innocence' and Regulating Sexuality." In *'Childhood' in 'Crisis'?* ed. P. Scraton. London: Bristol, 76–100.

Counihan, C. M. 1992. "Food Rules in the United States: Individualism, Control and Hierarchy." *Anthropological Quarterly* 65, no. 2: 55–66.

Crooks, D. L. 2003. "Trading Nutrition for Education: Nutritional Status and the Sale of Snack Foods in an Eastern Kentucky School." *Medical Anthropology Quarterly* 17, no. 2: 182–199.

Cullen, K. W., and D. I. Thompson. 2005. "Texas School Food Policy Changes Related to Middle School à la Carte/Snack Bar Foods: Potential Savings in Kilocalories." *Journal of the American Dietetic Association* 105, no. 12: 1952–1954.

da Silva Vargas, I. C., R. Sichieri, G. Sandre-Pereira, and G. V. de Veiga. 2011. "Evaluation of an Obesity Prevention Program in Adolescents of Public Schools." *Revista Saúde Pública* 45, no. 1: 1.

de Silva-Sanigorski, A., L. Prosser, L. Carpenter, S. Honisett, L. Gibbs, M. Moodie, L. Sheppard, B. Swinburn, and E. Waters. 2010. "Evaluation of the Childhood Obesity Prevention Program Kids 'Go for Your Life.'" *BMC Public Health* 28, no. 10: 288.

Donaldson, M. L. 1986. *Children's Explanations: A Psycholinguistic Study.* New York: Cambridge University Press.

Douglas, M. 1984. *Food in the Social Order.* New York: Russell Sage Foundation.

Fine, G. A., and K. L. Sandstrom. 1988. *Knowing Children: Participant Observation with Minors.* Newbury Park, CA: Sage Publications.

Flook, L., R. L. Repetti, and J. B. Ullman. 2005. "Classroom Social Experiences as Predictors of Academic Performance." *Developmental Psychology* 41, no. 2: 319–327.

Florencio, C. A. 2001. "Developments and Variations in School-based Feeding Programs around the World." *Nutrition Today* 36, no. 1: 29–36.

Foucault, M. 1975. *Discipline and Punish: The Birth of the Prison.* New York: Penguin.

Fox, S., A. Meinen, M. Pesik, M. Landis, and P. L. Remington. 2005. "Competitive Food Initiatives in Schools and Overweight in Children: A Review of the Evidence." *Wisconsin Medical Journal* 104, no. 5: 38–43.

Frank, B. 1991. "Straight/Strait Jackets for Masculinity: Educating for 'Real' Men." *Atlantis* 18: 47–59.

Frank, L. D., M. A. Andresen, and T. L. Schmid. 2004. "Obesity Relationships with Community Design, Physical Activity, and Time Spent in Cars." *American Journal of Preventive Medicine* 27, no. 22: 87–96.

Freedman, D. S., W. H. Dietz, S. R. Srinivasan, G. W. Berenson. 1999. "The Relation of Overweight to Cardiovascular Risk Factors among Children and Adolescents: The Bogalusa Heart Study." *Pediatrics* 103: 1175–1182.

French, S. A., and H. Wechsler. 2004. "School-based Research and Initiatives: Fruit and Vegetable Environment, Policy, and Pricing Workshop." *Preventive Medicine* 39, Suppl.: S101–107.

Galloway, T. 2006. "Obesity Rates among Rural Ontario Schoolchildren." *Canadian Journal of Public Health* 97, no. 5: 353–356.

———. 2007. "Gender Differences in Growth and Nutrition in a Sample of Rural Canadian Schoolchildren." *American Journal of Human Biology* 19, no. 6: 774–788.

Goldstein, H. 1986. "Gender Bias and Test Norms in Educational Selection." *Research Intelligence: BERA Newsletter* May: 2–4.

Goris, J. M., S. Petersen, E. Stamatakis, and J. L. Veerman. 2010. "Television Food Advertising and the Prevalence of Childhood Overweight and Obesity: A Multicountry Comparison." *Public Health Nutrition* 13, no. 7: 1003–1012.

Gortmaker, S. L., K. Peterson, J. Wiecha, A. M. Sobol, S. Dixit, M. K. Fox, and N. Laird. 1999. "Reducing Obesity via a School-based Interdisciplinary Intervention among Youth: Planet Health." *Archives of Pediatric and Adolescent Medicine* 153, no. 4: 409–418.

Greening, L., K. T. Harrell, A. K. Low, and C. E. Fielder. 2011. "Efficacy of a School-based Childhood Obesity Intervention Program in a Rural Southern Community: TEAM Mississippi Project." *Obesity* 19, no. 6: 1213–1219.

Hart, K. H., J. A. Bishop, and H. Truby. 2002. "An Investigation into School Children's Knowledge and Awareness of Food and Nutrition." *Journal of Human Nutrition and Dietetics* 15: 129–140.

Hasbrook, C. A., and O. Harris. 1999. "Wrestling with Gender: Physicality and Masculinities among Inner-city First and Second Graders." *Men and Masculinities* 1, no. 3: 302–318.

Hay, D. 1999. "School-Based Feeding Programs: A Good Choice for Children Health Canada." Health Promotion and Programs Branch, Childhood and Youth Division, Ottawa, ON.

Haydon, D. 1997. "'Crisis' in the Classroom?" In *'Childhood' in 'Crisis'?* ed. P. Scraton. London: Bristol, 101–123.

Heart and Stroke Foundation of Canada. 2006. "Tipping the Scales of Progress: Heart and Stroke Foundation of Canada Releases New Data and Recommendations on Tobacco, Obesity and Disease Prevention." Ottawa, ON.

Herman, K. M., C. L. Craig, L. Gauvin, and P. T. Katzmarzyk. 2009. "Tracking of Obesity and Physical Activity from Childhood to Adulthood: The Physical Activity Longitudinal Study." *International Journal of Pediatric Obesity* 4: 281–288.

Hesketh, K., M. Wake, E. Waters, J. Carlin, and D. Crawford. 2004. "Stability of Body Mass Index in Australian Children: A Prospective Cohort Study across the Middle Childhood Years." *Public Health Nutrition* 7: 303–309.

Hirsch, B. J., and D. L. Dubois. 1989. "The School-Nonschool Ecology of Early Adolescent Friendships." In *Children's Social Networks and Social Supports,* ed. D. Belle. New York: J. Wiley, 260–274.

Hoelscher, D. M., A. E. Springer, N. Ranjit, C. L. Perry, A. E. Evans, M. Stigler, and S. H. Kelder. 2010. "Reductions in Child Obesity among Disadvantaged School Children with Community Involvement: The Travis County CATCH Trial." *Obesity* 18, Suppl. 1: S36–44.

Hollar, D., S. E. Messiah, G. Lopez-Mitnik, T. L. Hollar, M. Almon, and A. S. Agatston. 2010. "Effect of a Two-Year Obesity Prevention Intervention on Percentile Changes in Body Mass Index and Academic Performance in Low-income Elementary School Children." *American Journal of Public Health* 100, no. 4: 646–653.

Hooper, M., and S. Evers. 2003. "What do Ontario Children Eat for Breakfast? Food Group, Energy, and Macronutrient Intake." *Canadian Journal of Dietetic Practice and Research* 64, no. 1: 28–30.

Ikeda, J. P., P. B. Crawford, and G. Woodward-Lopez. 2006. "BMI Screening in Schools: Helpful or Harmful?" *Health Education Research* 21, no. 6: 761–769.

Institute of Medicine. 2010. *Bridging the Evidence Gap in Obesity Prevention: A Framework to Inform Decision Making.* Washington, DC.

Irwin, C. C., R. L. Irwin, M. E. Miller, G. W. Somes, and P. A. Richey. 2010. "Get Fit with the Grizzlies: A Community-School-Home Initiative to Fight Childhood Obesity." *Journal of School Health* 80, no. 7: 333–339.

James, A. 1998. "From the Child's Point of View: Issues in the Social Construction of Childhood." In *Biosocial Perspectives on Children,* ed. C. Panter-Brick. New York: Cambridge University Press, 45–65.

James, J., and D. Kerr. 2005. "Prevention of Childhood Obesity by Reducing Soft Drinks." *International Journal of Obesity* 29, Suppl. 2: S54–57.

James, J., P. Thomas, D. Cavan, and D. Kerr. 2004. "Preventing Childhood Obesity by Reducing Consumption of Carbonated Drinks: Cluster Randomized Controlled Trial." *British Medical Journal* 328, no. 7450: 1237.

Jenks, C. 2000. "Zeitgeist Research on Childhood." In *Research with Children: Perspectives and Practices,* eds. P. Christensen and A. James. New York: Falmer, 62–76.

Johnson, C. C., D. Li, J. Epping, L. A. Lytle, P. W. Cribb, B. J. Williston, and M. Yang. 2000. "A Transactional Model of Social Support, Self-efficacy, and Physical Activity of Children in CATCH Texas." *Journal of Health Education* 31, no. 1: 2–9.

Jordan, E., and A. Cowan. 1995. "Warrior Narratives in the Kindergarten Classroom: Renegotiating the Social Contract?" *Gender and Society* 9, no. 6: 727–743.

Kipping, R. R., R. Jago, and D. A. Lawlor. 2010. "Diet Outcomes of a Pilot School-based Randomised Controlled Obesity Prevention Study with 9-10 Year Olds in England." *Preventive Medicine* 51, no. 1: 56–62.

Kovařík, J. 1994. "The Space and Time of Children at the Interface of Psychology and Sociology." In *Childhood Matters: Social Theory, Practice and Politics,* ed. J. Qvortrup, M. Bardy, G. Sgritta, and H. Wintersberger. Aldershot: Avebury, 101–122.

Krieger, N. 2005. "Embodiment: A Conceptual Glossary for Epidemiology." *Journal of Epidemiology and Community Health* 59: 350–355.

Kubik, M.Y., L.A. Lytle, P. J. Hannan, M. Story, and C.L. Perry. 2002. "Food-Related Beliefs, Eating Behavior, and Classroom Food Practices of Middle School Teachers." *Journal of School Health* 72, no. 8: 339-45.

Kubik, M.Y., L. A. Lytle, and M. Story. 2005a. "School-wide Food Practices are Associated with Body Mass Index in Middle School Students." *Archives of Pediatric and Adolescent Medicine* 159, no. 12: 1111–1114.

———. 2005b. "Soft Drinks, Candy, and Fast Food: What Parents and Teachers Think about the Middle School Food Environment." *Journal of the American Dietetic Association* 105, no. 2: 233–239.

Legislative Assembly of BC Select Standing Committee on Health. 2006. "A Strategy for Combatting Childhood Obesity and Physical Inactivity in British Columbia." Report, Victoria BC.

Lien, N., M. Bjelland, I. H. Bergh, M. Grydeland, S. A. Anderssen, Y. Ommundsen, L. F. Andersen, H. B. Henriksen, J. S. Randby, and K. I. Klepp. 2010. "Design of a 20-Month Comprehensive, Multicomponent School-based Randomised Trial to Promote Healthy Weight Development among 11–13 Year Olds: The Health in Adolescents study." *Scandinavian Journal of Public Health* 38, Suppl. 5: 38–51.

Lowe, C. F., P. J. Horne, K. Tapper, M. Bowdery, and C. Egerton. 2004. "Effects of a Peer Modeling and Rewards-based Intervention to Increase Fruit and Vegetable Consumption in Children." *European Journal of Clinical Nutrition* 58: 510–522.

Lubans, D. R., P. J. Morgan, D. Dewar, C. E. Collins, R. C. Plotnikoff, A. D. Okely, M. J. Batterham, T. Finn, and R. Callister. 2010. "The Nutrition and Enjoyable Activity for Teen Girls (NEAT Girls) Randomized Controlled Trial for Adolescent Girls from Disadvantaged Secondary Schools: Rationale, Study Protocol, and Baseline Results." *BMC Public Health* 10: 652.

Luepker, R. V., C. L. Perry, S. M. McKinlay, P. R. Nader, G. S. Parcel, E. J. Stone, L. S. Webber, J. P. Elder, H. A. Feldman, and C. C. Johnson. 1996. "Outcomes of a field trial to improve children's dietary patterns and physical activity: The Child and Adolescent Trial for Cardiovascular Health, CATCH collaborative group." *Journal of the American Medical Association* 275, no. 10: 768–776.

Lumeng, J. C., P. Forrest, D. P. Appugliese, N. Kaciroti, R. F. Corwyn, and R. H. Bradley. 2010. "Weight Status as a Predictor of Being Bullied in Third through Sixth Grades." *Pediatrics* 125, no. 6: 1301–1307.

Lytle, L. A., M. Z. Nichaman, E. Obarzanek, E. Glovsky, D. Montgomery, T. Nicklas, M. Zive, and H. Feldman. 1993. "Validation of 24-Hour Recalls Assisted by Food Records in Third-Grade Children." *Journal of the American Dietetic Association* 93: 1431–1436.

Lytle, L. A., J. Ward, P. R. Nader, S. Pedersen, and B. J. Williston. 2003. "Maintenance of a Health Promotion Program in Elementary Schools: Results from the CATCH-ON Study Key Informant Interviews." *Health Education and Behavior* 30, no. 4: 503–518.

Madsen, K. A., H. R. Thompson, L. Wlasiuk, E. Queliza, C. Schmidt, and T. B. Newman. 2009. "After-School Program to Reduce Obesity in Minority Children: A Pilot Study." *J Child Health Care* 13, no. 4: 333–346.

Mauthner, M. 1997. "Methodological Aspects of Collecting Data from Children: Lessons from Three Research Projects." *Children and Society* 11: 16–28.

Mayall, B. 1994. "Children in Action at Home and at School." In *Children's Childhoods: Observed and Experienced,* ed. B. Mayall. London: Falmer Press, 114–127.

———. 2000. "Conversations with Children: Working with Generational Issues." In *Research with Children: Perspectives and Practices,* ed. P. Christensen and A. James. New York: Falmer, 120–135.

Maynard, M. J., G. Baker, E. Rawlins, A. Anderson, and S. Harding. 2009. "Developing Obesity Prevention Interventions among Minority Ethnic Children in Schools and Places of Worship: The DEAL (DiEt and Active Living) Study." *BMC Public Health* 9: 480.

McCormack, L. A., M. N. Laska, C. Gray, S. Veblen-Mortenson, D. Barr-Anderson, and M. Story. 2011. "Weight-related Teasing in a Racially Diverse Sample of Sixth-grade Children." *Journal of the American Dietetic Association* 111, no. 3: 431–436.

McGaffey, A., K. Hughes, S. K. Fidler, F. J. D'Amico, and M. N. Stalter. 2010. "Can Elvis Pretzley and the Fitwits Improve Knowledge of Obesity, Nutrition, Exercise, and Portions in Fifth Graders?" *International Journal of Obesity* 34, no. 7: 1134–1142.

McKenzie, T. L., E. J. Stone, H. A. Feldman, J. N. Epping, M. Yang, P. K. Strikmiller, L. A. Lytle, and G. S. Parcel. 2001. "Effects of the CATCH Physical Education Intervention: Teacher Type and Lesson Location." *American Journal of Preventive Medicine* 21, no. 2: 101–109.

McKinley, M. C., C. Lowis, P. J. Robson, J. M. W. Wallace, M. Morrissey, A. Moran, and M. B. E. Livingstone. 2005. "It's Good to Talk: Children's Views on Food and Nutrition." *European Journal of Clinical Nutrition* 59, no. 4: 542–551.

Meigs, A. 1997. "Food as a Cultural Construction." In *Food and Culture: A Reader,* eds. C. Counihan and P. Van Esterik. New York: Routledge, 95–106.

Messner, M. A. 2000. "Barbie Girls Versus Sea Monsters: Children Constructing Gender." *Gender and Society* 14, no. 6: 765–784.

Moffat, T. 2010. "The 'Childhood Obesity Epidemic': Health Crisis or Social Construction?" *Medical Anthropology Quarterly* 24: 1–21.

Murnen, S. K., L. Smolak, and J. A. Mills. 2003. "Good, Thin, Sexy Women and Strong, Muscular Men: Grade-school Children's Responses to Objectified Images of Women and Men." *Sex Roles* 49, no. 9/10: 427–437.

Näsman, E. 1994. "Individualization and Institutionalization of Childhood in Today's Europe." In *Childhood Matters: Social Theory, Practice and Politics,* ed. J. Qvortrup, M. Bardy, G. Sgritta, and H. Wintersberger. Aldershot: Avebury, 65–187.

Neumark-Sztainer, D. 1999. "The Weight Dilemma: A Range of Philosophical Perspectives." *International Journal of Obesity* 23, Suppl. 2: S31–S37.

Neumark-Sztainer, D., M. Story, C. Perry, M. A. Casey. 1999. "Factors Influencing Food Choices of Adolescents: Findings from Focus-Group Discussions with Adolescents." *Journal of the American Dietetic Association* 99, no. 8: 929–934.

O'Dea, J. A. 2003. "Why Do Kids Eat Healthful Food? Perceived Benefits of and Barriers to Healthful Eating and Physical Activity among Children and Adolescents." *Journal of the American Dietetic Association* 103, no. 4: 497–501.

Ontario Ministry of Education and Training. 2005. "The Ontario Curriculum Grades 1-8: Health and Physical Education." Toronto, ON.

———. 2010. "Policy/Program Memorandum No. 150: School Food and Beverage Policy." Toronto, ON.

Opie, I., and P. Opie. 1992. "The Lore and Language of Schoolchildren." In *The Sociology of Childhood: Essential Readings,* ed. C. Jenks. London: Batsford Academic and Educational Ltd, 173–180.

Oswald, H., L. Krappmann, H. Uhlendorff, and K. Weiss. 1994. "Social Relationships and Support among Peers during Middle Childhood." In *Social Networks and Social Support in Childhood and Adolescence,* ed. F. Nestmann and K. Hurrelmann. New York: de Gruyter, 171–189.

Paluck, E. C., M. Allerdings, K. Kealy, and H. Dorgan. 2006. "Health Promotion Needs of Women Living in Rural Areas: An Exploratory Study." *Canadian Journal of Rural Medicine* 11, no. 2: 111–116.

Parcel, G. S., C. L. Perry, S. H. Kelder, J. P. Elder, P. D. Mitchell, L. A. Lytle, C. Johnson, and E. J. Stone. 2003. "School Climate and the Institutionalization of the CATCH Program." *Health Education and Behavior* 30, no. 4: 489–502.

Plachta-Danielzik, S., B. Landsberg, D. Lange, J. Seibert, and M. J. Müller. 2011. "Eight-Year Follow-up of School-based Intervention on Childhood Overweight: The Kiel Obesity Prevention Study." *Obesity Facts* 4, no. 1: 35–43.

Popkin, B. M. 2011. "Rank Prize Lecture: Contemporary Nutritional Transition: Determinants of Diet and its Impact on Body Composition." *Proceedings of the Nutrition Society* 70: 82–91.

Qvortrup, J. 2000. "Macroanalysis of Childhood." In *Research with Children: Perspectives and Practices,* ed. P. Christensen and A. James. New York: Falmer, 77–97.

Raynor, H .A., E. L. Van Walleghen, K. M. Osterholt, C. N. Hart, E. Jelalian, R. R. Wing, and G. S. Goldfield. 2011. "The Relationship between Child and Parent Food Hedonics and Parent and Child Food Group Intake in Children with Overweight/Obesity." *Journal of the American Dietetic Association* 111, no. 3: 425–430.

Reynolds, K. D., F. A. Franklin, D. Binkley, J. M. Raczynski, K. F. Harrington, K. A. Kirk, and S. Person. 2000. "Increasing the Fruit and Vegetable Consumption of Fourth-Graders: Results from the High-5 Project." *Preventive Medicine* 30: 309–319.

Robinson, S. 2006. "Victimization of Obese Adolescents." *Journal of School Nursing* 22, no. 4: 201–206.

Sadeno, C., G. Wolf, T. Drake, and M. Reicks. 2000. "Behavioral Strategies to Increase Fruit and Vegetable Intake by Fourth- through Sixth-Grade Students." *Journal of the American Dietetic Association* 100, no. 7: 828–830.

Sandler, I. N., P. Miller, J. Short, and S. A. Wolchik. 1989. "Social Support as a Protective Factor for Children in Stress." In *Children's Social Networks and Social Supports,* ed. D. Belle. New York: J. Wiley, 277–307.

Sargent, C., and M. Harris. 1998. "Bad boys and good girls: the implications of gender ideology for child health in Jamaica." In *Small Wars: The Cultural Politics of Childhood,* eds. N. Scheper-Hughes and C. Sargent. Berkeley: University of California Press, 202–228.

Schwartzman, H. B. 2001. "Introduction: Questions and Challenges for a 21st Century Anthropology of Children." In *Children and Anthropology: Perspectives for the 21st Century,* ed. H. B. Schwartzman. Westport, CT: Bergin and Garvey, 1–14.

Siega-Riz, A. M., L. E. Ghormli, C. Mobley, B. Gillis, D. Stadler, J. Hartstein, S. L. Volpe, A. Virus, and J. Bridgman. 2011. "The HEALTHY Study Group, Efficacy of a School-based Childhood Obesity Intervention Program in a Rural Southern Community: TEAM Mississi

Simpson, B. 1997. "The Body as a Site of Contestation of Power within the School Context." *Anthropology in Action* 4, no. 3: 13–19.

Singhal, N., A. Misra, P. Shah, and S. Gulati. 2010. "Effects of Controlled School-Based Multi-component Model of Nutrition and Lifestyle Interventions on Behavior Modification, Anthropometry and Metabolic Risk Profile of Urban Asian Indian Adolescents in North India." *European Journal of Clinical Nutrition* 64, no. 4: 364–373.

Story, M., D. Neumark-Sztainer, and S. French. 2002. "Individual and Environmental Influences on Adolescent Eating Behaviors." *Journal of the American Dietetic Association* 102, no. 3: S40–51.

Sugarman, S. 1987. "The Priority of Description in Developmental Psychology." *International Journal of Behavioral Development* 10: 391–414.

Toruner, E. K., and S. Savaser. 2010. "A Controlled Evaluation of a School-Based Obesity Prevention in Turkish School Children." *Journal of School Nursing* 26, no. 6: 473–482.

Towle, A., W. Godolphin, and T. Alexander. 2006. "Doctor-Patient Communications in the Aboriginal Community: Towards the Development of Educational Programs." *Patient Education and Counseling* 62, no. 3: 340–346.

U.S. Department of Health and Human Services, Office for Human Research Protections. 2004. "Code of Federal Regulations Part 46, Protection of Human Subjects, Section A: Basic Policy for Protection of Human Research Subjects." Washington, DC. Electronic document, accessed 31 May 2011, available from: hhttp://ohsr.od.nih.gov/guidelines/GrayBooklet82404.pdf

Urquhart, C. S., and T. V. Mihalynuk. 2011. "Disordered Eating in Women: Implications for the Obesity Pandemic." *Canadian Journal of Dietetic Practice and Research* 72, no. 1: 50.

van Strien, T., and F. G. Bazelier. 2007. "Perceived Parental Control of Food Intake is Related to External, Restrained and Emotional Eating in 7-12-Year-Old Boys and Girls." *Appetite* 49, no. 3: 618–625.

Voorhees, C. C., D. Murray, G. Welk, A. Birnbaum, K. M. Ribisl, C. C. Johnson, K. A. Pfeiffer, B. Saksvig, and J. B. Jobe. 2005. "The Role of Peer Social Network Factors and Physical Activity in Adolescent Girls." *American Journal of Health Behavior* 29, no. 2: 183–190.

Warde, M. J. 2001. "Childhood, School, and Family: Continuity and Displacement in Recent Research." In *Governing the Child in the New Millennium,* ed. K. Hultqvist and G. Dahlberg. New York: RoutledgeFalmer, 172–192.

Weems, L. 2003. "Between Deficiency and Excess: Representations of Substitute Teachers and the Paradoxes of Professionalism." *Journal of Teacher Education* 54, no. 3: 254–265.

Wesnes, K. A., C. Pincock, D. Richardson, G. Helm, and S. Hails. 2003. "Breakfast Reduces Declines in Attention and Memory over the Morning in Schoolchildren." *Appetite* 41: 329–331.

Williams, J., M. Wake, and M. Campbell. 2007. "Comparing Estimates of Body Fat in Children using Published Bioelectrical Impedance Analysis Equations." *International Journal of Pediatric Obesity* 2, no. 3: 174–179.

Williams, S. 2001. "Overweight at Age 21: The Association with Body Mass Index in Childhood and Adolescence and Parents' Body Mass Index, A Cohort Study of New Zealanders Born in 1972–3." *International Journal of Obesity and Related Metabolic Disorders* 25: 158–163.

Willis, P. 1977. *Learning to Labour: How Working Class Kids Get Working Class Jobs.* New York: Saxon House.

Worthman, C. M. 1999. "Epidemiology of Human Development." In *Hormones, Health and Behavior: A Socio-Ecological and Lifespan Perspective,* ed. C. Panter-Brick and C. Worthman. Cambridge: Cambridge University Press, 47–104.

Youniss, J. 1994. "Children's Friendship and Peer Culture: Implications for Theories of Networks and Support." In *Social Networks and Social Support in Childhood and Adolescence,* ed. F. Nestmann and K. Hurrelmann. New York: de Gruyter, 75–88.

Zittleman, K., and D. Sadker. 2002. "Gender Bias in Teacher Education Texts." *Journal of Teacher Education* 53, no. 2: 168–180.

PART

IV

Fat Etiologies, Stigma, and Gaps of Care in Biomedical Models of Obesity

CHAPTER 9

An Ounce of Prevention, a Ton of Controversy

Exploring Tensions in the Fields of Obesity and Eating Disorder Prevention

Lisa R. Rubin and Jessica A. Joseph

✛ ✛ ✛

In the United States, the past twenty-five years have been marked by preoccupation both with bodies that are "too fat" and bodies that are "too thin." This is particularly true for women, who still experience significantly greater pressure to achieve the thin ideal and exhibit higher rates of disordered eating (Smolak and Murnen 2001) and also experience more weight-based discrimination (Puhl and Heuer 2009). As concerns about "overweight" and "obesity"[1] increasingly take the center stage among public health concerns in the United States, and often share the stage at national and international eating disorders conferences, tensions among scientists and practitioners involved in the prevention and treatment of obesity, and those involved in the prevention and treatment of eating disorders are increasingly evident (Academy for Eating Disorders 2011). Whereas eating disorder experts raise concerns about widespread body dissatisfaction among women, a well-established risk factor for eating problems (Stice and Shaw 2002), for many engaged in the field of obesity prevention, body acceptance among those who are overweight is a significant concern. In this chapter, we map the underlying tensions, assumptions, and contradictions across eating disorder and obesity fields as they relate to concerns about dieting, body satisfaction, and body weight among girls and women. Further, we consider how these tensions influence the framing of body weight and shape concerns among Black women, a demographic group who have been found to have the highest prevalence of obesity (Flegal et al. 2010) and on average the highest levels of body satisfaction (Grabe and Hyde 2006), and who are thus often "caught in the cross-fire" of the tensions between these fields.

The tensions we discuss are now ubiquitous in the United States and certainly not limited to health experts. We see them play out at the level of cultural representation, as we fascinate over TV shows like *The Biggest Loser* while calling for greater representation of plus-size models (Bellafante 2010). They are played out among eating disorder practitioners who ask, "How did we get to size 00? And what does that say to young women?" without also interrogating why yesterday's size 8 has become today's size 0 among certain designers, a practice referred to as "vanity sizing" (Clifford 2011). Moreover, these tensions are played out behind the scenes in our research labs, for example among scientists who may question the value and meaningfulness of the BMI statistic (see Yates-Doerr, this volume), but still feel compelled to include it as a key outcome variable in their research to be competitive for research funds. Most importantly, these tensions are played out in the minds and bodies of everyday people, who struggle with the dual neoliberal imperatives to work at both self-acceptance and self-transformation.

A Weight-Centered Approach toward Health

According to current definitions of overweight and obesity, more than one-third of U.S. adults are considered overweight, another one-third of U.S. adults are considered obese, and almost 6 percent are considered extremely obese based on standardized height and weight measures (Flegal et al. 2010). Moreover, in the past twenty years, the prevalence of obesity has increased by almost 50 percent (from 23 percent in the years 1988–1994). These trends have fueled concerns of a growing "epidemic" of obesity, and calls for a "war on obesity." Since obesity was first coined as epidemic in 1998 by a team of researchers at the CDC (Oliver 2006), drastic concerns have been promulgated by obesity scientists, health care journalists, and public health messaging, as well as the diet industry, about the medical, social, psychological, and economic costs of obesity. As a recent report published by the Trust for America's Health (2011), funded by the Robert Wood Johnson Foundation, "F as in Fat: How Obesity Threatens American's Future" warns, "It's not just our health that is suffering: obesity-related medical costs and a less productive workforce are hampering America's ability to compete in the global economy" (Trust for America's Health 2011: 3). That overweight and obesity are overrepresented among the poor and ethnic minorities likely adds fuel to what some experts have described as the "moral panic" associated with obesity. As Campos et al. (2006) note: "Moral panics are typical during times of rapid social change and involve an exaggeration or fabrication of risks, the use of disaster analogies, and the projection of societal anxieties onto a stigmatized group" (Campos et al. 2006: 58). Indeed, as Austin (1999) concludes in her analysis of several foundational public health studies concerning overweight and obesity, nutritional public health "should be viewed first and foremost as an ideological project" (Austin 1999: 245) overdetermined by biomedical materialism (i.e., conception of reality as situated within biology) and concerns about "deviance."

Of course, overweight and obesity are certainly not limited to poor or ethnic minority groups, or even to a small, stigmatized subset of the population. Moreover, mounting evidence suggests that poverty, stress, and discrimination contribute significantly to the onset and maintenance of conditions often associated with obesity (Ernsberger 2009). However, despite recognition of the relationship between poverty, discrimination, and health outcomes, and increasing awareness of the role an "obesogenic" social environment (e.g., changes in diet and the built environment that have shifted traditional balances of energy intake and expenditure) may play in rates of obesity, recommendations for prevention and treatment have generally focused on individualized behavioral regimes of dieting and exercise (see Becker, this volume). These prevention recommendations often encourage individuals to reduce caloric intake and increase energy expenditures to achieve a lower weight status—or biomedical interventions such as medication or surgery.

This emphasis on behavioral and biomedical rather than social or political strategies to address a socially influenced, and as some argue socially constructed (Campos 2004), problem is consistent with larger trends in medicalization and biomedicalization. Sobal (1995) denotes the contemporary medicalization of obesity as a sickness or disease in and of itself, even in the absence of a specific biomedical pathology. Indeed, the term *obesity* is a medicalized term for a body mass index (BMI) of 30 or above (underweight = < 18.5 kg/m²; normal range, 18.5–24 .9 kg/m²; overweight, 25.0 to 29.9 kg/m²; extremely obese, 40.0 kg/m²). Criteria for defining overweight and obesity among children is more varied, and controversial, due to the fact that BMI and height are positively correlated among children, whereas they are unrelated in adults (a reason for its use). Whereas in 1994, youth with BMI's ≥ the 85th percentile, but < the 95th percentile, were considered "at risk of overweight," recent guidelines suggest that "individuals with BMI of ≥ 85th percentile but < 95th percentile or 30 kg/m² (whichever is smaller) now be considered overweight and that this has replaced the term "at risk of overweight" (Krebs et al. 2007: S194).

Researchers have long noted the capriciousness of BMI classifications. Cheryl Ritenbaugh, as early as 1982, noted the "downward drift" in weight classifications. Similarly, the cutoff between "normal weight" and overweight shifted in 1998 from 27 to 25 (Brody 1998). We have noticed a further downward drift recently, with studies using a BMI of 23 as their overweight cutoff point (e.g., He and Karlberg 2002), as well as with the medicalization of risk for overweight (Himes and Dietz 1994), followed by the latter reclassification of this same "at risk" group as overweight. This conceptual bracket creep, or the tendency for diagnostic criteria to expand over time, such that one no longer need manifest symptoms to be considered at risk for disease (Clarke et al. 2003), and the transformation of risk into a treatable health problem, or "diseaselike state in itself" (Fosket 2010: 331), is characteristic of general trends in biomedicalization. Biomedicalization is marked not only by such expanding definitions of disease, but also by the emphasis on the active patient, who is expected to take responsibility for his/her own health and health enhancements, thus deemphasizing societal contributions and societal responsibilities.

The medicalization of obesity as a disease encourages what Cogan and Ernsberger (1999) describe as a "weight-centered approach toward health" (Cogan and Ernsberger 1999: 188), an approach that is antithetical to that of most eating disorder prevention programs. Despite our collective so-called weight problem, the United States is as a nation preoccupied with slimness. Public health messages targeting overweight and obesity are inevitably framed by this perspective (e.g., emphasizing body weight versus body function) and interpreted through a contemporary cultural logic that prizes thinness. Thus, while public health messaging underscores the pursuit of thinness, for those in the field of eating disorder prevention the overvaluation of thinness and the emphasis on its pursuit is responsible not only for the late twentieth century's rise in eating disorders, but also for the more widespread problems of body dissatisfaction and dysfunctional eating behaviors, particularly among women.

The Health at Every Size (HAES) movement is at the forefront of challenges to mainstream biomedical weight-centered approaches, presenting an alternative paradigm for thinking about body size and health, one that is often aligned with the field of eating disorders prevention. Although a comprehensive review of the HAES movement is beyond the scope of this chapter, the HAES perspective has helped to illuminate some of the tensions, assumptions, and contradictions that characterize the fields of eating disorders and obesity. For example, HAES advocates highlight the quixotic nature of obesity treatment and prevention approaches, which "prescribe for heavier people what we diagnose as eating disorders in thinner people" (Burgard 2009: 47). Whereas restrained eating or compulsive exercising may signal disordered eating in a thin or "normal" weight woman, and body dissatisfaction a reason for concern and psychological intervention, such behaviors and cognitions are expected among the overweight and obese. In fact, as we illustrate in this chapter, the absence of body dissatisfaction has become a cause for concern among overweight.

Normative Discontent: Public Health Problem, or Remedy?

In their classic paper, Striegel-Moore et al. (1986) suggested that weight concerns and dieting are now so prevalent among females that discontent as well as disregulated and restrained eating are normative. While approximately 1–3 percent of U.S. adolescent females meet diagnostic criteria for an eating disorder, it is estimated that another 10–13 percent of adolescent and college-age females engage in disordered eating practices. Moreover, a much larger percentage of teenage girls report using unhealthy methods to lose weight including diet pills, vomiting, skipping meals, and eating very little (Irving and Neumark-Sztainer 2002). Based on these reports, eating disorders and dieting have, like obesity, also been described as epidemic (e.g., Gordon 2000).

Findings from Nichter's (2000) ethnography of "fat talk" and "diet talk" among teenage girls, however, encourage as much caution about the use of the term *epidemic* to describe dieting behavior as many have argued should be taken in the use of the term to describe obesity, while also emphasizing the ubiquity of body dissatisfaction, particularly among the White adolescent girls in her study. Nichter (2000) found that despite widespread engagement with diet talk and self-deprecating body talk, "their behaviors largely reflect health-oriented strategies" (Nichter 2000: 9). Girls talked about "watching what they ate" far more than dieting, which she concludes is a healthier practice, although rarely measured in the dieting literature. Nichter contends that ambiguity in the definition of dieting, as well as specific diet-related practices such as "fasting" (for how long?) and "skipping meals" (how many?) may skew evaluations of its prevalence, as her analysis of teenage girls' food records indicated relatively few self-reported "dieting days." Nine percent of all food records, collected on three randomly selected days each semester from each girl were judged to be dieting days, compared with the 40 percent of girls who self-reported dieting on the day of the survey. Of course, this finding again compels us to ask what constitutes dieting—is it defined by actual food intake or by the intention to restrict on a given day? Taken together, Nichter's findings highlight a central theme of this chapter as manifested among a sample of teenage girls; namely, that girls who want to be healthy may struggle to navigate conflicting messages—including anti-dieting and anti-obesity messages—of out what healthy eating entails. If experts cannot agree on what constitutes healthy eating behaviors, how can we expect the general public to make sense of such conflicting messages?

Beyond different conceptualizations of overweight and obesity as viewed through biomedical or psychosocial lenses, and different concerns regarding dieting—whether we are dieting too much or too little—one of the most important tensions between the fields of obesity and eating disorder prevention lies in their different approaches to body dissatisfaction. Among obesity researchers, body dissatisfaction has been characterized as appropriate and necessary to motivate weight loss; conversely, satisfaction with an overweight or obese body may be framed in terms of knowledge deficits, problematic body ideals, or as a matter of flawed/disordered perception. In contrast, among those working in the field of eating disorders prevention, body dissatisfaction often underlies disregulated eating in a variety of forms, including behaviors associated with severe underweight, and those associated with overeating and overweight. In other words, body dissatisfaction is conceptualized as a risk factor for disordered eating, rather than a motivator of positive health behavior change. Although it is generally acknowledged that eating problems are multi-determined, internalization of sociocultural messages that exult thinness has been found to foster body dissatisfaction, which in turn increases the risk for eating pathology (Stice and Shaw 2002).

In a provocative essay, Heinberg et al. (2001) suggest "mild to moderate levels of distress may be beneficial for average to above-average BMI's because it serves as a constant motivator to continue a healthy lifestyle" (Heinberg et al. 2001: 216). They hypothesize an inverted U-shaped curve to describe the relationship between body image distress and "healthy dieting behavior," which may be overlooked by previous research testing only linear relationships. While more research is needed that examines these relationships in a nonlinear model, research does suggest that overweight and obese individuals who are content with their weight (i.e., those with mild levels of distress) tend to experience fewer physically and mentally *unhealthy* days than those who are weight dissatisfied (Latner and Wilson 2011).

A study by Neumark-Sztainer et al. (2006) examined longitudinal associations between body satisfaction and weight-related health-promoting and health-compromising behaviors five years later among adolescents. They found that among females, lower levels of body satisfaction predicted dieting, "very unhealthy weight control behaviors" (i.e., taking diet pills, self-induced vomiting, laxatives or diuretic use), as well as lower levels of physical activity. Among males, lower satisfaction was also associated with dieting, unhealthy weight control behavior (i.e., fasting, eating very little food, skipping meals, smoking), as well as binge eating. These findings are particularly concerning, given that such dangerous weight loss strategies are generally ineffective at addressing overweight and obesity and pose significant health risks (Cogan and Ernsberger 1999). In fact, an examination of patterns of weight gain among a subsample of girls in Neumark-Sztainer et al.'s (2006) study with BMI's above the 85th percentile found that girls with the lowest levels of body satisfaction had the highest increment of weight gain (3 units versus 1 unit among girls with high levels of satisfaction) over a five-year period, suggesting that body satisfaction, rather than dissatisfaction, protected against significant long-term weight gain.

To underscore the argument that a little body dissatisfaction can be a good thing, obesity researchers point to study findings of overweight and obese individuals (usually women) that misperceive their weight status, inappropriately classifying themselves as "normal" or "acceptable," suggesting that such misclassifications drive obesity-related behaviors (Bennett and Wolin 2006). As noted earlier, judging these perceptions as misperceptions represents the contemporary BMI classification as a culturally shared, ahistorical, and true standard for judging "normal." However, as Tiefer (2004) suggests, "normal" can be defined in at least five ways: subjectively, statistically, idealistically, culturally, or clinically.

Whereas researchers may endorse clinical (or idealistic), notions of normal, the lay public may use subjective (do I feel normal?), statistical (am I heavier than the average?), or cultural (am I different from my community?) standards, all reasonable interpretations. Nonetheless, interventions that aim to improve accurate self-perception in relation to clinical norms among adults, or more accurate perception among parents of overweight and obese children, are increasingly common.

A study by Chomitz et al. (2003) examining the effectiveness of a personalized weight and fitness report card given to an ethnically diverse group of parents about their elementary school children highlights the possible iatrogenic effects of this type of intervention. Parents were randomly assigned to receive a personalized intervention that included the weight and fitness report card and general information on healthy living, general information only, or no intervention. There were no differences in preventive behaviors (e.g., limiting television, encouraging exercise, consuming fruits and vegetables) across the conditions. However, despite the inclusion of anti-diet information, almost 20 percent of parents in the report card group reported efforts to encourage dieting activities, items that included skipping meals or giving diet pills or supplements, underscoring Cogan and Ernsberger's (1999) claim that weight-centered approaches encourage both unhealthy and ineffective weight loss behaviors (see Galloway and Moffat and Trainer, this volume). Parents of overweight children in the report card and information condition did report more awareness of their child's weight status than those in the control group; however, it is noteworthy that this awareness was gendered, with parents significantly more likely to accurately identify weight status of their overweight daughters than sons and less likely to accurately identify weight status of their healthy weight daughters. These findings suggest that, even when unintended, obesity prevention messages are interpreted through existing cultural frames, including the gendered nature of weight concerns and an emphasis on thinness as a marker of health and beauty that is disproportionately applied to girls, even those as young as elementary school age.

Chomitz et al. (2003) designed their study to assess possible iatrogenic consequences, an important consideration for research in this area that may be overlooked in studies framed by a weight-centered, rather than health-centered, approach. Underscoring this point, a review by Carter and Bulik (2008) examined studies of childhood obesity prevention programs for the inclusion of measures of eating pathology and other psychological measures. Although they found little evidence of iatrogenic effects in the published research, they suggest these results should be interpreted cautiously, as no studies compared rates of eating disorders across invention and control groups and only a minority of studies even examined eating disorder symptomatology or related eating attitudes. Although mentioned in their introduction, their review did not address the impact of interventions on stigmatization, perhaps because it was rarely, if ever, assessed in the studies they reviewed. Thus, it is noteworthy that, in addition to diet-related behavior, Chomitz et al. (2003) examined children's discomfort in response to the intervention. Overall, parents of children in the report card condition were more likely to report that the information made their children uncomfortable, with a trend suggesting more discomfort among overweight children. Although not a direct measure of stigma, elementary school children's discomfort suggests an awareness of the negative social judgments associated with overweight.

Within the United States, the stigmatization of obesity is pervasive and increasing (see McCullough, this volume, Andreyeva et al. 2008; Latner and Stunkard 2003; Latner et al. 2007; Puhl and Heuer 2009). Puhl and Brownell (2001) illustrate how biases stymie access to employment and education among overweight and obese individuals, including hiring decisions, wages, and job promotions. Crandall's research (1995) found that fat female college students were less likely to receive financial support from their parents, even after controlling for income, family size, siblings in college, and ethnicity. Fat stigma may also be associated with increased fear of fat, anti-fat attitudes, and negative body image among overweight and obese individuals (e.g., Latner et al. 2007). Not only do such results indicate the potential psychological and economic ramifications of stigmatization, it also points out another unique characteristic of fat stigma: Overweight and obese individuals and those in their personal support networks (e.g., coworkers and family) may also stigmatize overweight and obesity.

Per less access to education and employment, it is no surprise that lower socioeconomic status is negatively correlated with adiposity among women, men, and youth (see Banks et al. 2006; Hanson and Chen, 2007; Sobal and Stunkard, 1989). While this might be explained by that fact that poverty creates an environment conducive to fostering obesity (e.g., less access to nutritionally dense food, more necessitated reliance on processed food, and less physical activity opportunities), an alternative hypothesis is that obesity and overweight stigmatization facilitates poverty (Ernsberger 2009). However, as Ernsberger suggests, the two explanations may be intertwined—resulting in a potential cycle of poverty and adiposity. In other words, stigmatization may help to drive those that are obese and overweight to lower socioeconomic status, whereas lower socioeconomic status may provide an environment that encourages adiposity.

Obesity prevention campaigns often use fat stigma in their public health messages, an approach that both perpetuates and legitimizes such stigma. For example, a recent New York City Department of Health and Mental Hygiene (2009) subway campaign to discourage consumption of sugar-sweetened beverages asks passengers, "Are you pouring on the pounds?" In the poster, soda being poured from a bottle to a glass turns into grotesquely represented human body fat, followed by the advisory message: "Don't drink yourself fat." These messages, like the "F as in Fat" report noted above, equate fat with failure and fat persons as abject (see Becker, this volume). Although attention grabbing, messages that perpetuate weight bias may actually worsen health outcomes for overweight and obese individuals, as weight bias may contribute to maladaptive eating patterns, and weight bias in health care settings contributes to delays and avoidance of preventive care (see McCullough, this volume; Puhl and Heuer 2009 for a review of obesity stigmatization and its consequences).

Black Women, Body Image, and Obesity

In the prior section, we outlined some of the general tensions between the fields of obesity and eating disorder prevention, including (1) the hegemony of the BMI and the medicalization of overweight and obesity and how this conflicts with the HAES/non-weight-centered approach that characterizes the eating disorder prevention field and (2) the simultaneity of relatively high levels of overweight and obesity, relatively high levels of body dissatisfaction, and the different strategies and concerns of obesity and eating disorders prevention communities to this seeming paradox. In this section, we address tensions as they play out in research pertaining to Black girls and women, whose seemingly more positive body image has, at times, been celebrated within the eating disorder prevention community, while being raised as a cause for concern within the obesity prevention community. These tensions are exacerbated by the fact that, by and large, neither of these bodies of research addresses the significant intra-group diversity in relation to body satisfaction among Black girls and women, nor the more nuanced and complex ways Black women experience their embodiment in relation to prevailing discourses of health and beauty ideals.

Across gender and ethnic groupings, rates of obesity are highest among Black women, with epidemiologic studies indicating a 49.6 percent prevalence of obesity. This compares with an obesity prevalence of 33 percent among White women and 43 percent among Hispanic women (Flegal et al. 2010). Nonetheless, studies also suggest that, on average, Black women are more satisfied with their bodies than are women of other ethnic groups, although the differences are generally small (Grabe and Hyde 2006). In a study of BMI and body satisfaction, Yates et al. (2004), note, "In this study, African American females presented the highest BMI of all female groups, and yet were relatively comfortable with body and self. These findings support other studies showing that African-American women are more realistic about the body and satisfied with a range of sizes" (Yates et al. 2004: 305). Taking into account findings from both quantitative and qualitative studies, researchers have put forth the buffering hypothesis, which postulates that aspects of African-American culture have "a protective effect to prevent or reduce body dissatisfaction or disordered eating" (Sabik et al. 2010: 141) by lessening the impact of the thin ideal, thereby reducing body dissatisfaction.[2] Those aspects that have been highlighted include larger body ideals and a broader view of what constitutes a "normal" body size (e.g., Allan et al. 1993).

Shifting to the obesity literature, these same values are reframed as risk. In a large-scale study of self-perception of overweight, Paeratakul et al. (2002) found that among Black women classified as overweight based on their self-reported BMI, only 46 percent perceived themselves as overweight (versus underweight or "about right"), compared with 65 percent of White women self-classified as overweight. Women of both groups classified as "obese" based on self-reported BMI were significantly more accurate. Based on their findings, the authors raise a warning flag about the health and behavioral implications of the "erroneous perception[s] of body weight" (Paeratakul et al. 2002: 345) among Black women, albeit acknowledging that the actual health or health behaviors of participants was not evaluated. The authors also did not examine the intersections of race/ethnicity and socioeconomic status despite collecting income and education information.

The framing of research studies suggests that "erroneous perceptions" are not just a problem for women, but also for their children, as indicated by the title of a study of low-income and predominantly Black mothers published in the journal *Pediatrics*, "Why don't low-income mothers worry about their preschoolers being overweight?" (Jain et al. 2001). Other studies describe mothers as *failing* to classify correctly their overweight children, as *lacking* an understanding of what overweight means, as *minimizing* weight concerns (Maynard et al. 2003), or as (problematically) determining that having a large body size was acceptable as long as children were healthy, active, and had good self-esteem (Jain et al. 2001). The tone of this work is that such misperceptions must be corrected, with an underlying assumption that more accurate perception will motivate health behavior change.

In their study, "Satisfied, or unaware? Racial differences in perceived weight status," which draws on "nationally-representative data" (Bennett and Wolin 2006: 1) from the National Health and Nutrition Examination Survey (NHANES) study, Bennett and Wolin (2006) note that when asked, "Do you consider yourself now to be overweight, underweight, or about the right weight?" Black participants were twice as likely to "misperceive" their weight as were White participants. Although the authors do not directly address their proposed question—satisfied or unaware?—their interpretation and recommendations suggest that a lack of knowledge or awareness is the answer. They speculate that "rather than considering their membership in BMI-defined categories, some Blacks might rely on social comparison to make judgments about their respective weight status" (Bennett and Wolin 2006: 4), suggesting that self-perceptions of normalcy ought to be determined primarily by clinical standards, rather than cultural ones.

However, there is a difference between knowing BMI-defined categories, but not using these as a basis for self-perception of one's normalcy or acceptability, and lacking knowledge or awareness. In fact, to better sort out the question of awareness versus satisfaction, researchers might consider also asking participants,

"Does my physician consider me to be overweight, underweight, or about the right weight?" While Bennett and Wolin (2006) recommend correcting misperceptions of weight status, they hypothesize "that some Black patients might be resistant to physician diagnoses of overweight" (Bennett and Wolin 2006: 4).

Here "resistance" is portrayed in a negative manner. However, resistance to externally imposed standards may in fact be the very factor that supports many Black girls and women's positive body and self-esteem. Indeed, sociologist and Black feminist scholar Collins (1986) contends that self-definition, or the ability to forge an identity other than one imposed by society, has been central to Black women's well-being. She explains, "When Black females choose to value those aspects of Afro-American womanhood that are stereotyped, ridiculed, and maligned in academic scholarship … they are actually questioning some of the basic ideas used to control dominated groups in general" (Collins 1986: S17). Instead of a lack of awareness, Black women respondents in these studies may be proclaiming their bodies "acceptable" regardless of, and perhaps in response to, definitions imposed by the medical establishment. As Shaw (2006: 128) writes: "In the contemporary African Diaspora, the fat black woman's body occupies a largely resistive and transgressive space, despite the fact, and because of the fact, that some of the earlier images and literary representations of that body, shaped mostly by white hegemonic culture, were part of an effort to diminish black womanhood."

Embodying Controversy

As often occurs with comparative research, findings of small group differences overshadow the (typically larger) intra-group diversity. Moreover, differences are reified—viewed as the result of stable, inner qualities of individuals—rather than understood in context (Hare-Mustin et al. 1994). While theory-based writings, such as those by Collins (1986) and Shaw (2006), are invaluable in illustrating the strategies Black women may draw upon to cultivate a positive body and self-image, like extant quantitative studies, they may not provide a full picture of the varied, complex and nuanced ways individual Black women negotiate prevailing discourses of beauty and health.

A recent study by Antin and Hunt (2011), which entailed interviews with African-American women ages eighteen to twenty-five living in low-income areas in the San Francisco Bay Area, may help move the literature beyond existing either/or frameworks of Black women's body acceptance and dissatisfaction. Among study participants, satisfaction and dissatisfaction with their bodies exists simultaneously, challenging research that "considers an individual's perception of her body as a single, fixed conceptualization" (Antin and Hunt 2011: 5). Participants reiterated extant findings about culturally produced body ideals: "[W]e feel beautiful no matter what our weight is or what our body image is ... because our families instill different morals and values in us" (Antin and Hunt 2011: 10). However, participants also expressed concerns about health and weight gain: "I'm getting older and I'm not going to get no smaller eating like I'm eating. Not that I want to get smaller, but I don't want to get bigger in my size, my weight" (Antin and Hunt 2011: 7). Moreover, instead of feeling protected from body dissatisfaction, some participants expressed dissatisfaction twofold: discontent from deviating from the (societal) thin body as well as from the (cultural) thick body.

Consistent with Austin's (1999) claims, noted earlier, that nutritional public health ought to be understood first and foremost as an ideological project, so too might the current concern for Black women's weight. Shaw (2006) contends that "fetishization of blackness and the black female body is a means of further installing blackness as anomalous and disorderly" (Shaw 2006: 49). Updating Austin's critique, we contend that the focus on Black women illustrates how racialized ideologies are embedded in the moralistic ideologies of deviance and difference she notes and disciplined through the materialist ideology of modern science she discusses.

Conclusions

Despite acknowledgement of the seeming paradox of a predominantly so-called overweight nation preoccupied with slimness, obesity prevention efforts rarely recognize the shared cultural context in which these problems develop: a milieu of relative abundance that simultaneously promotes self-indulgence while revering self-restraint. From a biomedical perspective, obesity, eating disorders, and unhealthy weight loss practices are generally "regarded as distinct, with different origins, courses, and approaches to prevention and treatment" (Irving and Neumark-Sztainer 2002: 300). The field of eating disorders has long held a broader, more integrated perspective on eating and weight concerns (see Orbach 1978), and its anti-dieting approach has been foundational to the development of the HAES movement. This movement represents an important response to the epidemiologic trend of increased obesity that coincides with, rather than undermines, eating disorder prevention efforts. The HAES movement offers a more holistic definition of health, one that includes psychological and functional well-being, rather than that which is encompassed by the obesity prevention/biomedical community's devotion to the BMI statistic. Body image, a hallmark concern among eating disorder professionals because of the well-documented associations between body dissatisfaction and eating pathology, and its relationship to mood and well-being, is emerging as new site of tension between the fields of obesity and eating prevention, as more theoretical and research attention is devoted to the "problem" of too little body image–related distress, particularly among Black women. Eating disorder professionals have warned that too much focus on the greater body satisfaction of Black women may conceal the extent of disordered eating, particularly binge eating and other disorders "not otherwise specified" (e.g., Striegel-Moore et al. 2000). Although body satisfaction may not necessarily be a panacea for eating problems among Black women, we concur with Wilson (2009), who contends "the goal of public health work should not be to convince a group of people that their sense of themselves is inherently unhealthy or problematic" (Wilson 2009: 61). More research is needed to examine concerns about eating disorders, overweight, and obesity among Black women from their own perspective, rather than one imposed by a dominant medical, or eating disorder, establishment.

Notes

1. From the obesity literature, we adopt the term *overweight* to describe individuals with a BMI of 25.0 to 29.9 kg/m², BMI of 30 or above as *obese*, and 40.0 kg/m² as *extremely obese* for the sake of clarity and consistency as we review existing research. However, on this first mention, we use quotations to distance ourselves from this particular terminology, as inherent to these terms are the assumption of a normal or correct weight, consistent with the weight-centered approach to health problematized here and elsewhere.

2. Although research has consistently documented that on average Black women reported greater weight-related and global body satisfaction (Roberts et al. 2006), Black women are certainly not immune from developing eating disorders, with some studies suggesting comparable rates of DSM-IV (APA 1994) eating disorder prevalence among white and African-American college women (Mulholland and Mintz 2001).

References

Academy for Eating Disorders. 2011. "International Conference on Eating Disorders." Available at http://www.aedweb.org/AM/, accessed June 29, 2011.

Allan, Janet D., K. Mayo, and Y. Michel. 1993. "Body Size Values of White and Black Women." *Research in Nursing and Health* 16, no. 5: 323–333.

American Psychiatric Association. 1994. *Diagnostic and Statistical Manual of Mental Disorders* (4th ed.). Washington, DC: American Psychiatric Association

Andreyeva, T., R. M. Puhl, and K. D. Brownell. 2008. "Changes in Perceived Weight Discrimination among Americans, 1995–1996 through 2004–2006." *Obesity* 16, no. 5: 1129–1134.

Antin, T. M. J. and G. Hunt. 2013. "Embodying both stigma and satisfaction: An interview study of African American." *Critical Public Health*, vol. 23: 1, 1–15. http://www.tandfonline.com/doi/abs/10.1080/09581596.2011.634784#.UYWbSSt37T8

Austin, S. 1999. "Fat, Loathing and Public Health: The Complicity of Science in a Culture of Disordered Eating." *Culture, Medicine and Psychiatry* 23: 245–268.

Bellafante, G. 2010. "Plus-Size Wars." *The New York Times,* July 28. Available at http://www.nytimes.com/2010/08/01/magazine/01plussize-t.html

Banks, J., M. Marmot, Z. Oldfield, and J. P. Smith. 2006. "Disease and Disadvantage in the United States and in England." *Journal of the American Medical Association* 295, no. 17: 2037–2045.

Bennett, G. G., and K. Y. Wolin. 2006. "Satisfied or Unaware? Racial Differences in Perceived Weight Status." *International Journal of Behavioral Nutrition and Physical Activity* 5: 1–5.

Brody, J. E. 1998. "Personal Health: New Guide Puts Most Americans on the Fat Side." *The New York Times*, June 9, available at http://www.nytimes.com/1998/06/09/science/personal-health-new-guide-puts-most-americans-on-the-fat-side.html?src=pm

Burgard, D. 2009. "What is Health at Every Size?" In *The Fat Studies Reader*, ed. E. Rothblum and S. Solovay. New York: New York University Press, 41–53.

Campos, P. F. 2004. *The Obesity Myth: Why America's Obsession with Weight is Hazardous to your Health*. New York: Gotham Books.

Campos, P., A. Saguy, P. Ernsberger, E. Oliver, and G. Gaesser. 2006. "The Epidemiology of Overweight and Obesity: Public Health Crisis or Moral Panic?" *Internal Journal of Epidemiology* 35: 55–60.

Carter, F. A., and C. M. Bulik. 2008. "Childhood Obesity Prevention Programs: How Do They Sffect Eating Pathology and Other Psychological Measures?" *Psychosomatic Medicine* 70: 363–371.

Chomitz, V. R., J. Collins, J. Kim, E. Kramer, and R. McGowan. 2003. "Promoting Healthy Weight among Elementary School Children via a Health Report Card Approach." *Archives of Pediatrics and Adolescent Medicine* 157, no. 8: 765–772.

Clarke, A. E., J. K. Shim, L. Mamo, J. R. Fosket, and J. R. Fishman. 2003. "Biomedicalization: Technoscientific Transformations of Health, Illness, and U.S. Biomedicine." *American Sociological Review* 68, no. 2: 161–194.

Clifford, S. 2001. "One Size Fits Nobody: Seeking a Steady 4 or a 10." *The New York Times*, April 24, available at http://www.nytimes.com/2011/04/25/business/25sizing.html.

Collins, P. H. 1986. "Learning from the Outsider Within: The Sociological Significance of Black Feminist Thought." *Social Problems* 33, no. 6: S14–S32.

Cogan, J. C., and P. Ernsberger. 1999. "Dieting, Weight, and Health: Reconceptualizing Research and Policy." *Journal of Social Issues* 55, no. 2: 187–205.

Crandall, C. 1995. "Do Parents Discriminate against Their Heavyweight Daughters?" *Personality and Social Psychology Bulletin* 21, no. 7: 724–735.

Ernsberger, P. 2009. "Does Social Class Explain the Connection Between Weight and Health?" In *The Fat Studies Reader*, ed. E. Rothblum and S. Solovay. New York: New York University Press, 25–36.

Flegal, K. M., M. D. Carroll, C. L. Ogden, and L. R. Curtin. 2010. "Prevalence and Trends in Obesity among US Adults, 1999–2008." *Journal of the American Medical Association* 303, no. 3: 235–241.

Fosket, J. R. 2010. "Breast Cancer Risk as Disease: Biomedicalizing Risk." In *Biomedicalization: Technoscience, Health, and Illness in the U.S.*, ed. A. E. Clarke, L. Mamo, J. R. Fosket, J. R. Fishman, and J. K. Shim. Durham: Duke University Press, 331–352.

Gordon, R. A. 2000. *Eating Disorders: Anatomy of a Social Epidemic, 2nd ed.* Oxford: Blackwell Publishers.

Grabe, S., and J. S. Hyde. 2006. "Ethnicity and Body Dissatisfaction among Women in the United States: A Meta-Analysis." *Psychological Bulletin* 132, no. 4: 622–640.

Hare-Mustin, R. T., and J. Marecek. 1994. "Asking the Right Questions: Feminist Psychology and Sex Differences." *Feminism and Psychology* 4: 531–537.

Hanson, M. D., and E. Chen. 2007. "Socioeconomic Status, Race, and Body Mass Index: The Mediating Role of Physical Activity and Sedentary Behaviors during Adolescence." *Journal of Pediatric Psychology* 32, no. 3: 250–259.

He, Q., and J. Karlberg. 2002. "Probability of Adult Overweight and Risk Change during the BMI Rebound Period." *Obesity Research* 10, no. 3: 135–140.

Heinberg, L. J., K. Thompson, and J. L. Matzon. 2001. "Body Image Dissatisfaction as a Motivator for Healthy Lifestyle Changes: Is Some Distress Beneficial?" In *Eating Disorders: Innovative Directions in Research and Practice,* ed. R. H. Striegel-Moore and L. Smolak. Washington, DC: American Psychological Association, 215–232.

Himes, J. H., and W. H. Dietz. 1994. "Guidelines for Overweight in Adolescent Preventive Services: Recommendations from and Expert Committee." *American Journal of Clinical Nutrition* 59: 307–316.

Irving, L. M., and D. Neumark-Sztainer. 2002. "Integrating the Prevention of Eating Disorders and Obesity: Feasible or Futile?" *Preventive Medicine* 34: 299–309.

Jain, A., S. N. Sherman, L. A. Chamberlin, Y. P. Carter, W. Scott, and R. C. Whitaker. 2001. "Why Don't Low-income Mothers Worry about Their Preschoolers Being Overweight?" *Pediatrics* 107, no. 5: 1138–1146.

Krebs, N. F., J. H. Himes, D. Jacobson, T. A. Nicklas, D. Styne, and P. Guilday. 2007. "Assessment of Child and Adolescent Overweight and Obesity." *Pediatrics* 12 (December): S193–S228.

Latner, J. D., M. Simmonds, J. K. Rosewall, and A. J. Stunkard. 2007. "Assessment of Obesity Stigmatization in Children and Adolescents: Modernizing a Standard Measure." *Obesity* 15, no. 12: 3078–3085.

Latner, J. D., and A. J. Stunkard. 2003. "Getting Worse: The Stigmatization of Obese Children." *Obesity Research* 11, no. 3: 452–456.

Latner, J. D., and R. E. Wilson. 2011. "Obesity and body image in adulthood." In *Body Image: A Handbook of Science, Practice, and Prevention,* eds. T. F. Cash and L. Smolak. New York: Guilford Press, 189–197.

Maynard, M. L., D. A. Galuska, H. M. Blanck, and M. K. Serdula. 2003. "Maternal Perceptions of Weight Status of Children." *Pediatrics* 111: 1226–1231.

Mulholland, A. M., and L. B. Mintz. 2001. "Prevalence of Eating Disorders among African American Women." *Journal of Counseling Psychology* 48, no. 1: 111–116.

Neumark-Sztainer, D., S. J. Paxton, P. J. Hannan, J. Haines, and M. Story. 2006. "Does Body Satisfaction Matter? Five-Year Longitudinal Associations between Body Satisfaction and Health Behaviors in Adolescent Females and Males." *Journal of Adolescent Health* 39: 244–251.

Nichter, M. 2000. *Fat Talk: What Girls and their Parents Say about Dieting.* Cambridge: Harvard University Press.

New York City Department of Health and Mental Hygiene. 2009. "Are you Pouring on the Pounds?" Available at http://www.nyc.gov/html/doh/html/cdp/cdp_pan.shtml, accessed July 11, 2011.

Oliver, J. E. 2006. "The Politics of Pathology: How Obesity Became an Epidemic Disease." *Perspectives in Biology and Medicine* 49, no. 4: 611–627.

Orbach, S. 1978. *Fat is a Feminist Issue: The Anti-diet Guide to Permanent Weight Loss.* Berkeley: Berkley Publishing.

Paeratakul, S., M. A. White, D. A. Williamson, D. H. Ryan, and G. A. Bray. 2002. "Sex, Race/Ethnicity, Socioeconomics, and BMI in Relation to Self-Perception of Overweight." *Obesity Research* 10, no. 5: 345–350.

Puhl, R. M., and K. D. Brownell. 2001. "Bias, discrimination, and obesity." *Obesity Research* 9, no. 12: 788–805.

Puhl, R. M., and C. A. Heuer. 2009. "The Stigma of Obesity: A Review and Update." *Obesity* 17, no. 5: 941–964.

Ritenbaugh, C. 1982. "Obesity as a 'Culture Bound Syndrome.'" *Culture, Medicine and Psychiatry* 6: 347–361.

Roberts, A., T. F. Cash, A. Feingold, and B. T. Johnson. 2006. "Are Black-White Differences in Females' Body Dissatisfaction Decreasing? A Meta-analytic Review." *Journal of Consulting and Clinical Psychology* 74, no. 6: 1121–1131.

Sabik, N. J., E. R. Cole, and L. M. Ward. 2010. "Are All Minority Women Equally Buffered from Negative Body Image? Intra-ethnic Moderators of the Buffering Hypothesis." *Psychology of Women Quarterly* 34, no. 2: 139–151.

Shaw, A. E. 2006. *The Embodiment of Disobedience: Fat Black Women's Unruly Political Bodies.* Lanham: Rowman and Littlefield Publishers, Inc.

Smolak, L., and S. K. Murnen. 2001. "Gender and Eating Problems." In *Eating Disorders: Innovative Directions in Research and Practice,* ed. R. H. Striegel-Moore and L. Smolak. Washington, DC: American Psychological Association, 91–110.

Sobal, J. 1995. "The Medicalization and Demedicalization of Obesity." In *Eating Agendas: Food and Nutrition as Social Problems,* eds. D. Maurer and J. Sobal. New York: Aldine de Gruyter, 67–90.

Sobal, J., and A. J. Stunkard. 1989. "Socioeconomic Status and Obesity: A Review of the Literature." *Psychological Bulletin* 105, no. 2: 260–275.

Stice, E., and H. E. Shaw. 2002. "Role of Body Dissatisfaction in the Onset and Maintenance of Eating Pathology: A synthesis of Research Findings." *Journal of Psychosomatic Research* 53, no. 5: 985–993.

Striegel-Moore, R. H., L. R. Silberstein, and J. Rodin. 1986. "Toward an Understanding of Risk Factors for Bulimia." *American Psychologist* 41, no. 3: 246–263.

Striegel-Moore, R. H., D. E. Wilfley, K. M. Pike, F. Dohm, and C. G. Fairburn. 2000. "Recurrent Binge Eating in Black American Women." *Archives of Family Medicine* 9, no. 1: 83–87.

Tiefer, L. 2004. *Sex Is Not a Natural Act and Other Essays, 2nd ed.* Boulder: Westview Press.

Trust for America's Health. 2011. "F as in Fat: How Obesity Threatens America's Future." Available at http://healthyamericans.org/report/88/, accessed July 8, 2011.

Wilson, B. D. M. 2009. "Widening the Dialogue to Narrow the Gap in Health Disparities: Approaches to Fat Black Lesbian and Bisexual Women's Health Promotion." In *The Fat Studies Reader,* eds. E. Rothblum and S. Solovay. New York: New York University Press, 54–64.

Yates, A., J. Edman, and M. Aruguete. 2004. "Ethnic Differences in BMI and Body/Self-Dissatisfaction among Whites, Asian Subgroups, Pacific Islanders, and African-Americans." *Journal of Adolescent Health* 34, no. 4: 300–307.

CHAPTER 10

Fat and Knocked-Up

An Embodied Analysis of Stigma, Visibility, and Invisibility in the Biomedical Management of an Obese Pregnancy

Megan B. McCullough

✦ ✦ ✦

I am a fat anthropologist and not an anthropologist who is fat. I state this bluntly, although if you had met me or seen me, you would already have decided that I was fat; were you inclined toward medical diagnostic terminology, you would have said to yourself I was obese. I understand the term *fat* to mean "anyone who sees themselves as larger, rounder or bigger than other people and who might be medically categorized as 'overweight' or 'obese'" (Wilson 2009: 54). For some weight gain is temporary or cyclical, and thus, the body is something one periodically works on. However, for me, being fat dominates my physical universe, and it has done so for years.

Being fat shapes my understanding of space and social relations; and it is a deeply integral, although not always a comfortable, way that I am in my own body. Fat dictates not only how I move through the world physically and emotionally, but also how I am seen and how I attempt to navigate and am managed, judged, and controlled by the spaces and landscapes of the social and moral world that I inhabit. As anthropology notes, it is difference and how much difference matters (materially, politically, economically, medically, and socially) that dictates how much of the social and moral world one feels entitled or privileged to construct. I would not want to minimize my own agency or social power as a white, middle-class woman; there are issues about fat that limit one's capacity to act.

I know that my body, and therefore my perceived character, is read in a number of cultural and biomedical ways that I cannot control but with which I am always forced to be in conversation or in argument or in despair about. Fat is not a stable category but rather a multivalent, flexible symbolic system that produces a multitude of meanings and practices that illustrate the way cultural forces shape private and public lives in distinct cultural ways (Becker 1995; Becker et al. 1999; Bordo 1993; Kulick and Meneley 2005; Sobo 1993). This chapter is about the impact and the reverberations the barrage of fat etiologies—ontological, social, moral, and biomedical—have on the body and the personhood of a fat, pregnant anthropologist and her relationship with her fetus.

This volume on obesity is challenging existing paradigms, theories, and approaches regarding obesity research in primarily cultural and biological anthropology and in allied fields such as psychology, sociology, public health, and biomedicine. Drawing on a different methodology, this chapter is a reflexive, narrative account of being both fat and pregnant. I see this approach as similar to that of other anthropologists who have analytically interpreted and used their personal experiences in anthropological ways and grounded their analyses within a larger disciplinary discussion (Ginsburg and Rapp 1999; Layne 2003; Martin 2009; Winkler and Winniger 1994).

Through a retelling of my pregnancy experience as both subject and anthropologist (Ginsburg and Rapp 1999), I will trace the discursive ways that obesity and pregnancy manifest as both high risk and morally troubling. Currently, obesity and pregnancy are characterized as serious health issues. Approximately 60 percent of American women of childbearing age are either overweight or obese (Sarwer et al. 2006: 720). Studies on obesity and pregnancy indicate that obesity in pregnancy leads to complications, illnesses, and diseases as well as increased risk for cesarean sections and poor childbirth outcomes.[1] Obese pregnancies demand a higher level of biomedical and reproductive management from medical practitioners and public health officials. Through the circulation of public health and medical studies, as well as the commentary and interpretations of such studies in the media, the public is invited to evaluate, judge, and socially police obese bodies. This reproductive management technique resides in the medicalization of reproduction and of obesity; the obese pregnant body, despite being statistically on the increase, is still seen as matter-out-of-place in "typical" obstetrical practices.

Drawing on the multivalent concepts of stigma, visibility, and invisibility, I ethnographically chart this discursive imbalance between an obese pregnant individual and her bodily experiences and the practices of pregnancy with the larger public and medical discourses about obesity and pregnancy (Goffman 1963; Kleinman 1988). Obesity is seen as an individual problem, and it incurs an uneven medical surveillance. The visibility of weight creates an invisibility of the person as such and fundamentally permeates the experience of pregnancy itself for obese women.

Although the obese-embodied experience of pregnancy can be joyful, there are medical and social discourses about obesity and pregnancy with which one must contend. These medicalized and moralized discourses often focus on how irresponsible or high risk the pregnancy could be, or is, rather than the cultural "norm," which is often characterized as happy and healthy (McNaughton 2011).

My concern here is to discuss reflexively how the fetus is both a valued product and a production made visible and therefore needing medical care through technologies (Morgan and Michaels 1999; Taylor 2008). I will examine how the fat maternal body is both rendered visible and invisible through reproductive surveillance. Even so-called normal pregnancy and birth are medicalized (Davis-Floyd 1997; Davis-Floyd 2003; Jordan and Davis-Floyd 1993; Rapp 2000), and regulation only increases in obese pregnancies. Visualization of the fetus has increased with biomedical research. The popularization and circulation of data about fetal development encourages American women, as citizen-subject-patients, to be vigilant about their health during pregnancy so as not to endanger the fetus.

Obesity is overly and overtly naturalized as a social and medical problem, whereas reproduction has also been naturalized in medical and social discourse as needing medical surveillance to produce successful births. Both these approaches obscure how fat women, how fat pregnant bodies, and how personhood exist in social life. I propose that a reflexive exploration of obesity and pregnancy can demonstrate that we need new understandings of the local body to better unpack the universalizing nature of the discourses of obesity, as well as the medicalization of specific categories of reproductive bodies as high-risk and morally questionable. I explore the cultural significance of the construction and the reading of the fat maternal body as irresponsible or troubling, which are expressed and performed in many obstetrical practices in the United States.

Stigma Embodied and Performed

After returning from fieldwork, I began to think about having children. I joined my husband in California, and to catch up on my health exams after fieldwork, I made an obstetrician/gynecologist appointment. After the exam, the doctor asked if I had any questions; I said I wanted to have children in a few years. I had barely gotten out the words when she announced that I was "too fat" to have a baby. She proceeded into a long tirade about my weight, my perceived faults (weight-based), the impossibility of me having a baby at my size, and the danger I would be placing any potential baby in, should I become pregnant. I have never had a new physician spend so much time with me before or since, but it was hardly a positive experience.

This gynecologist stated she would not even let me get pregnant or let me stay in her practice unless I lost 100 pounds. She made the definitive statement that I would have gestational diabetes and the baby would be unhealthy if I did not lose weight before pregnancy. She went on to offer dieting advice and she told me that all it took was self-control.

During this appointment I was rendered only a fat body that was unhealthy and morally dissolute if not also disgusting. This doctor made it clear that I needed to solve the problem of my fat, which was a problem with me—the body and the self were conflated and rendered a readable, simple symbolic system. Her discourse was a potent mixture of medical knowledge and commonplace cultural ideas of what fatness means and who fat people are (Ernsberger 2009). There certainly was the implication that I was lazy. I do not think I am the exception in either the realm of pregnancy care or primary care. Studies demonstrate that obese patients are stigmatized by health care providers (Drury et al. 2002; Puhl and Heuer 2010; Puhl and Heuer 2009; Puhl and Brownell 2001), and this results in obese patients going in for medical care less frequently or later than optimal for treatment. Medical care and medical practice are deeply cultural acts and cannot be divorced from the cultural and individual contexts in which the care is delivered.

Goffman (1963: 4) identified three types of stigma: abominations of the body, blemishes of individual character, and tribal stigma of race, nation, and religion. In the experience I describe above, I think we see abomination of the body as well as blemish of the individual character, or, in Goffman's terms, a spoiled identity (1963), in the doctor's treatment of me (Farrell 2011). Obese African-American women may embody all three types of stigma because as Rubin and Joseph (this volume), note they are caught between local values and popular culture's and biomedicine's characterization of large body size as unhealthy in combination with discriminatory constructions of race in the United States.

This doctor's performance of stigmatizing behavior is seen in her declaration that she would not "let" me become pregnant if I did not lose 100 pounds. The intensity of the surveillance, impossible though it would be to perform, carries a threat, as did her statement that if I did not lose weight and became pregnant she would not keep me in her practice. The obstetrician stigmatized my body in culturally readable ways, following a popular model in American media in which obesity is individualized. Individualizing this alleged social problem results in blaming the individual rather than looking at systemic forces or other complicating factors that contribute to obesity (Saguy and Almeling 2008). Her approach brings all sense of worth, all sense of personhood down to the body itself as symbolizing the whole person.

Anthropologists have long noted, the body is a both a reflection and construction of a culture's values and beliefs (Bourdieu 1992; Douglas 1970; Lock and Farquhar 2007; Sault 1994; Scheper-Hughes and Lock 1987). What is fascinating in the doctor's lecture is her emphasis on the idea that it is only my body and not my embodied self that is the proper symbolic form from which she can assess both my health and my worth. I understand an embodied self as phenomenological one. An embodied self is composed of mind, body, and the practice of social life—it is being in the world (Bourdieu 1992; Csordas 1993). Health and worth were intrinsically related in this doctor's response to me. The doctor's treatment, which focused almost entirely on my body as reflective of who I was and who I could be, demonstrates a larger concern in the United States with "body projects" that focus solely on the body and not other aspects of personhood (Brumberg 1997). If I lost weight, I would conform to standards of acceptability in both medical and social terms, and then my worth as a body, as a person, would increase.

My experience exemplifies how fatness and thinness are both naturalized and pathologized. The binary opposition of fatness and thinness reflects and reifies each. One has little meaning in the United States without the other since fatness and thinness shadow each other and one is always implied or almost present when there is a discussion of either. Embedded within this binary of fat and thin, the body, which can only be one or the other, stands in for the totality of the self. For a culture that often engages in the Cartesian mind/body split as an ontological belief and cultural practice, it is interesting that especially for fat individuals, as perhaps it is for others who are "different," the body is the self writ large and is therefore stigmatized.

My education and background also seemed to annoy the gynecologist. Several times she remarked how I must be intelligent. The implication seemed to be, if I were intelligent, why was I fat? In this schema, intelligence and educational level reflect self-discipline, hard work, and focus, and these characteristics should be writ upon the body. I felt this doctor struggled to understand how fat, which represents sloth and stupidity, could relate legitimately with intelligence and an advanced degree. The fact that my intelligence was embodied in fat seemed to make me a contradiction. My fat made me a "social problem" (Campos 2004; Spector and Kitsuse 2000). I lacked self-discipline and was therefore a betrayer of my class and not as intelligent as my degree suggested (Carr and Friedman 2005; Saguy and Gruys 2010).

There were also my doctor's concerns for my potential fetus. Medical studies and ideas circulating in the public sphere advance the idea that fat women who are pregnant are not only subjecting themselves to an increase in medical risk, but obese women are also placing their fetuses at risk (Oken 2009). The rate of miscarriage and stillbirth is higher for obese women. The fetus is visualized through biomedical studies which link obesity in pregnancy to increasing the risk of allergies, asthma, psychosocial consequences, and a variety of other illnesses and complications. Studies also show that obese mothers also increase the risk for obesity in their children's future (Durand et al. 2007). While the fetus is visualized as very vulnerable, it is also visualized as being a potentially obese person.

These implications increase the visibility of the obese pregnant body as not only a set of risks but also as a potential danger to the fetus. In the obesity as a form of endangerment model, obese pregnant women are morally irresponsible.

This concept of irresponsible mothering groups obese mothers in with other troubling kinds of mothers, such as those who smoke or use drugs and alcohol. Pregnant women in these deviant categories are more visible in the clinic through risk calculations which tend to judge the individual body and the individual's decisions as inherently right or wrong; in the case of obesity and pregnancy, the onus is often on the woman as morally suspect (Bell et al. 2009; Bell et al. 2011; Harthorn and Oaks 2003; Oaks 2001).

Thresholds of Visibility and Invisibility in the Clinic

In this section I wish to discuss briefly several ways in which my obese pregnant body was both rendered more visible due to my body size and yet also less visible and therefore less worthy of care during my first pregnancy. I will address how medical practices established the visibility of my fetus through technology and the complications obesity poses for such technology and therefore how the fat body/fat person poses a problem for medical practice.

After I moved to the Northeastern United States, I became pregnant. As soon as my over-the-counter pregnancy test indicated I was pregnant, I chose an obstetrician on my health plan. My main goal was to get into a practice that would not judge me based solely on my weight and that would support my choice to have a natural childbirth. The nurse taking my blood pressure on my first appointment did mention that a 300-pound patient had delivered a healthy baby vaginally just the month prior. She noted that the 300-pound patient was just so "proud of herself" and she "showed off her baby to the whole office." One of the complicated things about being fat, is that it is hard to gauge when something you encounter is about weight and stigma; signs from other people about one's body, especially if one has a stigmatized body, are often cloaked either intentionally or unintentionally. The narrative's meaning was unclear but left me uneasy. The doctor herself seemed kind enough, and when the nurse informed her of the questions I had been asking she gave me similar answers except when we came to the obesity issue. She then remarked that she dealt in *high-risk* pregnancies, so I should not worry. No one ever discussed gaining weight with me, but I did feel immediately rendered visible but desubjectivized with the implication that I was high risk based only on my weight.

Notions of risk permeate experiences in reproduction and in contemporary health projects; risk has become an important factor in the governance of reproductive health (Fordyce and Maraesa 2012). The doctor's comment began a long journey through two pregnancies in which risk was a field of meaning that I had entered because I was fat. My risk assessment was based solely on obesity. Lynn Freedman has written, "the seemingly neutrality of risk assessments…often hides the value-laden nature of the decisions they are used to support" (2005: 529). Within the economy of visibility, I understood my obese pregnant body to be hypervisible to my doctor and her staff. I embodied now, even more than before, as a non-pregnant fat person, a risk. (Cheyney and Everson 2009; Harthorn and Oaks 2003; McNaughton 2011)

While I did not feel pleased, I chose to stay with this practice because others had seemed even less of a fit. Within weeks of being pregnant, I began to have morning sickness, except I was sick most of the time. I found functioning difficult, as I needed a bathroom to be easily and instantly accessible. I mentioned the issue to my doctor and her staff but thought, as did they, that it was regular morning sickness. One nurse noted on the plus side that at least I would not gain much weight. However, the constant nausea continued, and due to the slow response of my obstetrician, I was ready to leave the practice by the fourth month. I continued to be sick until six months, was not sick the seventh month, and then was back to nausea for the remainder of the pregnancy.

When I became pregnant, the Institute of Medicine had not released its revised guidelines which stated that an obese woman should gain no more than 20 pounds while pregnant (Rasmussen et al. 2009). There was a tacit message that I should not gain much weight. Since I was not gaining much weight, my sickness was not seen as negative. What was most painful about the experience was not to be taken seriously—to be seen as having some sort of emotional reaction. Somehow my attempts to talk about what I was experiencing with my doctor were transformed into complaining. I almost stopped advocating for myself. The most pernicious thing was to wonder if my doctor and her staff were correct—that this was nothing out of the ordinary and I was somehow weak. Fat people are considered weak; if they were stronger, they would have self-control and not be fat.

The vomiting continued after the first trimester with no abatement, and I finally got my doctor and her staff to listen to me. She suggested antiemetics, and I was concerned about my fetus, but I finally agreed to them because I could not manage day-to-day living. I had further trouble with the first antiemetic because it made me vomit more severely. Calls to the nurse advised me to keep taking it, to give it time to work. I suspect I became hypervisible as a problematic patient. Eventually my situation was reviewed and I was switched to a different antiemetic. At this point I was disillusioned, and I switched practices to one much farther away, associated with a different hospital.

Nothing serious happened to me in the first medical practice, but what surprised me is how invisible my problem was because first it was seen as normal, and second, it was seen as almost helpful because it prevented much weight gain. Nurses praised this fact without ever talking to me directly about weight as a medical concern. The visibility of fat combined with stigma made my body something that was referred to indirectly but never discussed with me directly.

Medical Technologies, Medical Professionals, and Materializing the Fetus and the Fat Maternal Body

Arthur Kleinman's point that all levels of staff are participants in a patient's medical experience (1988: 259–265) is particularly germane here. I think the brilliancy of his idea rests on how he recognizes and calls attention to the obvious and notes the significance of observable everyday activity in medical practice to the patient experience. Kleinman also is quite clear in assessing the role of the medical hierarchy in creating great inequality among categories of service providers and how rankings and the treatment of those considered lowly by those considered experts has the unintended consequence of ricocheting onto patients and changing their medical experiences, from parking to the check-in desk and on through to the doctor (Kleinman 1988: 253–267). For the obese patient whose stigmatized body is understood to be open for comment on all levels of a medical practice, Kleinman's point is particularly salient. The issue of the use of medical technologies which materialize the fat maternal body and the fetal body are discussed here.

The quotidian events of a medical appointment are a different embodied and emotional experience for larger people. To begin with patient robes need to be larger, and if the room is out of larger robes, patients are given small robes and then sheets of plastic-coated paper to attempt to cover up what remains—usually they are best set over the lap. Blood pressure cuffs must be changed to a larger size for a more accurate measurement.[2]

Getting weighed is also a loaded ritual with fiddling on the scale and moving the weights up to the largest and heaviest weights. What happens in these small acts is that fat maternal body is made more visible—as out of the designated normal range—and this is performed and emphasized each weigh-in. I have on occasion gotten on the scale and turned my back to the numbers. I wanted to embody my pregnancy and feel where I was and not deal with the numbers. This choice on my part usually invited scorn and scolding or if not scolding, then biting comments. For example, "So we are not dealing with things today are we?" That one stuck in my mind especially because the nurse who said it was rather big herself. The introduction to this volume as well as the work of Yates-Doerr (this volume), questions the meaning of measurements by noting how measurements become fetishized in public health practice as an end in and of themselves. The data from scales is accepted as truth because scales do not lie, although they do vary considerably in accuracy and quality. This reality is not often incorporated in their use.

Eventually, learning that I had not gained weight actually helped me get attention for an issue that was being ignored. However, the subtle cues that take place during this measurement reinforce the fat maternal body as a problem and a shameful one. There is a sense that it is the measurement in medical practice that matters rather than the body/person. Measurement is often seen as some-how neutral, although the way this data is gathered, recorded, and interpreted by medical personnel is overlooked as a area of study by public health and biomedi-cal studies. The affect of this emphasis on measurement, for me at least, is that the complexities and emotional experiences of fatness is diminished, deemed less relevant or perhaps seen as something too messy to deal with during a weight in, and yet it is these times when fat people are very vulnerable. Seeing and com-municating with the *whole* person and not just his or her numbers could be an opportunity for further communication in medical settings, and respectful treat-ment invites a patient in to his or her own care rather than judges him or her for somehow failing at it.

Any patient who is in hospital robes is at a disadvantage in the clinical encoun-ter as that person is symbolically only a patient and not an entirely full, complex person (Lazarus 1988). Being in a hospital robe that does not fit leaves one dou-bly vulnerable. Many nurses are gracious in the performance of their duties, but I have had nurses sigh and say such things as "I don't have any extra large robes in here so you will have to make do with this and a sheet" or "I have to go and get the bigger blood pressure cuff from the other room," and the tone, set of the shoulders, and heavy footfalls indicate that this is an inconvenience at best and an inconvenience that is my fault. Since fat is often seen as an individual failing, some medical staff felt comfortable displaying their annoyance and disapproval. The visibly stigmatized body/person in such a social situation does not have many options for response to this constant low level mistreatment. Every response can cost the stigmatized individual social and emotional capital, and often the price might be even worse medical care. The visible stigmatized individual is left with, as Goffman notes, "anxious unanchored interactions" (1963: 18).

Work in anthropology has noted that materializing and visualizing the fetus has a complicated impact on women and women's autonomy in the United States (Casper 1998; Casper and Moore 2009; Morgan and Michaels 1999; Rapp 2000; Taylor 2008). This may be culturally troubling because visualizations often work to construct the fetus as a person and a person whose interests may not be in line with the maternal body. The maternal body is often not complexly viewed as an entity with her own personhood; women are more than a host for the fetus

This American ritual of materializing and individualizing the fetus becomes particularly problematic for heavy women when technological practices are im-bued with sociomedical beliefs and moral discourses in ways that further stig-matize. I have been told that because I am fat it might be hard to hear the fetal heartbeat. I have been told that I because I am fat I may not be able to feel my fetus move. In ultrasounds, I have had medical technicians tell me that it is dif-ficult for them to get good pictures or to sigh and remark that size makes their job more difficult. Ultrasounds can be less effective in obese women. However, other statements are pernicious myths, particularly the idea that large women cannot feel their fetus move.[3] Moreover, all fat bodies are not the same, and what is true for some fat bodies is not true for all. Lock's concept of local biologies applies here—fat people have their own genetic, environmental, and medical histories as well as their own social and cultural histories. For some fat women ultrasound may present no issues. The issue for the fat pregnant woman is the assumption that there will be a problem (Lock 1993).

If technologies that visualize the fetus are used to discipline women in the United States, then these technologies are doubly used to stigmatize and discipline obese women. Prenatal testing visualizes the fetus for the prospective parents by mapping out the fetuses' genetic "health" (Rapp 2000). I wanted to know if I was bearing a Down syndrome child or a child with other possible fetal anomalies. The choice to find out and the results had me, as Rapp points out in her pioneering work, navigating through various moral boundaries and intersections (social, legal, medical, religious) to make an "informed decision." I had an amniocentesis since that was what was available to me at the time. However, I know that currently many obese women are not offered less invasive nuchal scans, as this route is perhaps less effective given their respective size.[4] Amniocentesis has its own risks, such as miscarriage, cramping and vaginal bleeding, needle injury, and leaking amniotic fluid, among others. I am not contesting that a nuchal scan might not be ineffective for obese women, as this is possibly the case. What I note is that a stigmatized and medically troubling body often leads to obese pregnant women to experience treatments, tests, and technologies that are in many ways increasingly more invasive. The delivery of more invasive technologies can feel more punitive on both a physical and an emotional level.

Additionally, medical visualizing technologies emphasize that a fetus's and a woman's interests are not aligned, especially because fat women are regarded as choosing to put their fetuses at higher risk. While there may be medical evidence for this, there is no reason to use medical technologies to treat fat women poorly. I believe this also increases anxiety among heavy women. Women feel increased pressure to place the fetus first in their technologies of care, and anthropology has noted both the growth and the impact of this culturally. Heavy women feel this pressure as well, but they face an impossible task wherein they are supposed to privilege the fetus but because of their fatness, they are also endangering the fetal subject, which makes them morally troubling as maternal.

Invisibility and Visibility in the Public Sphere

The maternal body is a shifting, changing symbol in American public life. There is an emphasis on showing off one's bump, and there is a whole new celebrity culture around revealing and consuming images of celebrity's pregnancies and maternity clothing. As fat bodies are not considered attractive, fat women are not encouraged to show off their pregnancies and maternity clothing for fat women is difficult to find. For the most part, the fat maternal body is invisible in the public sphere. It registers as simply fat. And therefore it is visible as a stigmatized visual sign (Rothblum and Solovay 2009).

I found that even in the waiting room at my obstetrical practice, my body rarely figured as pregnant. Many pregnant women chatted in the waiting room, and I rarely chatted but occasionally did so. Most women assumed I was there for an annual exam. On several occasions when I clarified that I was pregnant, there would be an uncomfortable pause and often the conversation would end or switch tracks, as a social mistake had occurred. In public, I was just viewed as fatter, which provoked comments on occasion in grocery stores, etc.

Only once toward the end of my second pregnancy was I recognized as pregnant in a well-known coffee chain. A woman sitting near the pick-up line remarked to me that she hoped I was not drinking caffeine because it was not good for the baby. At first I was stunned that I had been recognized as being pregnant. Then I found myself feeling normal in that people felt free to police me as pregnant and not fat. Lastly, I decided that I resented being policed for being pregnant as much as I resented being policed for being fat. I told her it was decaffeinated. I was struck that I was always in the defensive position in that I had to answer accusations of fatness and pregnancy. One could not leave such an accusation alone, as that leaves one in a morally questionable space—a weak social position. I left rather bemused by the collision of visibility, invisibility, and stigmatization that involves American women's bodies in diverse ways whether they are fat or pregnant or fat and pregnant.

Giving Birth and the Aftermath

I was a week past my due date and had experienced no signs of labor. I had not even experienced any Braxton Hicks contractions. I had to go in for a sound test where they blasted loud noise to my fetus, and he certainly startled. And that proved he could still move, as he had not been moving much. I agreed to an induced pregnancy after my due date passed by over a week and my fetus was not moving much nor had I experienced any signs of labor. At this point my complex and nuanced anthropological worldview was being overwhelmed by months of nausea, the discomfort of the end of pregnancy, and a pregnancy that involved a tremendous amount of emotional work to maintain a sense of my personhood and my body in the face of repeated acts of discrimination. I was beginning to be scared because my baby was hardly moving. Ultimately, I learned that this was so because he had twisted the umbilical cord around his neck repeatedly and he was not able to unwind himself. Fetuses can tangle and untangle themselves even during birth, but my son was not able to do this.

I was induced. I reported to the hospital with my partner at 7:00 A.M. for induction where Cervidil in a tampon-like form was placed on my cervix to try and "ripen" it. I was hooked up to a fetal monitor despite my protests. The midwife checked my baby by ultrasound, and he seemed fine. The cord around his neck was not visible. By 3:00 P.M. my water broke. Meconium was present, which can happen with induction, and it can happen in any case for a variety of other reasons. I was then hooked up to pitocin and in for a long night. Pitocin was hard to keep up with physically. I was not to push, but I could never catch up to the pitocin to breathe through it. This was very painful. I had two doses of opiates over the long night but was unable to rest. I walked.

I did tell the midwives that although I studied reproduction and I understood that other cultures understood labor pain differently as "good pain," I was not a fan of pain and not particularly stoic. I was never anything but honest in my assessment of myself. Two of the midwives I saw most often in the practice stated that it was important not to judge a laboring or birthing woman. That comforted me when I heard it, but it did not seem to apply during actual labor. After close to twenty-plus hours of pitocin, I still had not progressed and I was only about 4 cm dilated—exhausted and in pain from the pitocin and from trying not to push. My partner walked me to the restroom, and there my midwife came in and asked me if I was person who held onto things. I said yes, and then I said I had no idea and asked what this was about. Then she asked me if I had been sexually abused and if therefore, I was holding the baby in. Little did I know but my doula was asking my mother the same question at the same time. Because labor had been nonprogressive despite many interventions, I was being questioned about how I was perhaps unconsciously holding on to the baby. I have not been sexually abused. I understand that studies support a correlation between obesity and sexual abuse and that there is a correlation between sexual abuse and longer, more difficult labors. However, this is one of the situations where I was again left wondering how much my treatment here had to do with my body size.

Obesity is read as a body in distress. Fat is often understood in the United States as a sign of being emotionally troubled. Fat in the United States is, I argue, seen as a somatic idiom of distress (Nichter 1981) and a symbol of maladaptive coping mechanisms. So my fat and my slow labor were both read by the midwife treating me as an idiom of distress from the past and therefore a somatic body/ mind memory of sexual abuse. My caregivers seemed genuinely frustrated with me and with my labor. Even though I felt hardly conscious, I strongly stated that I had not been sexually abused and although under the duress of pain, exhaustion, and questioning, I had said I was person "who held onto things," I was retracting my confession. I stated that I could not believe this approach would be helpful for anyone who had been sexually abused. The midwife assured me that it was. And my partner, who had been fuming about the whole thing, then asked the midwife to leave. Soon after that my mother announced that she was calling the obstetrician if the midwife would not due to my obvious non-progressive labor. I got an epidural and a caesarian section during which the pregnant obstetrician announced that my son had the cord wrapped tightly around his neck and that he could not have been delivered vaginally. She later postulated that the pitocin had been pushing him down and then he would be pulled back up by the umbilical cord—hence the signs of fetal distress that showed up on the fetal monitor. Perhaps it also speaks to how programmed I had become at this point, that I started to believe that the fetal monitor might not be working very well, not only because they have a high rate of false positives, but because I was fat and therefore it might not work very well on me. Upon learning about the cord and the doctor's belief that my son would never have descended, I loudly announced, "It was not my fault!" and I was met with silence by my midwife.

Do I think my obesity played a role here? I do. I think I was seen as weak and too sensitive to pain. I was seen as not working hard enough, and finally I was seen as emotionally distressed and unconsciously holding on to my child and resisting labor. This is all a matter of interpretation, but since fat played a role in every facet of pregnancy and every facet of my life, I think it was a factor here. The stigmatized fat maternal body here was rendered very visible to judgment and evaluation during childbirth, and yet the complexity of my body and my personhood remained invisible. Fat appears so visible and easy to read and yet by doing this, medical practitioners of all levels do not read bodies in a manner that is richly symbolic. I am not condemning the way medical care views bodies so much as pointing out its limitations. I recognize that doctors are trained to read bodies differently in ways that demonstrate evidence of competence in medical practice, which is the goal of medical education (DelVecchio Good 1998).

During my medical care and birth, my fat body provoked a negative somatic mode of attention (Csordas 1993) in many of my caregivers. Csordas defines somatic modes of attention as a "culturally elaborated ways of attending to and with one's body in surroundings that include the embodied presence of others" (Csordas 1993: 138). The very negative ideas about fat as enunciated and performed through various social processes, including medical practices which are also social processes, came to be mirrored on my body and therefore my body embodied ontological resonances of stigma, of a polluted identity.

My fat represented not only weakness and moral corruption but also contagion—the visceral, unconscious, and conscious responses to my body contribute not only to my bodily memory and my embodiment but also to the bodily responses of my care givers who seemed to find my body a failure and also possibly repulsive. I argue that the ways their bodies attended to my body created an exchange between bodies that was negative and not about care or healing but rather about stigmatizing my body as a troubling one without an easy solution. Since obesity cannot be solved as a medical problem easily or quickly, fat embodiment becomes that much heavier as it bears the weight of the medical and social gaze as a spoiled body and a spoiled person (Goffman 1963).

Conclusion: Carrying the Weight

Jessica Hardin and I organized a session on obesity for the American Anthropological Association Meetings in 2010. Initially, discussion afterward appeared to be taking in our overall themes such as: (1) fat and obesity are categories that need to be reexamined, (2) that culture is often used to "dress" a body size study or intervention but that it was not deeply contextualized and incorporated in studies of obesity, and that (3) measurements and rubrics of obesity needed to be examined for the meanings they created and promulgated. Measurements matter as much for their accuracy and how they are valued and what this valuing does to the whole experience of those who are obese. Soon, however, discussion shifted away from the issues we hoped to raise in the panel and moved quickly instead to the topic of measurement and how to do effective measurements. This is a traditional and well-trodden way of discussing obesity. It is important. Such data are needed in global health. Yet I suggest that measurement-centric approaches have their limits, especially because they lack real analysis of meaning.

The work I have done here in ethnographically exploring embodiment, stigma, visibility, and invisibility of the fat maternal body cannot be captured in measurements. Nevertheless this approach does raise questions about how risk is assessed, how fetuses are visualized, how beliefs about maternal behavior change the fetus as a product of pregnancy, and how stigmatized fat maternal bodies are medically treated and the impact of this treatment.

In a preliminary phone interview with Dr. Naomi Stotland, an assistant professor in the Department of Obstetrics, Gynecology, and Reproductive Sciences at UCSF and an expert in obesity and pregnancy, she explained how she had just completed her first qualitative study of providers to survey what type of advice they give their patients on weight gain and health during pregnancy (Stotland et al. 2010). Stotland et al. (2005, 2010) and Jackson et al. (2011) note that medical staff are concerned about weight gain in their obese patients during pregnancy and many are struggling with how to provide helpful advice to patients. Her work suggests that it will be important to study the relationship between provider advice and pregnancy outcomes.

This issue has become more crucial with the new weight gain guidelines issued by the Institute of Medicine (Rasmussen et al. 2009). I think the question of how to talk to obese pregnant women about weight and weight gain alone graphically illustrates one of the crucial problems with medical care of fat pregnant women, which is that there are a set of beliefs about obesity and these beliefs need to be uncovered and analyzed. I suggest that the set of issues raised by medical providers about weight and pregnancy outcomes are important but should not be the only focus.

Whether practitioners discuss weight with clients directly or not, my narrative illustrates that this discussion about weight, health, and the value of certain maternal bodies over others is already taking place. It would be more valuable for medical practitioners to acknowledge how much they are cultural actors who are in a position of power to reinforce very negative ideas about fat women advertently or inadvertently.

It is not that quantitative studies on obesity are not useful, but the addition of qualitative data is essential for a rigorous, methodological approach to combating obesity and obesity and pregnancy. Many fat women may disagree with me, but I think Kleinman's idea (1988) that doctors should collect mini-ethnographic narratives of illness may be of help here. I think that fat patients need to construct a fat narrative that is short and makes cogent personal and medical points to humanize themselves for medical professionals. It will be uncomfortable, but as I note the discussion about fat is already taking place, and it behooves all involved to address the issues more directly to deliver more effective and more respectful medical care. Additionally fat patients can be encouraged to construct a fat narrative in an appointment or over the course of several. Medical caregivers need to understand what food means to people, how they use it, what stresses are in their life, the addictive nature of habits, and the immense difficulty of losing weight and keeping it off for any extended amount of time. Anne Becker eloquently speaks to the medical research in this area and how much it contradicts what the diet industry and popular media promulgate about the possibilities of weight loss (Becker, this volume).

Caregivers can impart knowledge about the health risks of obesity to fat pregnant women or to fat women wanting to become pregnant but should do so with sensitivity and respect, getting to understand the local moral worlds of their patients. Medical knowledge is generated in a cultural context (including biomedical research and medical practice as cultural contexts), and advice for patients should not be given as if the clinical encounter took place in a "culture of no culture" (Gershon and Taylor 2008); this is simply not the case. Obesity is often seen as a disorder derived from ignorance. "If people were informed they would not eat this or that" is how the thinking goes. I support nutritional education for obese patients and obese pregnant patients but noncompliance is not about only lack of information alone, it is also about cultural beliefs about food, habit, practice, and care taking activities. Many people eat in an attempt to care for themselves emotionally, and many people feed others in an attempt to demonstrate care. If food is in complex ways a manifestation of love and care then any health intervention that does not understand the cultural and contextual particulars of food will not succeed.

Obese pregnant patients carry a range of "weights" beyond physical weight. Due to the lived realities of class, race, and gender in the United States, some obese pregnant women carry more of the weight of stigma, visibility, and invisibility than others. Obese pregnant women also carry the weight of a judgmental gaze about their fitness as mothers and the anxiety that their children will also be obese and therefore future burdens to American health care. My health care during pregnancy as a fat woman was poor, damaging, and demoralizing. Others have developed very clear suggestions for fat women to advocate for themselves, which is appropriate given our consumer model of health care, and while I believe this is laudable and important work, for me bigger cultural questions remain.[5] Given that fat is so stigmatized, how can fat women effectively advocate for better care and what are the cultural, social, economic, political, and medical costs of advocating? It is significant that medical care is trying to solve the obesity epidemic but most of my experiences as a fat pregnant woman in medical care conflated my fatness with any health issue I was experiencing. That is not effective medicine.

Studies on obesity and pregnancy indicate that obesity in pregnancy leads to complications, illnesses, and diseases in pregnancy as well as increased risk for cesarean sections and poor childbirth outcomes. I do not contest this, but I am concerned with how much difference, difference makes in the actual practice of health care. The valences of the weight of stigma, visibility, and invisibility impact the kinds of care obese women receive. What kinds of care are obese African-American women or Hispanic women receiving? What about obese lesbian mothers? How does race and gender intersect with sexuality in the treatment of an obese pregnancy? What are the life circumstances that lead women of all kinds and creeds to over eat? What is going on in the lives of fat pregnant women? Studies on the complications of obesity in pregnancy have proliferated in the past thirty years with a series of compelling conclusions (Reece 2008; Smith et al. 2008). A large portion of current public health research is concentrated on describing and attempting to explain health disparities but often miss what Williams aptly terms the "social imbeddedness" of health (Williams 2002). What are the consequences both long and short term of such destructive and punitive treatment of any and all obese mothers and their fetuses? Treating obese women as weak and blameworthy will not improve health statistics. If the concern is the relationship between maternal fat and birth outcomes, perhaps the medical establishment should also be concerned about the correlation between stigmatizing treatment of obese pregnant women and birth outcomes. Problematic statistics in the area of bariatric pregnancy may also be an indicator of the dysfunction of the medical system and not just the dysfunction of the fat maternal body. This is precisely why obesity and pregnancy need to be better theorized and studied in a cross-cultural and interdisciplinary way (see Unnithan-Kumar and Tremayne 2011), and it is also important that anthropology offer some qualitative data to assist in the training of medical professionals so that better care is provided for obese pregnancies and better understanding is afforded to fat mothers.

Notes

1. The complications related to obesity and pregnancy include issues of fertility, spontaneous abortion, stillbirth, gestational diabetes mellitus, preeclampsia, congenital malformations, preterm delivery, cesarean section, hypertension, toxemia, urinary infections, labor induction, and increased length of hospitalization (Sarwer et al. 2006).
2. The cuff issue is one that childbirth educator, blogger, writer and plus-sized mother, Pamela Vireday (2002, 2008, 2009, 2012) writes on.
3. Vireday (2009, 2012) again is useful here.
4. A nuchal scan is a sonographic ultrasound scan that assesses the amount of fluid behind the neck of the fetus—also known as the nuchal fold or the nuchal translucency. Fetuses at risk of Down syndrome tend to have a higher amount of fluid around the neck. Its high-definition imaging may also detect other less common chromosomal abnormalities.
5. The Our Bodies, Ourselves blog has an article on obesity and pregnancy by Pamela Vireday (2008) that details ways that women of size can advocate for themselves. She spends time deconstructing diagnoses that obese women frequently receive. An example would be the diagnosis of "soft tissue dystocia" in which women's vaginas are claimed to be "fatty" and therefore a c-section must be performed.
6. Please see endnote 1.

References

Becker, A. E. 1995. *Body, Self, and Society: The View from Fiji.* Philadelphia: University of Pennsylvania Press.

Becker, D. M., L. R. Yanek, and D. M. Koffman. 1999. "Body Image Preferences among Urban African American and Whites from Low-Income Communities." *Ethnicity and Disease* 9, no. 3: 377–386

Bell, K., D. McNaughton, and A. Salmon. 2009. "Medicine, Morality and Mothering: Public Health Discourses on Alcohol Exposure, Smoking around Children and Childhood Overnutrition." *Critical Public Heath* 19, no. 2: 155–170.

Bell, K., A. Salmon, and D. McNaughton. 2011. "Introduction." In *Alcohol, Tobacco and Obesity: Morality, Mortality and the New Public Health,* ed. K. Bell, A. Salmon, and D. McNaughton. London: Routledge.

Bordo, S. 1993. *Unbearable Weight: Feminism, Western Culture, and the Body.* Berkeley, Los Angeles, and London: University of California.

Bourdieu, P. 1992. *The Logic of Practice.* Stanford: Stanford University Press.

Brumberg, J. J. 1997. *The Body Project: An Intimate History of American Girls.* New York: Random House.

Campos, P. F. 2004. *The Obesity Myth: Why America's Obsession with Weight Is Hazardous to Your Health.* New York: Gotham Books.

Carr, D., and M. Friedman. 2005. "Is Obesity Stigmatizing? Body Weight, Perceived Discrimination, and Psychological Well-being in the United States." *Journal of Health and Social Behavior* 46: 244–259.

Casper, M. J. 1998. *The Making of the Unborn Patient: A Social Anatomy of Fetal Surgery.* New Brunswick, NJ: Rutgers University Press.

Casper, M. J., and L. J. Moore. 2009. *Missing Bodies: The Politics of Visibility.* New York: New York University Press.

Cheyney, M., and C. Everson. 2009. "Narratives of Risk: Speaking across the Hospital/Home-birth Divide." *Anthropology News* 50, no. 3: 7–8.

Csordas, T. J. 1993. "Somatic Modes of Attention." *Cultural Anthropology* 8, no. 2: 135.

Davis-Floyd, R. E., ed. 1997. *Childbirth and Authoritative Knowledge: Cross-Cultural Perspectives.* Berkeley: University of California Press.

———. 2003. *Birth as an American Rite Of Passage.* Berkeley: University of California Press.

DelVecchio Good, M. 1998. *American Medicine: The Quest for Competence.* Berkeley: University of California Press.

Douglas, M. 1970. "The Two Bodies." In *Natural Symbols: Explorations in Cosmology.* New York: Pantheon Books.

Drury, C. A. A., et al. 2002. "Exploring the association between body weight, stigma of obesity, and health care avoidance." *Journal of the American Academy of Nurse Practitioners* 14, no. 12: 554–561.

Durand, E. F., C. Logan, and A. Carruth. 2007. "Association of Maternal Obesity and Childhood Obesity: Implications for Healthcare Providers." *Journal of Community Health Nursing* 24, no. 3: 167–176.

Ernsberger, P. 2009. "Does Social Class Explain the Connection Between Weight and Health?" In *The Fat Studies Reader,* ed. E. Rothblum and S. Solovay. New York: New York University Press, 25–36.

Farrell, A. E. 2011. *Fat Shame: Stigma and the Fat Body in American Culture.* New York: New York University Press.

Freedman, L. P. 2005. "Human Rights and the Politics of Risk and Blame: Lessons from the International Reproductive Health Movement." In *Perspectives on Health and Human Rights,* ed. S. Gruskin. New York: Routledge, 527–537.

Fordyce, L. and A. Maraesa, eds. 2012. *Risk, Reproduction and Narratives of Experience.* Vanderbilt University Press.

Gershon, I., and J. S. Taylor. 2008. "Introduction to In Focus: Culture in the Spaces of no Culture." *American Anthropologist* 110, no. 4: 417–421.

Ginsburg, F., and R. Rapp. 1999. "Fetal Reflections: Confessions of Two Feminist Anthropologists as Mutual Informants." In *Fetal Subjects, Feminist Positions,* ed. L. M. Morgan and M. W. Michaels. Philadelphia: University of Pennsylvania Press, 279–295.

Goffman, E. 1963. *Stigma: Notes on the Management of Spoiled Identity.* New York: Simon and Schuster.

Harthorn, B. H., and L. Oaks. 2003. *Risk, Culture, and Health Inequality: Shifting Perceptions of Danger and Blame.* Westport, CT: Praeger.

Jackson, R. A., et al. 2011. "Improving Diet and Exercise in Pregnancy with Video Doctor Counseling: A Randomized Trial." *Patient Education and Counseling* 83, no. 2: 203–209.

Jordan, B., and R. Davis-Floyd. 1993. *Birth in Four Cultures: A Crosscultural Investigation of Childbirth in Yucatan, Holland, Sweden, and the United States.* Prospect Heights, IL: Waveland Press.

Kleinman, A. 1988. *The Illness Narratives: Suffering, Healing, and the Human Condition.* New York: Basic Books.

Kulick, D., and A. Meneley, eds. 2005. *Fat: The Anthropology of an Obsession.* New York: Penguin.

Layne, L. L. 2003. *Motherhood Lost: A Feminist Account of Pregnancy Loss in America.* New York: Routledge.

Lazarus, E. S. 1988. "Theoretical Considerations for the Study of the Doctor-Patient Relationship: Implications of a Perinatal Study." *Medical Anthropology Quarterly* 2, no. 1: 34–58.

Lock, M. 1993. *Encounters with Aging: Mythologies of Menopause in Japan and North America.* Berkeley: University of California Press.

Lock, M. M., and J. Farquhar, eds. 2007. *Beyond the Body Proper: Reading the Anthropology of Material Life.* Durham, NC: Duke University Press.

Martin, E. 2009. *Bipolar Expeditions: Mania and Depression in American Culture.* Princeton, NJ: Princeton University Press.

McNaughton, D. 2011. "From the Womb to the Tomb: Obesity and Maternal Responsibility." *Critical Public Health* 21, no. 2: 179–190.

Morgan, L. M., and M. W. Michaels, eds. 1999. *Fetal Subjects, Feminist Positions.* Philadelphia: University of Pennsylvania Press.

Nichter, M. 1981. "Idioms of Distress: Alternatives in the Expression of Psychosocial Distress, a Case Study from South India." *Culture, Medicine and Psychiatry* 5: 379–408.

Oaks, L. 2001. *Smoking and Pregnancy: The Politics of Fetal Protection.* New Brunswick, NJ: Rutgers University Press.

Oken, E. 2009. "Excess Gestational Weight Gain Amplifies Risks among Obese Mothers."

Puhl, R. M., and K. D. Brownell. 2001. "Bias, discrimination, and obesity." *Obesity Research* 9, no. 12: 788–805.

Puhl, R.M., and C. A. Heuer. 2009. "The Stigma of Obesity: A Review and Update." *Obesity* 17, no. 5: 941–946.

———. 2010. "Obesity Stigma: Important Considerations for Public Health." *American Journal of Public Health* 100, no. 6: 1019–1028.

Rapp, R. 2000. *Testing Women, Testing the Fetus: The Social Impact of Amniocentesis in America.* New York: Routledge.

Rasmussen, K. M., and A. L. Yaktine, eds. 2009. "Committee to Reexamine IOM Pregnancy Weight Guidelines Institute of Medicine." *Weight Gain During Pregnancy: Reexamining the Guidelines.* Washington, DC: National Academies Press.

Reece, E. A. 2008. "Perspectives on Obesity, Pregnancy and Birth Outcomes in the United States: The Scope of the Problem." *American Journal of Obstetrics and Gynecology* 198, no. 1: 2327.

Rothblum, E., and S. Solovay, eds. 2009. *The Fat Studies Reader,* New York: New York University Press.

Royce, T. 2009. "The Shape of Abuse: Fat Oppression as a Form of Violence against Women." In *The Fat Studies Reader,* ed. E. Rothblum and S. Solovay. New York: New York University Press, 151–157.

Saguy, A. C., and R. Almeling. 2008. "Fat in the Fire? Science, the News Media, and the 'Obesity Epidemic.'" *Sociological Review* 23, no. 1: 53–83.

Saguy, A., and K. Gruys. 2010. "Morality and Health: News Media Constructions of Overweight and Eating Disorders." *Social Problems* 7, no. 2: 231–250.

Sarwer, D. B., K. C. Allison, L. M. Gibbons, J. T. Markowitz, and D. B. Nelson. 2006. "Pregnancy and Obesity: A Review and Agenda for Future Research." *Journal of Women's Health* 15, no. 6: 720–733.

Sault, N., ed. 1994. *Many Mirrors: Body Image and Social Relations.* New Brunswick, NJ: Rutgers University Press.

Scheper-Hughes, N., and M. M. Lock. 1987. "The Mindful Body: A Prolegomenon to Future Work in Medical Anthropology." *Medical Anthropology Quarterly* 1, no. 1: 6–41.

Smith, S. A., T. Hulsey, and W. Goodnight. 2008. "Effects of Obesity on Pregnancy." *Journal of Obstetric, Gynecologic, and Neonatal Nursing* 37, no. 2: 176–184.

Sobo, E. J. 1993. *One Blood: The Jamaican Body.* Albany: State University of New York Press.

Spector, M., and J. I. Kitsuse. 2000. *Constructing Social Problems.* New Brunswick, NJ: Transaction Publishers.

Stotland, N. E., J. S. Haas, P. Brawarsky, R. A. Jackson, E. Fuentes-Afflick, G. J. Escobar. 2005. "Body Mass Index, Provider Advice, and Target Gestational Weight Gain." *Obstetrics and Gynecology* 105, no. 3: 633–638.

———. 2010. "Preventing Excessive Weight Gain in Pregnancy: How Do Prenatal Care Providers Approach Counseling?" *Journal of Women's Health* 19, no. 4: 807–814.

Taylor, J. S. 2008. *The Public Life of The Fetal Sonogram: Technology, Consumption, and the Politics of Reproduction.* New Brunswick, NJ: Rutgers University Press.

Unnithan-Kumar, M., and S. Tremayne. 2011. *Fatness and the Maternal Body: Women's Experiences of Corporeality and the Shaping of Social Policy.* New York: Berghahn Books.

Vireday, P. 2002. "Are You a Size-Friendly Midwife?" *Midwifery Today: The Heart and Science of Birth,* available at http://www.midwiferytoday.com/articles/size_friendly.asp, accessed August 5, 2012.

———. 2008. "Women of Size and Cesarean Sections: Tips for Avoiding Unnecessary Surgery." *Our Bodies Ourselves Health Resource Center: Pregnancy and Birth,* available at http://www.ourbodiesourselves.org/book/companion.asp?id=21&compID=125, accessed August 5, 2012.

———. 2009. *The Plus-Size Pregnancy Website.* Available at www.plus-size-pregnancy.org, accessed August 5, 2012.

———. 2012. *The Well-Rounded Mama.* Available at http://wellroundedmama.blogspot.com/, accessed August 5, 2012.

Williams, D. R. 2002. "Racial/Ethnic Variations in Women's Health: The Social Embeddedness of Health." *American Journal of Public Health* 92, no. 4: 588–597.

Wilson, B. D. M. 2009. "Widening the Dialogue to Narrow the Gap in Health Disparities: Approaches to Fat Black Lesbian and Bisexual Women's Health Promotion." In *The Fat Studies Reader,* ed. E. Rothblum and S. Solovay. New York: New York University Press, 54–64.

Winkler, C., and K. Winniger. 1994. "Rape Trauma: Contexts of Meaning." In *Embodiment and Experience: The Existential Ground of Culture and Self,* ed. T. J. Csordas. Cambridge: Cambridge University Press, 248–268.

Acknowledgments

The productive session of the American Anthropological Association in 2010 was marvelous, and I would like to thank all participants, Anne Becker, Emily Yates-Doerr, Sarah Simpson Trainer, Rochelle Rosen, and, of course, my co-organizer, Jessica Hardin. Leslie Carlin also deserves thanks for her efforts on the volume's behalf. Last, but certainly not least, I would like to lovingly thank Ann and Richard Lozeau for continued support and assistance. Thanks also to my life partner and best friend, Stephen Rybicki, and our wonderful boys.

Afterword

Stephen T. McGarvey

✤ ✤ ✤

The increase in individual and population levels of body weight and adiposity throughout the world over the last several decades presents challenges to holistic anthropology, public health, psychology, and related population and clinically oriented disciplines. This volume intelligently and insightfully addresses those challenges. The emphasis in this work, which ranges from the context of measurements to public health messaging to actual medical care, is on missing the essential individuality of the persons involved and actively denying, or passively subverting, opportunities for improved well-being and health. Work by Jessica Hardin and Rochelle Rosen on Samoa, Sarah Trainer's work in the UAE, and Hanna Garth's work on Cuba deal with specific societies and their particular historical contexts in describing and analyzing large body size and the presence there of stigmatizing forces, generational differences, and difficulties in negotiating and accommodating body size differences. These specific case studies offer fresh ways of viewing large body size and obesity in ways that offer optimism for improving respectful interactions and procedures by medical and public health institutions by taking the detailed individual person into account.

Across all the scholarly areas represented, the papers call for more careful attention to these changes in body size and fatness by broadening studies to embrace the heterogeneities of causes and consequences of adiposity and employing more intensive methods with a focus on detailed perception of the large body–sized. The following are some key themes worth highlighting:

1. Public health and epidemiology in their central population-based perspectives are perceived as predicting scenarios that apply to all without enough regard to the individuals and enough detail about levels of risk, competing causes of death and disability, and translating into lay terms how group level predictions can be applied for specific individuals. Darlene McNaughton

and Emily Yates-Doerr critiqued the overly simplistic public media and sometimes clinical presentation of obesity risk assessment in light of the complex pathophysiology of adipose biology, insulin resistance, and type 2 diabetes. The way forward must be to have a concrete focus on defined groups, critical reviews of published studies, and in-depth collaborations across many fields. Additionally Anne Becker makes the case for the significance of local context, which can assist researchers and health practitioners collect and use statistical data in dynamic and insightful ways.

2. Social institutions such as schools conform to the broader worries about overweight and translate these concerns into gender- and age-specific informal and formal advice and lessons. Negative fat stigma may be introduced and created, as well as perpetuated. The work of Tracy Moffat and Tina Galloway on a school nutrition program in Canada is a stand-out contribution in this area.

3. Medicalization of body size has led unfortunately all too frequently to a narrow communication set between individuals and clinicians with a high potential for unintended and, sadly, seemingly purposeful stigmatization. Ignoring key social and cultural differences and their influence on knowledge and ideas about body size, obesity, and health carries a heavy societal and individual penalty on the goals of open discussion of information and its tailored interpretation. More nettlesome is the issue of individuals being stigmatized as having varieties of moral failings. Much more research and practice is needed on ways to inform, support, and help individuals with demonstrable risk toward self-aware and even self-managed changes. This goes beyond good patient-doctor communication or cultural competence and includes the intensive knowledge of people and their histories, and the purposeful production of sensitive and respectful human biological health education and information. Lisa R. Rubin and Jessica A. Joseph and Megan McCullough's work in this volume illustrate this need for a new approach to health behavior change in both research and medical care.

Broader consideration of the chapters produced the following recommended action items for the multiple disciplines with interests in body size, obesity, and health. These are not new recommendations, but readers I hope will be motivated to further specify and elaborate nuanced ways to carry forward scholarship. We must ask specific questions about mechanisms both biological and sociobehavioral while imbedding both in a solid cultural and historical context of clearly defined populations and their likely increasing diversities. There is a need for integrated intensive studies of the lived daily lives of people defined both by experts and most importantly by people themselves. Such studies will allow us to develop deep understanding of individuals and contribute to the individual ethnographies we wish our medical providers had in our charts. We need in-depth education of the general public and health specialists about the biology and health of body weight and adiposity as a source of empowerment to facilitate self-directed changes or management and to engage in candid conversations with public health and medical personnel.

This education should have as a goal an increased skepticism and self-reflection about media messages and interpersonal conversations about body size and health that locate and maintain the primacy of the individual, not the mass and not the narrow professional concerns. Perhaps such an enterprise would increase the ability of all of us to interpret with the respectful help of care providers the public health consensus as it might apply to us. Similarly in populations for which no consistent evidence is available about body size and health and, thus, evidence-based recommendations, we would call for the expansion of professional training of individuals from those groups and cautious extrapolations from other evidence. In short, a key implication of my reading of these chapters is the call for the use of the full set of multidisciplinary perspectives toward the complete ecology of the cultures of body size and obesity.

We will not stem the technological and evolutionary biology tides that have combined to raise Homo sapiens' levels of body size and adiposity in any near-time future. Thus, a sober analysis of particularistic historical scenarios, human biologies, and culturally embedded factors of these unprecedented changes is required so that we can understand the ways in which body size has literally and figuratively become embodied.

Contributors

✛ ✛ ✛

Anne E. Becker, MD, Ph.D., SM, is the Maude and Lillian Presley Professor of Global Health and Social Medicine at Harvard Medical School, where she is vice chair of the Department of Global Health and Social Medicine. She is also director of the Eating Disorders Clinical and Research Program at Massachusetts General Hospital. An anthropologist and psychiatrist, Dr. Becker studies the impact of social and cultural environment on mental health. Her book, *Body, Self, and Society: The View from Fiji,* probes the cultural mediation of self-agency and body experience, and her NIMH-funded research has investigated the impact of rapid social change on eating pathology and other youth health risk behaviors in Fiji. She is the immediate past president of the Academy for Eating Disorders, an associate editor of the *International Journal of Eating Disorders,* and serves on the American Psychiatric Association's DSM-5 Eating Disorders Work Group.

Tracey Galloway received her Ph.D. in 2008 from McMaster University, where she studied patterns of growth and nutrition in rural Canadian schoolchildren. She held a postdoctoral fellowship at the Dalla Lana School of Public Health, University of Toronto, and from 2009–2011 was International Polar Year Research Fellow in Nutritional Anthropology at McGill University. Tracey is assistant professor of human biology in the Department of Anthropology at University of Manitoba in Winnipeg, Canada. Her research examines obesity and chronic disease risk among Aboriginal Canadians, particularly the Inuit inhabitants of Canada's circumpolar regions. Current projects include international comparison of obesity prevalence among Inuit children and evaluation of nutrition and physical activity interventions designed to promote healthy weights.

Hanna Garth is a Ph.D. candidate in anthropology at UCLA. She is broadly interested in studying how people use food systems. Her research focuses on how marginalized communities access food in resource poor settings. Her most recent project analyzes the ways in which the changing food rationing system in Cuba affects household and community dynamics and in turn individual subject positions. Hanna is also conducting a study of several Los Angeles–based food justice organizations that are part of a growing social movement for improving equal access for diverse low-income communities in Los Angeles. In addition to her work in Cuba and Los Angeles, Hanna has conducted research in the Philippines, Chile, Peru, and Houston, Texas.

Jessica A. Hardin is a Ph.D. candidate at Brandeis University. Trained as a cultural and medical anthropologist her research focuses on how metabolic disorders, including diabetes, hypertension, and cardiovascular diseases, are spiritualized in their etiologies by evangelical Christians in independent Samoa. Additionally, her research focuses on how changing food environments influence the value and meaning of foods and body size. She has conducted research with Samoans in independent Samoa, American Samoa, Hawaii, and California. She has lectured at Brandeis University and the National University of Samoa as well as worked as an applied anthropologist at the Institute for Community Health in Cambridge, Massachusetts. For more information visit her personal website: http://www .jessica-hardin.com

Jessica A. Joseph is a Ph.D. candidate in clinical psychology at The New School for Social Research. Her research interests include motherhood, the maternal body, and psychological outcomes in relation to social constructions such as gender, power, culture, and oppression; gender diversity in psychology pedagogy; and fat studies. Her research has been published in *Sex Roles* and presented at the Association for Women in Psychology's annual conference. Her master's thesis examines how pregnant women experience their bodies in a discursive environment; her dissertation will explore how mothers navigate child feeding decisions while suffering from depression and anxiety. She is currently an American Psychological Association Division 35 campus representative.

Megan B. McCullough, Ph.D., is a medical anthropologist whose research focuses on provider behavior change, the context of health care practices, pharmaceutical care, embodiment, and patient-centered experiences of chronic conditions. Her research career began with an in-depth exploration of the sociocultural context of indigenous women's health, reproductive health and well-being in Aboriginal Australia. She has conducted extensive fieldwork in North Queensland, Australia. She has increasingly become invested in exploring clinical pharmacists as health providers, pharmaceutical treatments for chronic conditions, and the cultures of health practice. Additionally, she is interested in health disparities, obesity, stigma, and structural competence in health care. Presently she is a Research Health Scientist at the US Department of Veteran Affairs. She is a visiting scholar at Brandeis University and holds a Ph.D. in anthropology from New York University.

Stephen T. McGarvey is the director of the International Health Institute and professor of epidemiology at Brown University. McGarvey earned a Ph.D. in anthropology from Pennsylvania State University and an M.P.H. in epidemiology from Yale University. McGarvey is concerned with issues of human population biology and global health, specifically modernization-related socioeconomic and behavioral changes, genetic and environmental influences on obesity and cardiovascular disease risk factors, tropical parasitology and child nutritional status and health, with research in Samoa, the Philippines, South Africa, and Ghana. He has worked among Samoan communities for more than thirty-five years. He is leading a behavioral intervention to improve diabetes care using community health workers in American Samoa and directs genetic epidemiology research on cardiometabolic conditions in Samoa. He is an elected fellow of the American Association for the Advancement of Science and on the editorial board of the *American Journal of Human Biology.*

Darlene McNaughton is a social anthropologist in the Discipline of Public Health at Flinders University, Australia. Her research interests and publications have focused on the nature of subalternity and stigma, the anthropology of biomedicine, indigenous notions of well-being, and the cultural dimensions of public health discourses on obesity, diabetes, and dengue fever. She has undertaken long-term ethnographic research in Aotearoa-New Zealand, India, western Cape York Peninsula, and northern Queensland, Australia. For further details see her personal blog: darlenemcnaughton. wordpress.com.

Tina Moffat is an associate professor in the Department of Anthropology at McMaster University. Her research focuses on child health and nutrition in relation to environmental health and urban ecosystems. She has authored and co-authored numerous scholarly journal publications on child growth and infant feeding in Nepal and nutritional well-being and obesity among North American children. She is co-editor with Dr. Tracy Prowse of *Human Diet and Nutrition in Biocultural Perspective. Past Meets Present* (Berghahn Books).

Rochelle Rosen, Ph.D., is a medical anthropologist and an assistant professor (research) at the Centers for Behavioral and Preventive Medicine at The Miriam Hospital and in the Department of Behavioral and Social Sciences of the Warren Alpert Medical School. She is also affiliated faculty at the International Health

Institute of Brown University. Her research interests are focused in two areas: (1) HIV prevention for women via vaginal microbicide acceptability; and (2) preventive health care issues in the South Pacific island of American Samoa. She has a particular specialty in using qualitative research methods for translational health research in behavioral medicine.

Lisa R. Rubin, Ph.D., is assistant professor of psychology at The New School for Social Research and practicing clinical psychologist in New York City. Her research and clinical interests concern the interface of objectification and medicalization processes in women's health care, particularly in relation to body image and obesity, reproductive health and assisted reproductive technologies, and psycho-oncology. She is particularly interested in how processes of objectification and medicalization are enacted, how they intersect with gender and racialized ideologies, and how they are resisted or otherwise negotiated across individuals and within social groups. She is a graduate of the Women's Therapy Centre Institute's postgraduate training program in cultural, relational psychoanalytic approaches to eating and the body.

Sarah Trainer recently received her Ph.D. from the University of Arizona and is currently an instructor there. Trained as a medical and biocultural anthropologist, her research interests focus on the interplay between local and global influences, the effects of these interactions on women's health, global trends in chronic disease, and obesity linked (among other variables) to development and urbanization, and transnational flows of ideas, foods, eating patterns, and people. She explored these issues most recently in her dissertation, the research for which was based in the United Arab Emirates in the Arab Gulf. She has other ongoing, long-term projects in Arizona, with current research exploring the interplay between the "foodie movement" in the United States and domestic trends in chronic disease, and obesity.

Emily Yates-Doerr is a postdoctoral fellow in the health care and body division at the Amsterdam Institute for Social Science Research. She is part of a European Research Council–funded study that interrogates eating in practice (http://eatingbodiesfluidnetwork.wordpress.com/). Her previous research, which was carried out in a region of the Guatemalan highlands where malnutrition was a longstanding concern, examined the emergence of public health programs aimed at obesity prevention. This work analyzes how obesity in Guatemala has been scientifically established, how obesity science circulates within people's lives, and how matters of everyday dietary practice in turn shape the process of scientific knowledge production about obesity. She holds a Ph.D. in anthropology from New York University. Her work has been published in *Medical Anthropology Quarterly, Food Culture & Society, Cambridge Anthropology,* and *Anthropology Today.*

Index

✛ ✛ ✛